VALUES IN
MODERN
MEDICINE

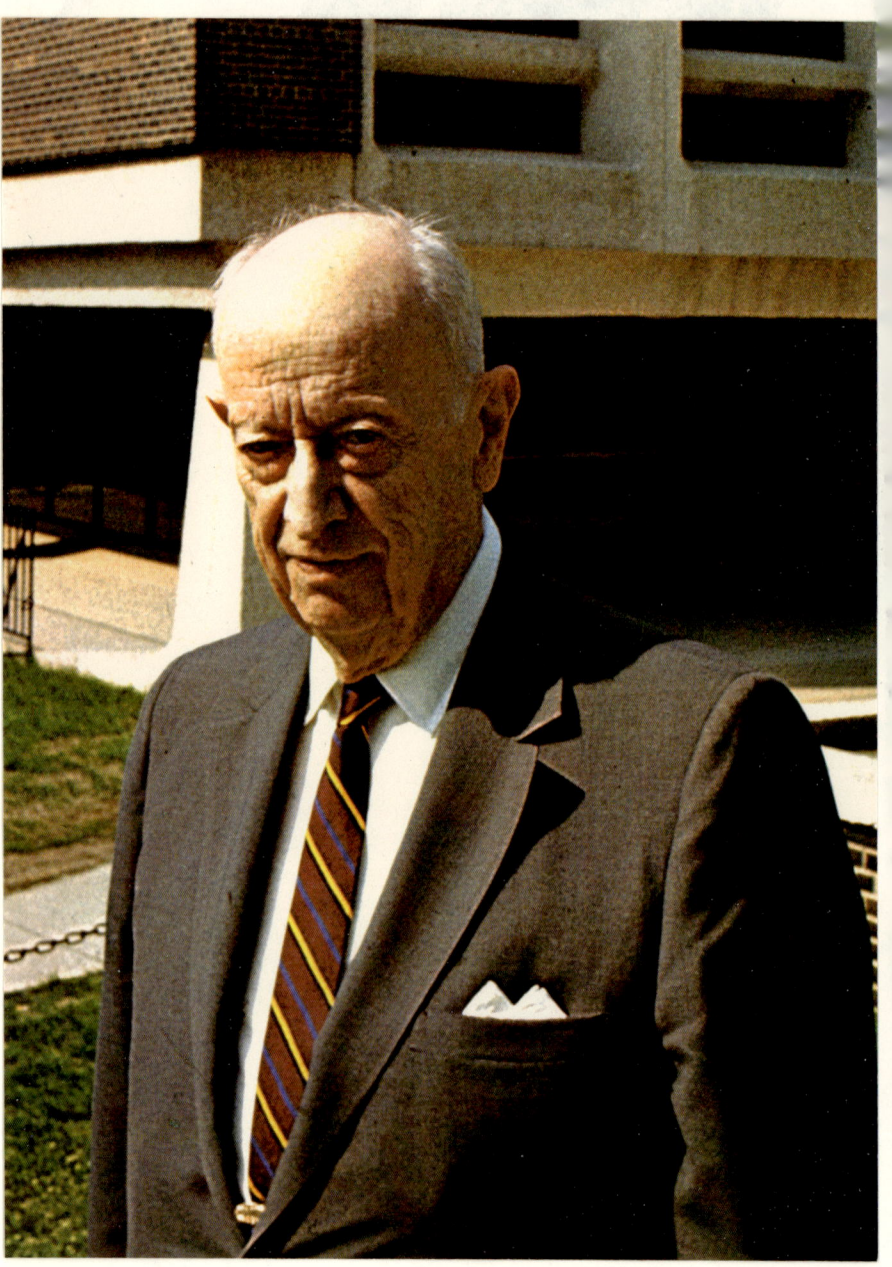

William Shainline Middleton

VALUES IN MODERN MEDICINE

Published for

The Wisconsin Medical

Alumni Association

The University of Wisconsin Press

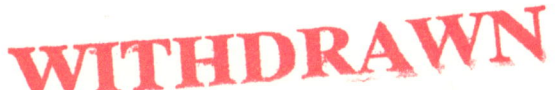

Published 1972
The University of Wisconsin Press
Box 1379, Madison, Wisconsin 53701

The University of Wisconsin Press, Ltd.
70 Great Russell Street, London

First printing

Printed in the United States of America

For LC CIP information see the colophon

ISBN 0-299-06220-1

To M. H. W. M.

CONTENTS

MEDICAL PRACTICE

RANDOM REFLECTIONS

ILLUSTRATIONS

PREFACE

During my sixty years in the practice of medicine I have witnessed momentous changes. In a considerable measure science has replaced empiricism in precept and practice. Yet the art of medical practice perforce still bridges many gaps left by the limitations of the current knowledge of the human being in health and disease. This biologic variable contributes materially to the difficulty in the solution of the unanswered questions. Over the years unusual opportunities have been afforded me to observe these matters at first hand. Furthermore, medicine is belatedly taking its appropriate place in the social evolution of our times. Whether in the classroom or in professional meetings the discussion of cogent issues has been undertaken. From a number of papers published in the medical journals, a representative group has been selected and herein assembled.

Autobiography has been categorized as a form of self-adulation. The same characterization can scarcely be leveled at the collection here offered. Admittedly, the experience of long years in academic, military, and government service will have been sublimated in a credo as expressed in certain of these essays. For example, "Tangible and Intangible Values in Modern Medicine" arose from the intimate interchange at the bedside and in the classroom, where the emergence of the inquiring young mind afforded the supreme reward of the teacher. Then, "Books and Physicians" bespeaks the innately pervasive design of the physician to broaden his intellectual horizon.

In general these essays on widely diversified subjects are reproduced in a single volume to render them more accessible as an invitation for kindred spirits to partake and a challenge for inquisitive souls to debate.

W.S.M.

PHILOSOPHY

TANGIBLE AND
INTANGIBLE VALUES IN
MODERN MEDICINE

"Time is like a river made up of events which happen, and a violent stream; for as soon as a thing has been seen, it is carried away, and another comes in its place, and this will be carried away too."
MARCUS AURELIUS

While the philosopher may weigh human affairs and values in their appropriate perspective against the backdrop of the ages, nature has circumscribed the visual field of ordinary man. Each generation, yes, each individual, is inclined to consider his period the most progressive of all time. The admonition "All the present time is a point in eternity," is either totally ignored or discounted as a vagary of another era. For a certain psychology some useful purpose may be served by assuming that medicine has advanced at an unprecedented pace and has attained a remarkable pinnacle of perfection in our day. Upon such mental pabulum, however, is bred a sense of complacency that invites a decline of the curve of progress for the future. The present vantage point of medicine has not been gained in a single decade or generation. It represents the accumulation and the sublimation of past centuries. The recent acceleration of scientific progress in medicine stems from a remarkable growth in knowledge in the contributory sciences and from the improved channels of communication for its application to practice.

Lest we assume that the ledger is entirely on the credit side, let us investigate certain of the potential hazards of the present situation. Into medical thought have been transferred a host of new devices for

Presented at Medical Convocation, University of Iowa, June 10, 1954. Reprinted from *The Pharos of Alpha Omega Alpha* 18 (November 1954): 1–8.

the study of problems. Complicated chemical and physical principles are involved. Special techniques require highly developed skills and involved apparatus. For example, in the utilization of radioactive isotopes for the investigation of metabolic processes in the mammalian body the tagged element is produced in atomic piles at the Oak Ridge and Argonne National Laboratories under governmental control. Its distribution is limited to authorized workers whose use of the radioactive isotopes is carefully monitored to assure protection. Upon the administration of the tagged element, its dispersion and distribution through the body may be accurately established by the Geiger counter or the scintillation counter and scanner. Few clinicians are trained in this field and physicists are assuming an increasing responsibility for the technical aspects of these observations. This liaison is a natural and welcome outgrowth of the stupendous development in this area; but medicine must not relinquish leadership in the laboratory or in the clinic. We need more physicians with physical training as well as more physicists with a medical outlook.

In the great growth of scientific medicine, research has taken an increasingly important place in medical planning. Federal and private foundation funds have greatly augmented the effort. Indeed, under the generally accepted pattern of fixed projects, the temptation to exploit such sources of revenue may at times prove too inviting for the hard-pressed administration of the medical school to resist. Sound financing will dictate the protection of the basic staff of a medical school by maintaining its responsibility for the salaries of the key faculty members. Furthermore, the budget for research should bear a definite relationship to the total figure for medical education to avoid potentially serious dislocations on readjustments periodically necessitated by waves of enforced economy. Otherwise, the total financial structure of the medical school may collapse under the impact of an economic tidal wave. Nor may we overlook the actual cost of such accepted research projects to the institution. Costs ranging from 8 to 50 percent of the respective grants are quoted for these overhead services. If these figures be reduced to a working level of 20 percent, the camel of research grants may still prove an expensive guest in certain academic tents. At least the time for careful bilateral reassessment is long overdue, and it may properly begin in our state-supported institutions where such programs are on a relatively sound basis.

The pressure of World War II materially accelerated and exploited certain areas of research applicable to medicine. To cite an isolated example, penicillin, which had been discovered in 1928 by Alexander Fleming, was brought to clinical light and maturity by Howard Florey and the Oxford group in 1940. The catalyst of war greatly expedited its clinical availability by consolidating the efforts of widely dispersed groups of research workers. Such instances of the established value of teamwork and coordinated research in the solution of scientific problems and in the application of derived data might be multiplied many times. However, this expedient presents a very obvious danger common to mass production in general. Even with the best of intentions, promising young men may become links in a conveyor belt, the product of which is stereotyped publication and the reward a listing among three to six collaborators. Significantly few epochal discoveries in science have resulted from a fusion of minds. Conversely, how desolated would be our medical past, if the independent works of Harvey, Pasteur, Koch, Roentgen, and Kendall, to mention only a few of the great contributors to our scientific growth, had awaited intellectual companionship. The intricacies of modern science may require a pooling of individual skills; but in such amalgamations let us attempt to keep the spark of independent thinking alive.

In a period of intense research activity a critical viewpoint, however honestly motivated, may be unwelcome. Yet, the time is indeed ripe for self-analysis of our methods and results. Let me bespeak a stimulation of the inquiring mind always. I would buy the man with an idea any time. We can ill afford research puppets, whose intellectual processes are responsive only to the strings of expediency. Too much potential talent is sacrificed on the altar of the fixed contract. From the administrative standpoint it would appear that the first requisitions of every man with a research problem are a Beckman spectrophotometer and a biochemist! Perhaps one may rate the level of research activity of a medical school by its Beckman index. Wisconsin has thirty-two! Independent thought is as refreshing as it is rare in most laboratories and clinics. Osler wrote: "He who follows another sees nothing, learns nothing, nay, seeks nothing." Too frequently the worker is so submerged in the application of a special technique or the mastery of an intricate instrument that he is oblivious of the new vistas that are opened to him. This criticism may even more fairly be levelled at the clinician whose senses should be particularly attuned to the phenomena of nature. With the evolution of newer methods of precision, the modern physician has too frequently become an interpreter of records, tracings, and laboratory returns. Justice Cardozo said: "There is an accuracy that defeats itself by overemphasis of details." Then perforce the research neophyte may feel the urge for publication. Printer's ink is still one of the most insidious and possessive poisons known to man. Fortunate is the young worker whose sponsor is a lover of trees.

Among other factors, the impersonality and the detachment of modern medicine have done much to jeopardize the traditional patient-physician relationship. Instead of further limiting or restricting the place of medicine in the social fabric, the future will undoubtedly witness a serious broadening of medicine's sphere. By common consent, medicine is the instrument of society in the protection of a common commodity, health. To take our proper position in the body politic, we must appreciate the fact that we are partners, not sole proprietors, in a common cause. Organized medicine has not always maintained an unselfish, statesmanlike attitude in this respect. The future pattern was clearly forecasted by Henry Favill (1908) in an address to the alumni of Rush Medical College: "The time is already here when to be only a practicing physician is a discredit. Not only has the medical profession to furnish its full quota to the army of social service, but in many respects it must point out the way. The pathology of society is as much the function of the medical man as the pathology of human disease." With the growing appreciation of the influence of environment and social forces upon disease expression Favill's position becomes more cogent. It is impossible to divorce the mission of modern medicine from its sociologic implications. By the same token, this renewed interest in the important interfaces of medicine and social forces carries no suggestion of the governmental control of medical practice.

As a natural outgrowth of the appreciation of medicine's place in the social pattern comes an increasing emphasis on the prevention of disease and disability. Physicians prate glibly of the age of prevention but crave more desperate surgical risks and more seriously ill patients. In the abstract we are for preventive medicine; but recruitment for this field has been very inadequate. Candidly, medicine is still psychologically geared for the care of the sick and disabled; prevention is a dream of the future. Enormous strides have nevertheless been made in the prevention of infectious diseases and in the limitation of industrial hazards. The scourge of the exanthemata has passed from the civilized world. The devastations of Asiatic cholera and bubonic plague are now geographically circumscribed. The threat of diphtheria is limited. Typhoid fever and bacterial pneumonia are almost deceased diseases. The pall of tuberculosis is lightened upon the land, and syphilis no longer carries its stigmata to the second generation. So the list of infectious diseases controlled or literally vanquished by prophylactic or therapeutic measures grows to a point where in the foreseeable future their impact upon the health and the life of the American people will be negligible. Less spectacular but none the less significant has been the improvement in the industrial health of the nation. Hygienic conditions have been vastly improved to the mutual advantage of labor and industry. Toxic hazards have largely been eliminated. Great strides have been made in the alleviation of dust exposures. Safety measures for the protection of workers receive the continued attention of representatives of labor, industry, medicine, engineering, and insurance carriers. When the millennium of universal health and deferred disintegration is reached, preventive will have largely displaced curative medicine. Medicine will then look for new worlds to conquer.

Entrance upon a career in medicine affords a stimulating, yet arresting, prospect. No thoughtful young man can view his responsibilities lightly. The master Osler wrote: "Give him good methods and a proper point of view, and all other things will be added as his experience grows." A wholesome respect for nature and nature's handiwork will engender a deep humility. Henley expressed his opinion of the attributes of a physician:

> Faultless patience and unyielding will,
> Beautiful gentleness and splendid skill.

To such high qualifications should be added unusual powers of discernment. To many men is given the ability to observe and to note objective phenomena. Fortunate is the individual who, while making the same observations, is able to assign the values and the relations that bring order and perspective to the composite picture.

In the professional life ahead I ask for you time for contemplation. Drinkwater phrases my thought:

> Lonely is the man who understands.
>   Lonely is the vision that leads a man away
> From the pasture-lands,
>   From the furrow of corn and the brown loads of hay
> To the mountain-side,
>   To the high places where contemplation brings
> All his adventurings
>   Among the sowers and the tillers in the wide
> Valleys to one fused experience,
>   That shall control
> The courses of his soul,
>   And give his hand
> Courage and continence.

The American pace of life is so driving that it virtually kills living. At this early stage in your development you will do yourself a great service by budgeting your day to afford an hour for reflection. Self-analysis will lead to a more effective utilization of the rest of your waking hours, while contemplation and discernment will give you a better sense of values. For example, it is a national habit to refer to the high standards of living in the United States and as a corollary to belittle the mores of foreign countries. When we take the trouble to evaluate our national virtues we are struck by the fact that our assets are largely physical. We have more automobiles, telephones, radios, television sets, washing machines, refrigerators, and other accessories catering to human comfort, than any other country. But who was our last great author? What outstanding artist or musician has represented us in the last fifty years? Have we had a real philosopher in recent years? Is our way of living in a spiritual sense superior to that of materially less favored peoples?

The medical profession exacts the highest ethical standards. Service to mankind is the cornerstone upon which medical ethics is built. Exploitation of the sick and disabled is as repugnant as it is indefensible in medical practice. "Medicine exists for the benefit of the afflicted and not the afflicted for the benefit of medicine" (Middleton). The Golden Rule clearly states our credo. The best interests of the patient are protected by our adherence to its tenets. You have just completed the vital undergraduate phase of your medical training at considerable expense to yourself and your family. A fair competence is assured you in the practice of good medicine. Do not attempt to recoup your fortunes by inordinate and unfair charges. Do not fall into the temptation of "keeping up with the Joneses." With the high moral standards of the individual practitioner there can be no compromise. When Christiana commented upon the poor state of the road over the Slough of Despond, the Old Gentleman answered: "Yes, too true; for many there be that pretend to be the King's laborers, and they say they are for mending the King's highways, who bring dirt and dung instead of stones, and so mar instead of mending." Intellectual integrity begins at home. You may dissemble in your associations with your fellow men, at a cost; but you must live and sleep with yourself. One of the human frailties that affords the entering wedge to intellectual trimming is rationalization. In the long run you are much further on the road to spiritual equilibrium if you wrestle with the devil in the open. Assuredly, your stature among your medical conferes is greatly improved by forthright candor. Confidence begets confidence and shortly the warmth of comradeship transforms the entire atmosphere of professional association.

As a natural consequence to peace of mind will come serenity and tranquillity. In these days of turmoil and unrest, such objectives are especially coveted. Clearly they are attainable only when one is master of himself and his destiny. It is difficult to be serene and contained with the Selective Service breathing down your neck; but at least you may set this state of mind on an attainable pinnacle to be sought when the pressure is removed. Indeed, these attributes may properly be coupled with "that gentleness and compassion for his suffering fellow man without which no man . . . need hope to be a great physician" (Brown). Trousseau wrote: "There are no diseases, only sick people." If you herewith dedicate yourselves to the service of mankind, major problems become minor and minor difficulties disappear. The present position of medicine is defensive, because the leaders in organized medicine were outmaneuvered. In a rearguard action we hesitatingly adopted the programs of hospitalization insurance and of prepayment medical care. We are housecleaning in areas of patent abuse. Grievance committees are adjusting differences between the public and the profession. The future is brighter by reason of improved public relations. There remain areas of further reconciliation that must be attained to regain a fuller measure of the old patient-physician relationship. In this effort a marriage of the art and the science of medicine is essential. "The understanding of truth, the appreciation of beauty, sympathy with those who suffer and aspire and love, such are the things that give life its meaning, and of these science knows nothing" (Compton).

The physician should cultivate his avocations as sedulously as his profession—albeit on a quantitatively reduced scale. May I suggest relaxing recreations against the day when your shadow lengthens behind you. Strenuous physical sports carry with them certain hazards. Then, too, the rise of successive generations to take your measure in tennis by the simple expedient of drop shots over the net or deep lobs to the base line bespeaks an exasperating collusion not covered in Potter's *Gamesmanship.* Swimming and hiking have the virtue of complete control. You may modify the effort to your capacity and reserve. Gardening has many staunch devotees in the medical profession. Interestingly these physicians are inclined to specialize as sharply in floriculture as in their practice. Aside from the "high breathlessness about beauty that cancels lust and superstition" (Santayana), gardening brings to them a surcease from the trials of the sick room, operation clinic, and the office. They are for the time at peace with the world. The toughest officer in the Medical Department of the Regular Army was clay in my hands when I learned that he was an iris fancier with some 120 varieties in his collection. Climatic obstacles are accepted challenges. A hobby may grow into a remunerative business venture, as in the case of a prominent specialist of our community whose orchid culture has now assumed very profitable commercial proportions. Beware the lure of the gentleman-farmer role, however, unless you have the background of farming. Many of my medical friends not so endowed pay exorbitant prices for the beef and other commodities thus derived.

Bird watching is one of the most engaging of all outdoor pursuits—and you meet many fine people who are similarly attracted. How fascinating it is to observe the migratory birds, to register the successive waves of warblers, to settle the neighborhood rumor of a flight of "parrots" by recognizing cedar waxwings! One nature study leads naturally to another. So an absorption in the flora and the fauna of an area may follow an initial limited interest. The earth, the sky, and *The Sea Around Us* have their fascination. The great natural scientist, Joseph Leidy, once said: "How can life be tiresome so long as there is still a new rhizopod undescribed?" So absorbing may the wonders of nature become. The Nimrod and the follower of Izaak Walton will find relaxation in the field or the stream; but you must use reason in adjusting the effort to your accustomed pace. Do not let the sport possess you. The American holiday commonly involves a change of scene. Whether it be summer or winter, the highways, railways, and airways will be crowded with the mingled passengers from the North going South, and those from the South coming North. How fortunate that human beings are so eager for different greener pastures. The diversity of climate and scenery in North America affords you a wide choice of vacation opportunities for any period or purse.

Foreign travel has always had its attraction. Unfortunately, its expense and the detachment from the growing family have usually meant a deferment until the children have grown. May I urge that you indulge in this extravagance early so that its memories may be with you for many years. A lack of facility in a foreign language should not deny you this privilege. You will experience every courtesy and helpful attention. If Great Britain or Europe be your objectives, the ties of language, literature, art, and history will render every moment a source of fascinating interest. Particularly will you find relaxation and pleasure off the beaten path; but in the interest of marital peace, arrange for a token stay in Paris and London, or Rome and Madrid! A personal car is the most convenient mode of transportation, although it lacks the intimacy and the economy of the bicycle.

The habits of your later years are in the formative stage at this time. If music has been a relaxation, do not neglect it. Its technical appreciation and performance are unexcelled sources of recreation. In many communities physicians have banded together for vocal or instrumental music. Chamber music has afforded an artistic outlet for many talented physicians that should be encouraged. The muscial programs of the radio and television supply a portion of this need to the less endowed. Records of operas, symphonies, and separate musical numbers are available to all. The opportunity to listen to the major musical organizations in opera or concert is otherwise largely limited to the metropolitan areas. Art has a growing representation in the profession. From a study of art many physicians advance to active participation in painting, etching, and other media of expression. Photography has always attracted a large segment of our profession. While writing has been a common outlet for American physicians in the past, few contemporaries are so engaged. Usually our recent representatives have contented themselves with literal translations of technical subjects for the lay reader. Few have thereby increased their professional stature. Philately and other collections are diverting avocations. Woodworking and other handicrafts are engaging pastimes for other physicians; and so the list of hobbies of professional men might be extended interminably.

The habit of reading should be assiduously cultivated, for it offers an ever present source of mental refreshment and diversion. Obviously, the selection of subjects varies widely with different individuals. Aside from medical literature, one's reading interest may follow any one of a series of channels. Biography is a common field of incidental reading among physicians. For example, Abraham Lincoln has been a subject of sustained interest to me for many years. Medical history and biography are natural outlets. The novel may have passing appeal. Indeed, a number of physicians find a remarkable surcease from the cares of the working day in perusing the pulp mystery or detective stories. More substantial sources include Shakespeare, Bunyan, Epictetus, Marcus Aurelius, the Bible, and a host of others. After an evening of heavy or technical reading, there is no better relaxation than a change of pace in reading some nonmedical subject—and the wife may therein accommodate you by reading you to sleep! Do not underestimate your literary taste. Set its standards high rather than low, and the interest will be maintained.

Choose your friends well and hold them. May you "enjoy the trust of pure women, the respect of intelligent men, and the love of little children" (Stanley). One of the rewards of teaching is the recurring contact with young men. My father in medicine, Doctor David Riesman, when asked the secret of his sustained mental vigor, said: "I have always maintained contact with 'young men' of all ages." May you retain your mental youth always!

THE STUFF OF A MEDICAL CAREER

"Solicitude for your welfare . . . urge[s] me on an occasion like the present, to offer to your solemn contemplation, and to recommend to your frequent review, some sentiments."
GEORGE WASHINGTON, "Farewell Address"

Dean Doan, members of the Faculty, students all, ladies and gentlemen: For the curious-minded, education is a continuing process from the cradle to the grave. Aspiring to careers in medicine and nursing, you young men and women have grounded your education on the bedrock of sound primary and secondary schooling. On this firm basis you have poured the foundations of your collegiate studies. We may assume that they are firmly set. We are come together on this momentous occasion to lay the cornerstone of your professional careers. So significant is your design for human service that this ceremony may appropriately be designated as your consecration. From time to time in the years ahead you will pause in the pursuit of your sacred responsibilities to rededicate yourselves to your lofty mission, for: "Once one puts his hand to the medical plow, he is not fit for the Kingdom of Heaven unless he looks ever forward" (Waring).

Academic tradition has established a certain protocol for such occasions that shall be observed mainly in the breach. As Samuel Johnson wrote: "Age looks with anger on the temerity of youth, and youth with contempt on the scrupulosity of age." LaRochefoùcauld gave the French accent, "Les vieillards aiment à donner de bons préceptes pour se consoler de n' etre plus en état de donner de mauvais examples." (The old love to give good advice to make up for their inability to set bad examples.) In bespeaking your indulgence may I remind you, "A few

Convocation Address, College of Medicine and School of Nursing, Ohio State University, September 28, 1959. Reprinted from *Health Centre Journal* (Ohio State University) 10 (January 1960): 2.

bees in the bonnet may be permitted to grey hairs; but a swarm is a sign of senility" (Forbes).

You have undergone long hours, yes, some years, of ordered preparation for a professional education in esoteric fields. Beyond the classroom, laboratory, and conference you have worked diligently to master subjects whose application to your ultimate objective at the moment appeared very remote, to say the least. The while you have sensed the atmosphere of pedagogic unrest that now permeates the halls of higher learning. In the anxiety to afford students of nursing and medicine the firmest foundation for their professional careers, for many years disproportionate emphasis has been given to the natural sciences. In this design the humanities and the social sciences have suffered serious shrinkage and dislocation. Presently educators in the general colleges throughout the land are attempting to retrieve lost ground by affording a balanced nonvocational background to the students with nursing and medical aspirations.

By the same token there is considerable disquietude in our respective interdependent professional schools. Nursing education is at the crossroads between vocational and academic objectives. Moreover at the present time there are at least ten experimental patterns of curricula in the medical schools of this country. These variants range widely from mere temporal readjustments to radical functional realignments. Integration is a shibboleth to medical educators who among other objectives champion vertical or horizontal orientation to facilitate instruction and comprehensive grasp of related subjects. In medical practice it is a truism that where there are many remedies, there is no cure. The manifold approaches to the important problems of medical and nursing education are a healthy sign of life in dynamic professions. Years of trial and error will be required to establish the correct curricular formulae—and then changing times and requirements of practice will dictate new studies! Meanwhile you are the guinea pigs. The traditional conservatism of Ohio State University is your protection against uncontrolled experimentation.

Undoubtedly your greatest asset upon entrance to your new curricula will prove to be the disciplines of the primary and secondary school carried into college. You have learned to study. Your hard-earned ability to assess the problem at hand and to come to grips with its essentials will spare needless peregrinations and meanderings in fruitless academic byways and brambles. To most of you the entire vocabulary of nursing and medicine will be startlingly new and foreboding. Years ago myology was one of the first subjects of our medical course. I recall vividly my secret pride in the memorization of the name of one of the smallest muscles in the body, *levator labii superioris alaeque nasi!* Oliver Wendell Holmes gave proper weight to this new task that confronts you: "even the learned ignorance of a nomenclature is something to have mastered, and may furnish pegs to hang facts upon, which would otherwise have strewed the floor of memory in loose disorder." Although this medium may now appear a strange and formidable code of communication among the select initiates, shortly it will have become your invaluable instrument of professional expression. Perchance you have had a sound background of Greek and Latin. If so, your introduction to medical terminology will prove an easy one; if not, you would profit immeasurably by a study of medical derivatives from these sources.

Medicine is distinctly individualistic in its outlook. The parameters of its social interests are singularly restricted. In its evolution from the mysticism and empiricism of an earlier day our profession has emphasized the responsibility of the individual nurse and physician. To the common mind the private duty nurse and the family physician exemplify the quintessence of personal service to the sick and afflicted. At the same time, the astounding growth of medical science and knowledge has initiated an ever extending wave of specialization that has profoundly affected nursing and medical practice. Preoccupied with our exacting responsibilities, we are inclined to overlook our appropriate place in the modern social fabric. We have assumed that the health of the people is our exclusive vested interest. In high places we have cavalierly treated as intruders other social agencies which are in truth partners in the common cause of guarding the public weal. In a reconstructed viewpoint we must realize we are servants and not masters in the protection of the health and the welfare of the people. In your personal and public professional relationships always bear this sacred trust in mind.

In the transition from the campus of the college to your present professional surroundings and exactions make a real effort to maintain some thread of intellectual continuity by study or practice in such nonscience fields as literature, history, or music. Upon assuming administrative duties in the University of Wisconsin (1935), my first proposal to the Medical Faculty was the introduction of required cultural courses into the curriculum. After an animated discussion the compromise of a nonscience elective carried. Thereupon unanticipated resistance was encountered in the reluctance of the College of Letters and Science to participate in the program. However, the soundness of such inclusions is gaining increasing support in academic circles. Culture is no obstacle to professional growth and development. Budget your time so that recreation is not neglected. Cultivate the simple pleasures and outlets. Allow full range to the appreciation of nature through your God-given senses. The trials of the classroom and clinic are quickly effaced by an hour of bird watching. The chagrin of an indifferent report or an unsatisfactory examination fades into insignificance on the tennis court or golf course. The natural effort of walking and swimming, coupled with the resultant deeper breathing, is an effective tranquilizer! Do not permit your spiritual life to undergo atrophy of disuse. To the physician and the nurse Divine guidance and support are sustaining sources of strength. Husband your resources for the long pull ahead. The self-disciplines imposed at this period will carry you well on the road to success, while your less resolute fellows fall by the way through their excesses.

Your generation is favored by a radical and rational change in the general educational pattern. The essential ingredients, i.e., "intelligent, receptive students; inspired, well motivated teachers; and ready, open channels of communication" (Middleton), remain unchanged. A growing appreciation of the stultifying hazards of the passive role of the student has led to a much sounder approach in the teaching-learning mechanism. For this reason the traditional lecture and the dramatized clinic have largely been displaced by the intimate seminar, round table, and bedside conference. The laboratory exercise takes an ever-increasing role in cross fertilization. No longer can it be said that: "the hungry sheep look up and are not fed; for the bread of the wards they are given the stones of the lecture-room and amphitheatre" (Osler). As party of the first part the student is now an active participant in his own education.

In this day of frenetic activity one is reluctant to characterize the qualifications for any human endeavor without conventional psychological tests. Yet no studies available to us will measure certain qualities of personality, intellect, and character that are so essential to the nurse and to the physician. Perhaps Warren came close with: "the bold spirit that prefers hazard to security and conflict to peace; the eager mind intent upon far horizons; the steadfast will that accepts victory without vanity, and defeat without regret; and the heart so possessed of its dream as to be cleansed alike of pride and malice and deceit." From long contacts with young minds, most impressive are the inquiring, independent thinkers. Not the "smart alecky" nor the supercilious; but the student who is not satisfied with the inconclusive answer. Such restless souls are our hope for the future. Their discontent assures studied progress instead of passive acceptance of the status quo. These rare spirits are marked for higher goals. By the same token the instructors are reciprocally put on their mettle. They will not stoop to sophistry in their interchange. In such an atmosphere of mutual respect the teacher takes the thoughtful student to the "Delectable mountains" and the latter in turn breathes the rarefied air of independent thought that will be his passport to the community of scholars. From these stimulating intellectual contacts flow the true fruits of Socratic instruction. The emergence of the alert minds of youth from such an exposure is one of the imponderable rewards of real teachers.

The primary function of a school of nursing and of a medical school is professional education. True, medical service of a high order is rendered in the associated university hospital; but its very existence depends upon the necessity for clinical training in your education. Actually, in effect, the University Hospital is the largest laboratory on the Ohio State Campus, the laboratory for the bedside training of nurses and physicians! Research is an important byproduct of the College of Medicine. Without the burgeoning force of research in your midst, moreover, the lamp of education and learning would burn dimly. Neither the responsibility for medical service nor the necessity for an active research program should distort the relative importance of these elements in our thinking and staffing for medical and nursing education. Fortunate is the university whose teachers of nursing and medicine possess research capabilities as well. Here productive scholarship may be measured, first, by the superior quality of its graduates and, second, by its conspicious scientific contributions.

Medical education has suffered immeasurably from the old adage that teachers are born, not made. All instructors resent Bruce's paraphrase of Shaw's devastating denunciation: "Those who can, do. Those who cannot, teach." Nevertheless there has been too ready acceptance of the inheritable order of pedagogy. The idiosyncrasies and mannerisms of the master are consciously or subconsciously absorbed by the junior staff. They walk, talk, dress, and act like the chief! Such foibles are human; but until recently there has been no serious study of the basic structure of medical education from a technical standpoint. Yet great strides have been made in fundamental pedagogical theory and practice in recent years. (The University of Buffalo, under the leadership of Dr. George E. Miller, is making a major contribution through constructive cooperative studies and a series of summer workshops in this area.)

However elevated may be the position and standing of a faculty, its effectiveness in medical education is, in the last analysis, weighed by the intimate interpersonal relations of its individual members with students. The erudition of a given teacher has but little influence upon the development and the ultimate career of his students unless his rapport with them be close. By the same token his reciprocal growth from such contacts will be sacrificed if he denies to himself refreshment from this source. There are rare members of our faculties who thrive academically or scientifically in the cloistered cell of the library and laboratory— and starve their souls. Austerity and native shyness may clothe a warm personality. The perceptive student soon penetrates this protective shell to the mutual benefit of both of the contracting parties. On the other hand the "sacerdotal cloak of orthodoxy" (Cannon) may prove impenetrable and militate against ready interchange. Furthermore the student is the first to expose the sham and dross of hypocrisy. The best teachers are profound and sustained students of their respective subjects. Their enthusiasm is infectious. They direct rather than dictate thought. From their vantage point of knowledge and experience they invite the exploration of new approaches by every expedient at the beck of the alert student. Individually his intellectual curiosity will stimulate you to pursue your independent paths of inquiry and study. His untrammeled integrity will engender your warm confidence and enhance your self-assurance. As a true teacher he will "carry from the altars of the past the fire and not the ashes" (Seneca).

"Seek facts and classify them and you will be the workman of science. Conceive or accept theories—and you will be their politicians" (Arthus). In this atmosphere you will maintain your ideals. When their leavening force is lost, principles are compromised and the spirit is embittered. "What America needs is more loafers, or rather dreamers, to save her from herself!" (Duhamel). Maintaining objectivity you will bring substance to your dreams through achievement. Convention may set reasonable limitations to your designs, but nothing can constrict the vision of the open mind. Bias and prejudice warp human judgment. Your sights will be set above such delimiting factors. Periodic withdrawal, physical or psychological, from the pressure of the daily task will afford a proper opportunity for contemplation. With such a perspective in life comes serenity of the mind.

Ambition is the birthright of every intelligent man and woman; but it must never be permitted to become all-pervasive and all-possessive, lest it consume you. Even at this early period you will have set certain pinnacles of success. It may be a position of responsibility and prominence to which you aspire. Again there may be some admired individual whom you would emulate. Human values change with the point of view. A presently vaunted station may shrink into insignificance upon closer scrutiny or with the passage of time. Your idol may prove to have feet of clay. You are building the edifice to house important careers in American society. Do not dwarf your growth by fixing its limits before the supporting walls are poured or laid. Too many professional lives are curtailed because the footings are too shallow for added stories. If your basic education has been broad, your perspective will be immeasurably extended. With the unfolding of new vistas in nursing and medicine your youthful enthusiasm will be fired by the boundless opportunities for growth through human service. Then, perforce, you will agree with Stevenson, "for to travel hopefully is a better thing than to arrive, and the true success is to labour."

May yours be the good and full life!

ADDRESS OF WELCOME

Ladies and gentlemen, friends, in the absence of President Fred it is my privilege and pleasure to welcome you to the Symposium on the Use of Isotopes in Biology and Medicine. This intellectual feast has been provided by a grant from the Wisconsin Alumni Research Foundation. The wide range of subjects on the program, together with their manifold scientific implications, is an adequate brief for the desirability of such a presentation. Your full delectation of this repast will be ample reward for your host, the University of Wisconsin, and for the Committee that has labored so faithfully and effectively in its preparation.

Your presence bespeaks a serious interest in the remarkable developments in the area of atomic energy. The very word, atom, has been shorn of its connotation of indivisibility. Nuclear fission is a fait accompli. Even the lay imagination has been captured by this revolutionary discovery. More important is its impact upon scientific thought and endeavor. Throughout the civilized world research workers are applying this new tool to a host of problems in biology and medicine, among related and diversified subjects. Beyond a peradventure, time and the judgment of history will relegate the application of this newly discovered force in the violence of warfare to a position of subsidiary importance as compared with its contribution to the sum of human knowledge. By this same token the Symposium in Madison may become more significant than the extravaganza at Bikini.

Two groups of our lineal forbears are watching this newer growth

Presented at Symposium on Isotopes in Biology and Medicine, University of Wisconsin—Madison, September 10, 1947.

with particular interest and absorption. The first of these curious-minded students of nature sought the philosopher's stone. By its virtue the baser metals were presumed to be transformed to gold. Precious stones might be derived from ordinary rock. Medically this thesis envisioned "potable gold" (*aurum potabile*) as the elixir of life. This panacea promised the cure of all diseases and the indefinite extension of life. So flagrant were its excesses that the Church issued two famous bulls (1317 and 1326) forbidding the practice of alchemy. Certainly Roger Bacon, Paracelsus, John Dee, Leonhard Thurnheysser sum Thurn (the original "gold bricker" who plated tin with gold), the Rosicrucians, and a host of fellow alchemists are viewing the wonders of the modern transmutation of metals with envious eyes.

Our more acceptable forefathers (scientifically speaking) are gathered about Robert Boyle in The Invisible College convening at Gresham College, as was their wont before the foundation of The Royal Society (1660). To their meetings were submitted all questions that excited the intellectual curiosity of these natural philosophers. Of this remarkable number Robert Hooke, warped of mind and crooked of body, is notable as secretary and gadgeteer extraordinary. He devised Boyle's air pump with which certain fundamental experiments on respiration were performed. Through him international scientific correspondence was maintained on an extended, if tardy, plane. One of the participants in this interchange was Antony van Leeuwenhoek. With his own hands this self-trained scientist ground the lenses for over 247 simple microscopes. His contribution opened the broad vista of microscopy to innumerable seekers for the truth. The tradition of intellectual curiosity took root in the United States through the foundation of the American Philosophical Society (1743). The most eminent of American natural scientists, Joseph Leidy, thrived in its atmosphere. In a day before narrow specialization his interests ranged from parasitology to paleontology. His authoritative work, *Fresh Water Rhizopods of North America*, was completed with a $50 microscope at the cost of $222 to the Geological Society. If science requires a further lesson in humility, the brilliant contributions of the Curies laboring in the shed of the School of Physics in Rue Lhomond, Paris, should suffice. From the Elysium of departed scientists all those kindred spirits will be listening to our deliberations with rapt attention.

The scientific horizon has been extended. New techniques require new and complicated apparatus. Much of this material is expensive and invites the monetary participation of private and governmental agencies. Science is a jealous mistress. You cannot buy brains and ideas. You may merely implement them. In the subsidy of research the munificent benefactors should be spiritual partners as well as material contributors. The modern urge to capitalize upon research by practical returns has tempered the zest for abstract fundamental study for truth itself. In taking our youth to the "Delectable mountains" let us not forsake the guides, Knowledge, Experience, Watchful, and Sincere.

In this season of our scientific triumph let us also reflect upon our responsibilities. The United States Atomic Energy Commission has demonstrated commendable insight and vision in rendering isotopes available for scientific research not only in this country but also to the world at large. John Hay won everlasting distinction as a statesman by his attitude toward China after the Boxer Rebellion (1900). The Fulbright Bill is heartening evidence that the "open door policy" still applies in education and science. By its provisions the United States of America gives notice of its material support of Pasteur's philosophy, "Science has no country."

BOOKS AND PHYSICIANS

"Reading maketh a full man, conference a ready man and writing an exact man."

BACON

The common bond of attachment to books brings us together today; but to assume that this devotion is universal in the medical profession recalls a revealing exception in the enlightened community of Madison some years ago. A financially successful physician was building a pretentious home on University Heights and one of my associates in the Medical Faculty was inspecting the ground floor. "This room will make a splendid library," he exclaimed. "Library!" rejoined the other. "I read *a* book once. This is our card room."

Medicine has been a favorite subject of authors in all periods of history. While there has been a sprinkling of Molieres and Le Sages, the profession has been almost fulsomely praised by the majority of writers. In our weaker moments we have accepted Robert Louis Stevenson's evaluation of physicians as "the flower of our civilization." Certainly, the account of the physician in Ian Maclaren's *Beside the Bonnie Brier Bush* is a tonic that every practitioner should read at least annually for the good of his soul.

Physicians are human beings subject to all the frailties of the species. Particularly are they susceptible to the insidious toxin known as printer's ink. Indeed, once impregnated with this habituating agent, physicians have been known to desert practice, home, and family in pursuit of the will o' the wisp of the printed page. In many instances the prospect of permanency of their writing is in inverse proportion to the weight of the ink consumed in its preparation. Yet, there have been

Presented before Association of Hospital and Institution Libraries, Sheraton Park Hotel, Washington, D.C., June 26, 1959. Reprinted from *The Pharos of Alpha Omega Alpha* 22 (October 1959): 211–16, 240.

many lasting contributions of physicians to general literature. In my judgment, Sir Thomas Browne so distinguished himself with *Religio Medici* and *Urn Burial*. John Brown, better known for "Rab and His Friends," has my vote for immortality in his *Horae Subsecivae*. So we might extend the list to include Goldsmith, von Haller, Coombe, Lamb, and others. John Keats did not quite make the grade after his apprenticeship at Guy's nor did Charles Darwin complete the medical course at Edinburgh.

Oliver Wendell Holmes brings the subject to our own shores. In medicine he will always be cited for his forceful and clamant charge of the communicable order of puerperal fever. Before Semmelweis and against the opposition of Hodge and Meigs of Philadelphia he held the accoucheur responsible for childbed fever. Holmes's literary excursions led Osler to term him "the greatest Brahmin among them"; yet, after a generation of assiduous cultivation, his *Autocrat of the Breakfast Table* leaves me strangely cool. On the other hand, "The Chambered Nautilus" is a priceless literary gem.

By a singular coincidence, the second notable American litterateur, S. Weir Mitchell, turned to Holmes for advice when first touched by the compulsive urge of the pen. The latter, in a thoughtful answer, advised Mitchell to put aside belles lettres until he was fifty years old. While this advice was not fully followed, many of his best novels were written in his later years. *Hugh Wynne, Free Quaker* ranks among the finest historical novels in the English language. *The Red City* is a stirring story of the yellow fever epidemic of 1793 in Philadelphia. With Matthew Carey's *A Brief Account of the Malignant Fever* and J. H. Powell's *Bring Out Your Dead,* this historical novel affords a vividly comprehensive grasp of this tragic chapter of American medical history. Written with Victorian purity, Mitchell's novels have undergone an eclipse of general interest. Perhaps one cogent reason is his avoidance of the sordid aspects of life, to which his practice in neuropsychiatry so singularly exposed him. Yet, he was certainly most human in his professional relations, as the following incident would indicate: Dr. Mitchell was called to New York City in consultation to see a woman who had been bedridden for five years. After taking a complete history and convincing himself that the patient was a malingerer, he asked the physician and the attendant to leave the room. Thereupon, he very ostentatiously locked the door and put the key in his pocket. Then, as the patient watched him anxiously, he took off his coat, vest and necktie. Seating himself on a chair, he methodically took off his shoes. Standing up, he proceeded to unbutton his shirt. Unable to contain herself longer, the patient asked, "What are you going to do?" When Dr.

Mitchell said, "I am going to get into bed with you," she screamed and ran to the door!

S. Weir Mitchell communed with the muses in poetry on occasion. His "Ode on a Lycian Tomb" is deemed his best effort; but from our viewpoint, "Books and the Man," in honor of William Osler, is particularly interesting in that it bridges another stream of literary continuity. A single verse conveys the warmth of personal relations between these two fine medical figures:

> Do you perchance recall when first we met,
> And gaily winged with thought the flying night
> And won with ease the friendship of the mind?
> I like to call it friendship at first sight.

Dr. Osler basked in the sun of Mitchell's favor in Philadelphia. Their friendship thrived in an atmosphere of mutual understanding and reciprocal esteem to the end of Mitchell's life (1914). The period of my medical education at the University of Pennsylvania (1907–11) and internship at Philadelphia General Hospital (1911–12) found the aura of Osler's influence still brilliant. The spell of his personality was heavy on American medicine. His idiosyncrasies were still voiced or copied by his younger associates of the Philadelphia period. In the old Post House at Blockley (Philadelphia General Hospital), now the Osler Memorial Building, there is a soapstone slab on which he had performed necropsies. No house officer of our day considered his training complete without similar exposure! Of Dr. Mitchell the picture is clearer. Although he was no longer teaching, on special occasions he attended the meetings of the College of Physicians of Philadelphia. His stooped person, with a cape rather than a topcoat, met with respectful deference on all hands. Responding with a slight nod, in every movement and reaction detached from his surroundings, he was a wraith from the past that he had lived so fully and captured so abundantly in his writings, professional and literary. His observations of peripheral nerve injuries in the Civil War (with Morehouse and Keen) are classical.

Although a spate of publications may be cited in protest, the temptation to expand the literary activities of medical men is readily resisted. Sir Arthur Conan Doyle, a graduate physician, was unable to earn a livelihood in the practice of medicine. The amazing deductive powers of his teacher, Dr. Joseph Bell, led Doyle to use him as the prototype for his master detective, Sherlock Holmes. In more recent years, Maugham and Cronin, among others, have deserted medicine for literature.

"Of the making of many (medical) books there is no end" (Ecclesiastes 12:12). If general literature has its attraction for physicians, medical expression through the printed page far transcends in number and volume this modest outlet. The National Library of Medicine, the groundbreaking for whose first adequate home was appropriately celebrated June 12, 1959, houses 695,076 volumes. Its accession rate is approximately 12,000 volumes a year. Its journals number 12,723. The Medical Section of our Central Office Library has a modest listing of 19,536 medical books with an annual accession of 181. Its current medical journals total 397 (in English, 382; in foreign languages, fifteen).

Medical librarians are of inestimable assistance in organizing such vast stores of knowledge in the libraries. In fact, we have maintained, "Books are the lifestream of the Medical School and the Library is its heart." The same principles apply to the hospital libraries. These sources of support to research and the practice of medicine are useful and effective just in so far as they are accessible and assimilable. After skilled librarianship has organized and catalogued the books and the journals, the consumer, undergraduate, graduate, and staff, must be trained in their appropriate use. Indeed the rudiments of such methods should be a part of every student's equipment. The teaching-learning process requires some measure of facility in this technique at every level of modern education. If deficient, it must be augmented upon entrance to the medical school. Certainly, the first-year medical student will be better prepared for the long pull ahead if this tool is sharpened and realigned to the special requirements of his esoteric field. The catalogues and indices peculiar to medicine will thereby become trusted allies instead of casual and baffling acquaintances in his future career.

In my visits to stations of the field, I have carefully reviewed the cataloguing, control of withdrawal, utilization of space, adequacy of stacks, work areas, and reading room facilities of the hospital libraries. All of these details relate to the tools of your profession. Then, I remove a series of medical books from the shelves. If you have observed carefully, you will have noted that I select textbooks applying to the basic sciences as well as clinical subjects. The withdrawal cards afford an excellent index of the intellectual curiosity of the staff. I have often wished that I might pursue this aspect to its logical conclusion of the occasion and the application of the information sought. It is not enough that our medical libraries are used. Let us ask to what purpose.

Familiarity with the medical literature is essential to progressive medical practice. Obviously it is impossible for any physician to keep abreast of the great volume of new developments in all aspects of research and clinical medicine. Even were it desirable, such an ambitious design would defeat its own ends in the hopeless confusion invited by the dissipation of interest and energy. Necessarily a lag must occur in the development of standard textbooks. In many respects their information is three to five years old when they emerge from the publishing house. Hence, reference to such sources is recommended primarily to medical students and such graduates as must have immediate access to an authoritative statement of an accepted position. From this base the more advanced student and graduate will seek the latest developments in a given subject through appropriate channels. As a teacher, I never came before a class of medical students without consulting the latest number of *Reader's Digest, Newsweek, Time* and *Ladies Home Journal!* Seriously, while personally eschewing these media of lay communication, one must admit that their plane is much higher than a generation past. By the same token, the laity is much better informed in medical matters. Since medical periodicals are the natural channels of professional interchange and since they are too numerous and too diversified for inclusive consumption, the physician must perforce discriminate among them according to his needs. At the same time he must avoid too restrictive a literary diet. A balanced ration for a family counsellor would add a journal on pediatrics, on surgery, and on obstetrics to two or three general medical journals for adequate coverage. The specialist would, on the other hand, be well advised to read two or three general medical journals in addition to his several special periodicals.

The habits of medical reading are singularly individualistic. Hence one is loath to impose his pattern upon others. In the first place, budget your time. An hour or two regularly assigned each day is more rewarding than longer periods of sporadic reading. If time permits, a given order is followed. The reading of the abstracts, book reviews, and editorials usually precedes a perusal of the articles, which are selectively chosen from personal interest. When time is afforded, the author is given the courtesy of careful reading. When time presses, the conclusion only is read; and if provocative, the entire article is studied. Incidentally, the title may capture the interest, whether the subject be one of pressing notice or not. A number of years ago (1937) the appeal of the title, "Some Clinical Caprices of Hodgkin's Disease," quickly exhausted my supply of reprints. Conversely, a redundant or an abstruse title may dissuade the prospective reader. To the uninitiated, mere publication in a standard medical journal is too often deemed the sine qua non of professional acceptance and authority. Time and acquaintance will spare certain compromises of this order. Prompt abstraction of significant reports and articles with the maintenance of an adequate card index by system and disease will preserve the immediate reaction and render the composite experience more accessible.

Private libraries are a source of sustained interest. Many years ago I was calling on a prominent New Yorker. To await the gentleman I was ushered into his library. The setting was most impressive. Comfortable armchairs and a davenport, beautifully upholstered in a soft brown leather, were perfectly lighted by individual floor lamps. The massive mahogany desk was immaculate and it was properly appointed with a heavy bronze desk set. The library itself was imposing in the matching brown leather of the bindings. From the floor, shelf after shelf mounted twelve feet to the ceiling on three sides of the room. A heavy oriental rug completed the scene of opulent culture. Time lagged and I naturally wandered to the books. The *Complete Works* of William Makepeace Thackeray first confronted me. One by one, I took them down. Three-quarters leather, gilded edge—not a leaf cut! So I passed to Dickens, Browning, Shakespeare, and a dozen other authors, all with the same result, uncut, untouched. If there is possible a greater sin than misuse of books, it is unuse!

In singular contrast to this ornamental library, I would take you into two private libraries where the love of books prevailed. In both instances, the terms, "collector" and "collection," were actively eschewed. Special interests led both men to extremes in the acquisition of coveted volumes; yet both were, in the finest sense of the term, medical bibliophiles. Doctor David Riesman, Philadelphia clinician extraordinary, had a profound interest in medical history. Indeed so deep were these roots that few of his clinical conferences escaped such notice. Furthermore, he imbued generations of medical students at Pennsylvania with a consuming interest in this rewarding field of study. From medicine and medical history, his absorption ranged to papal affairs, astronomy, and atomic physics. His library was a peaceful haven for the busy teacher-clinician. A step or two elevated the shelves from the study proper. Vivid in my mind is the leather upholstered armchair that Doctor Riesman regularly used. On one arm of the chair were two worn bands, where the Doctor rested his legs as he sat sideways to read!

Transplantation from Philadelphia to Madison (1912) found me early drawn to the circle that Dr. William Snow Miller had welded into a medical history seminar. An anatomist whose classical work, *The Lung*, remains the standard source reference on this structure, he had long been interested in the history of medicine. The members of the seminar were encouraged to follow their own bent and to develop independent interests. His personal library, which by careful accessions came to hold unusual preeminence in certain directions, was the rallying point for the seminar. Dr. Miller's priceless library found periodic exploitation in his "Fifty Feet of Anatomy," when on broad stretcher tables the works of the masters were displayed. Among the most valuable incunabula in this library, now owned by the University of Wisconsin, are the many editions of Vesalius. On each card in the index catalogue, Dr. Miller entered the cost of the book. From time to time, the quotations of the catalogues of book dealers would be compared. The regularity of enhanced prices bore testimony to his keen insight into values in this specialized field. The active participation of seminar members sustained their interest. From this origin similar foci for the study of the history of medicine have developed in Oregon, California, and Texas.

> Show me his friends and I the man shall know;
> This wiser turn a larger wisdom lends:
> Show me the books he loves and I shall know
> The man far better than through mortal friends.
>
> (Mitchell)

The physician's interest in books is natural. His application is not limited to their production. Furthermore, his reading should not be restricted to medical texts and journals. By his very preoccupation in technical and professional matters involving life and death, general literature affords a release and relaxation in its broader cultural outlook. Personal tastes and circumstances materially modify the selection of a physician's collateral reading; nor would I presume to stand in judgment of my fellow's choice. Yet, the lasting influence of certain works bespeaks a quality that is lacking in too many books with an ephemeral popularity. In *Pilgrim's Progress,* John Bunyan has allegorically met most of the problems of daily life. Lewis Carroll affords a philosophical outlook on life in *Alice's Adventures in Wonderland.* The profound truths of human relations are forcibly brought home in the Books of Psalms, Proverbs, and Ecclesiastes, of the Old Testament. Indeed, every excursion into The Holy Bible is a rewarding experience. Marcus Aurelius, Epictetus, Cervantes, and Chaucer are provocative bedtime consultants of long standing. Aside from medical history, which is a continuing challenge, biography and general history have an unusual personal attraction. Abraham Lincoln has been a lifelong subject of study, who still eludes definition in certain areas. Robert E. Lee and Thomas J. Jackson, each with his unusual but distinctive strength and weakness, continue to grow in stature in their respective capacities. Our present station has afforded an excellent opportunity for a closer study of the campaigns of the calamitous Civil War. A most

significant account of that conflict is found in Freeman's *R. E. Lee.*
His *Lee's Lieutenants* is a fitting companion book. The remarkable
resurgence of interest in the Civil War is evinced by a number of recent significant books on its various phases. Among these, three have
separate places. In a documented human approach Glenn Tucker relates the events leading to *High Tide at Gettysburg.* In his gripping
This Hallowed Ground, Bruce Catton makes his audience live the
stirring, stumbling events that were to end in *A Stillness at Appomat-
tox.* The unexcelled command of the English language that characterizes the speeches and writings of Winston Churchill has lent unusual
zest to the reading of his account of World War II. In this respect,
even his titles invite close scrutiny of the contents. So the list might be
extended when every commanding general or flag officer in that War
needs must write his personal account of its events. *The Memoirs of
Montgomery of Alamein* might better have concluded with the *memories* of that decisive engagement!

Both writing and books have a further unusual but cogent place in
medicine. If the reflection of a sound literary background be accepted
as a major asset for the cultured gentleman, then to no career is it more
essential than to that of the practicing physician. His intimate contacts
with the patients and the family, his community relationships, and his
professional responsibilities require the closest measure of rapport with
people. At the same time, in recent years, overemphasis upon scientific
qualifications for entry into medical schools has seriously compromised
a basic interest in and a grasp of the humanities among physicians. Our
medical schools and universities are frantically attempting to turn back
the tide that they initiated through their fixed requirements in the sciences for admission. In our professional relations the therapeutic value
of reading is repeatedly invoked. The Twenty-Third Psalm is one of
the finest tranquilizers for the troubled soul. Barrie's *Courage* is a tonic
for the faint of heart. Eve Curie's life of her mother, Marie Curie, is
one of the finest biographies of modern times. In her account of the
conquest of apparently insuperable obstacles by the elder Curies, the
downtrodden and oppressed will take renewed hope. So the list might
be extended. From the resources of his own reading the perceptive
physician may unobtrusively lead his patient to the fountains of literary
strength that will bring new courage and life. Term it what you will,
discriminating, purposeful reading is good medicine!

RANDOM SAMPLING
WITHOUT RESORT
TO REASON

INTRODUCTION

The year that the Congress inserted the words "including medical research" into our license to practice medicine (38 U. S. C. 4101) is worth remembering. It became the year of virgin birth, or rebirth, for Veterans Administration research as it was the occasion of the Tenth Annual Veterans Administration Research Conference, begun at Memphis December 16, 1958. And that was the day of two distinctive birthday addresses full of promise for the newborn. The publication of these two papers by separate authors in this one issue is contrary to the custom of the Editor of this distinguished series of bulletins, and he asks an explanation. The answer is popular demand by all those who heard these talks—and what more can an Editor ask?

Really, there was only one subject—that of creativity—albeit, by two very different men, and the two titles they used coalesced naturally into the one title used above. The one, the preeminent clinician-teacher, represented our internal support, evaluation, and direction, as Chief Medical Director. The other, the distinguished chemist and science administrator, represented our outside contacts, critics, and guidance, as Chairman, Division of Medical Sciences, National Research Coun-

Presented to Tenth Annual Veterans Administration Research Conference in Memphis, December 16, 1958. Reprinted from Veterans Administration, Department of Medicine & Surgery Medical Bulletin MB-3, February 6, 1959.

cil, National Academy of Sciences. In those who know these two, there is no thought even of possible collusion. But those who know the Chairman of the Conference, Dr. Martin M. Cummings, may entertain a suspicion of intuitive telepathy. However that may be, one talk begins with the questioning "Why?" of the child, and the other ends with the knowing "Why not?" of the young lady of Kent.

RANDOM SAMPLING   (W. S. M.)

Emerging in the light of day after nine months of intrauterine darkness, the newborn baby is confronted by a world of new impressions, visual, auditory, gustatory, olfactory, indeed perceptive in all modalities.

Throughout time parents, psychologists, and people in general have observed and discussed the ramifications of the mental processes of the curious-minded infant and child. Science has carefully studied the responses of infants and children to stimuli, natural and unnatural; but as yet we have not fathomed the direction and the depth of thought in these developing personalities. With the extending world of the youngsters come myraids of new impressions, freshly rediscovered by succeeding generations. From their natural curiosity arises the incessant repetitious question, "Why?" The rebuffed and disillusioned child comes to accept the conventional, if incomplete, answer with resignation. The curious-minded one continues to seek the answer and through his "Whys?" becomes the research worker and the productive scholar.

In numerous periods of history, students have considered themselves favored as living in a golden age of achievement. From the vantage point of fifty years in medicine, I would agree that we are presently in one of the most exciting and prolific eras of medical and scientific development. Nor am I speaking of mere publications, important as they are in the dissemination of information. (At heart, I am a conservationist and love trees!) New and revolutionary developments in the fundamental sciences are now promptly transferred to the clinical laboratory and sickroom. Communications are easy and not infrequently two-way streets. A remarkably profitable partnership has been developed between the laboratory and the clinic. Its dividends are so conspicuous that this union will be strengthened in the future.

Most significant has been the cultivation of group research. Perhaps the diversity of skills in modern techniques of chemistry, physics, and biology necessitates the concatenation of such congeries of stars. However, many publications have long lists of authors whose individual part can be little more than nominal. Weigh carefully this proposition from two angles. If there be seven coauthors, did each one contribute his seventh? Or, what is more important, did each one obtain one-seventh of the profit from his investment of time and energy? Without decrying group research, by contrast epochal contributions in the natural sciences and medicine have almost without exception been the product of a single inspired mind. My concern is less that initiative suffer by company than that independent thought be submerged in the community of interest and activity. This reservation will not apply to cooperative studies which have proved so effective in the Veterans Administration. Indeed we have an opportunity as well as an obligation to exploit this area in the interest of the American veteran and humanity at large. In the salubrious climate of such clinical observations basic and applied research will thrive and its fruits will enrich medicine not only as an art but as a science.

In this iconoclastic period, a materialistic public pictures the scientist as a removed individual, detached from the realities of life and devoid of many of the natural amenities and inhibitions of the common man. Oliver Wendell Holmes once characterized his associate, Louis Agassiz, thus: "Professor Agassiz would grasp truth by the throat and choke her until the sphincters relax!" Actually, medical research thrives in an atmosphere of quiet and serenity. Some of the most significant contributions to my intimate knowledge have emerged from thoughts that arose in periods of quiet contemplation. My associate, the late Dr. Arthur L. Tatum, conceived the probable usefulness and availability of mapharsen (arsenoxide) with his feet on the desk as his chair was tilted back to strike an even balance between appropriate oxygenation and stagnation of the cerebral circulation! Dr. Tatum reasoned, "If arsphenamine is oxidized in the body, why not use this product therapeutically?" Meta-amino parahydroxy phenylarsine oxide (mapharsen) was the direct result of daydreaming, constructive contemplation, if you prefer. Dr. William B. Castle related to me the circumstance of his discovery of the intrinsic factor. He was shaving one morning when he sharply recalled the impending appearance of his new chief, Dr. George R. Minot, at the Thorndike Memorial Laboratory. Thought he, "Now my new chief is coming and I have not a single idea in my head." Like a flash there occurred to him the fact that the single least common denominator for all patients with pernicious anemia was an absence of free hydrochloric acid in the gastric contents. When Dr. Castle reported to Dr. Minot, he suggested the classic experiment of feeding ground beef to normal subjects, abstracting the gastric contents after a period of digestion, and then giving the product after further incubation with hydrochloric acid to known subjects of pernicious anemia. The resultant remissions revolutionized medical thought of the pathogenesis of pernicious anemia and indeed, in many respects, initiated a new era of hematologic research and practice.

Time for contemplation. Reflect on your problems of the day. My father in pathology, Dr. Allen J. Smith, once said, "When your results are 50 percent correct, examine the methods. When your results are 100 percent right, examine yourself." Assess dispassionately the gain of the day. Review objectively your results. Certainly, at times you will experience a sense of frustration that would make Sisyphus a piker. You will recall this character in mythology who with great effort pushed the stone to the top of the hill, only to have it roll down each time. The counterpart in entomology is termed the dung-beetle. While we want no dung-beetles, there will be periods of frustrating discouragement. Such is the time for a modification of the approach or a change of scene. Even Louis Pasteur went on a holiday. When he returned, the chicken cholera cultures that had been ineffective became highly protective either through the deterioration or the inactivation of the virus; and the problem of the control of the disease was resolved.

Years ago, in Dr. Allen J. Smith's laboratory of pathology at the University of Pennsylvania, I spent many hours of interesting study of the possibility of the extramedullary production of eosinophiles. The steps and results of these experiments are inconsequential since I did not prove our thesis; but forty-five years later the technique is still vivid in my memory. Indeed, within the past five years I have had occasion to apply it in an entirely different relation. And the eosinophiles of the horse are most beautiful for study! Rarely is thoughtful research unproductive in the long run.

Deliver me from the too clean laboratory! Bear in mind that I am referring not merely to order as such. Justice Cardozo once said: "There is an accuracy that defeats itself by overemphasis of details." I am never quite comfortable in a laboratory where every bit of apparatus, every beaker, every test tube is spick and span. Few active laboratories can ever be accused of such regularity. The sense of disorder, however, usually obtains only in the mind of the casual intruder who has not looked behind the scene. Properly, we should realize that the apparent disarray reflects the peregrinations of an active mind. Such minds will improvise and blaze new trails rather than await the bulldozer, the roller, and the roadmaker of the gadgeteer.

Research is a state of the mind. Charcot once said: "Without incessant scientific renewal, [medical practice] becomes an obsolete routine." Research is truly the lifestream of medicine; the fire that sublimates ideas, whether in the clinic or in the laboratory. As clinicians, we turn to research for the advancement of our practice. With its support in the close relationship of the laboratory and the clinic, we shall go forward together.

WITHOUT RESORT TO REASON   (R. K. CANNAN)

My task, I take it, is to tune my preoccupations to your occupations.

Within the context of this Conference, your occupation is the conduct of research. Mine, and that of my companions on this platform, is the administration of research.

Your responsibility is to serve your own imagination; to pursue ideas and to discipline them. Ours is to give coherence to your ideas, and power, and thereby to ready them for the service of society.

Your interest is constrained within the clinic and the laboratory. Ours is required to roam over the whole national medical scene. We are concerned with the Art of the Possible; you with the Cultivation of the Improbable.

On this accounting it would seem that our job specifications and our territorial responsibilities are far apart. And yet we know that our affairs are considerably muddled up together.

It is well, therefore, that we should get together from time to time and compare notes in a search for a common understanding and a common purpose. This morning I would like to open the door to such a discussion with a few quite general reflections.

My thesis may be stated in three propositions:

Firstly, society has, rather suddenly, come to recognize that science is the very bulwark of national welfare and of national security;

Secondly, as a consequence, science, which over the centuries had been essentially a pastime for amateurs, is rapidly becoming professionalized;

And finally, the community of scientists is having some difficulty in feeling at home in its new relationship to organized society. Both sides recognize that the traditional treaty of segregation is out of date but the process of integration is requiring some uncomfortable readjustments. Perhaps you will agree that the root of the difficulty is the reconciliation of the eighteenth-century idea of science as the pursuit of knowledge for its own sake with the "hard and stubborn fact" of the twentieth-century that science has become the servant of society. We welcome the additional patronage that is coming our way but we would like very much to retain our amateur status.

Over the ages society has evinced only a fitful interest in science. Its impulse has been to restrain as often as to encourage. And yet, on the whole, its attitude has been benevolent.

As long as he remained in his ivory tower the scientist was tolerated as an amiable eccentric to be classed with poets, jesters, and mystics and was left to his own devices. He was even granted a share in that modicum of the surplus wealth of the country that the aristocracy was willing to contribute to the pursuit of culture. But indulgence in science remained a highly individual cult—amateur, academic, and remote from human affairs.

As the nineteenth century moved into full orbit this attitude began to change. Society came to realize that the fast-developing technologies of the physical sciences were a potential source of new power—new power to control man's environment to his own advantage.

Science began to be recognized as a potent servant of progress and society promptly moved in, adopted it, and proceeded to organize it.

As Alfred North Whitehead has cogently phrased the situation: "The greatest invention of the nineteenth century was the invention of the method of invention."

In its beginning this social augmentation of power was confined to the physical sciences and professionalization developed through the instrument of private enterprise. Somewhat later, geology and biology in their turn refined their technologies to practical ends of engineering, agriculture, and public health, and they too soon found themselves being socially organized. In these areas, however, it is to be noted that it was government rather than private enterprise that took the initiative and developed the professional patterns.

Turning to the world today there is certainly no need to elaborate the argument that atomic energy, rocket engines, and electronic brains have added orders of magnitude to man's command of power and that society is up to its neck in the fearful business of bringing these under control.

We are accustomed to blame international communism for the frenetic pace of the scientific effort of the last decade. But this is true, I think, only of its hysterical component. The statisticians tell that, throughout the last 100 years, the pace of scientific investigation has been increasing exponentially and the number of scientists has been doubling every ten years or so. In other words, if we accept this statistic we may conclude that about 90 percent of the world's total output of scientists is alive today.

The truth is that science is expanding because man has ordered it so —because he is insatiable for power. He has recognized science as the means to this end and has made its promotion a matter of national policy. His attitudes have swung full circle from tolerant indifference to unreasoned adulation. Scientists are a sort of priesthood that has the low-down on nature and life. They possess a mystique called the scientific method that can solve all problems. They can do most anything. Their statements are always "true."

Surely science is unique amongst human endeavors in that it is only its successes that are publicized.

This has been an overlong preamble. I apologize. My weakness always has been that I choose a canvas too large for my brush. Let us bring the story closer to home.

In the profound social reorientation of science during the last 100 years medical research might well have been left to languish in neglect along with the humanities. Until the last few years it has, indeed, retained its amateur status. But, all the time, it was quietly refining its techniques until, with the advent of the last war, it became evident that medicine had finally developed a coherent technology of diagnosis and therapy that gave promise of a longer life and better health. Longer life and health with which to enjoy the good life that material progress had made possible. Consequently society, largely through government, has now moved in on medical research and is proceeding to organize and to professionalize it.

All this has happened in a bare ten years or so. Whether we measure in dollars, in numbers of projects, in growth of laboratories, or by a census of the personnel involved, the expansion of effort has been prodigious.

The resources of medical research in this country have doubled in the last five years. In the past fifteen years they have increased fivefold.

In this same fifteen years the participation of Government has increased fiftyfold, so that, today, two-thirds of the pooled research budgets of the medical schools of the country derive from sources within the federal government.

This is socialization at a gallop. This is why administrators and their committees figure so prominently on your horizons.

Whether we like it or not, those who control the purse strings of research are in a position to exert a profound influence on the trends of investigation and also on the attitudes of investigators.

The history of the current forms of research administration is an interesting one. The salient fact is that these forms were, in large measuure, fashioned by scientists themselves.

When government first sought to mobilize scientists in a big way to meet the needs of the last war it established OSRD. The responsibility for organizing this agency was given over to scientists who naturally built on designs that were familiar to them in their erstwhile dealings with philanthropic foundations.

The method of project research was adopted and vastly expanded. Investigators who thought they had an idea were invited to submit proposals which were evaluated and grants were made on the advice of committees whose membership was drawn largely from the ranks of academic medicine.

With the termination of the war this type of machinery was adopted by ONR, VA, HEW, and NSF and has become the settled national policy. Moreover it is interesting to note that the majority of the executive officers with whom decision lies are men with a background of research experience.

There is good evidence that the scientific community has taken kindly to this method of operation. It meets immediate needs and has been singularly successful in protecting the scientist from the logrolling and political influence that he most feared.

Some of those whose business it is to take the long view have, however, had misgivings. There is a feeling that the dominance of "project research" is not designed, over the long pull, to maintain the intellectual climate most beneficent to creativity.

Let me repeat my earlier statement that the difficulty we face is the reconciliation of the pursuit of knowledge for its own sake with the accumulation of knowledge for service.

The hackneyed expression of this dilemma is the need to maintain a healthy balance between basic and applied research. Unfortunately disputants seldom agree on definitions and argument becomes sterile.

There is, however, a related antimony that I like better. Let me try it on you.

Albert Einstein has distinguished Science Existing from Science in the Making. "Science Existing," he wrote, "is the most logically consistent discipline known to man. Science in the Making, on the other hand, is as subjective and as psychologically conditioned as any branch of human endeavor."

May I add that these two disciplines are distinguishable both in their grammar and their logic. One uses the Present Indicative, the other the Future Imperfect. One employs the Logic of the Discovered and the other the Logic of Discovery.

Research in the Logic of the Discovered *can* be planned and organized. A defined body of knowledge *can* be taken and a logical series of experiments can be designed which will exploit this knowledge to its foreseeable limits. Planned research can take a set of postulates and drive them home to their logical conclusions. It can do this with exhaustive thoroughness, economy, and speed. Project outlines can be prepared on a rational design well suited to scientific evaluation by a committee of experts. The role of this kind of a project is to consolidate ground already won.

The Logic of Discovery is a different kind of construction. Its purpose is to seek new worlds to conquer. It is something realized in the imagination and not in fact. It is highly subjective and personal. Man sees things as he is and not as they are. It is a very human enterprise, rough, confused, naive, and colored by habit, fancy, and prejudice. It is compounded of error, astonishment, invention, and understanding. It takes leaps in the dark, plays hunches, and learns by mistakes.

The peculiar characteristic of Science in the Making is a willingness to believe that things are other than they seem. It is alert for the Unexpected. "Every new idea," wrote Whitehead, "has a certain air of foolishness." He meant only that it was novel and unfamiliar. The Logic of Discovery is designed for the manipulation of the unfamiliar.

Perhaps it is for this reason that it is ill-adapted for the writing of plausible projects. It is a logic that becomes fully articulate only in its outcome.

"How do I know what I think until I see what I do?" protested the old lady in one of E. M. Forster's novels.

Let me make myself plain that when I distinguish two logics of science I am not contrasting two types of scientists. In the pursuit of his ideas every investigator has recourse to both languages. He supplements reason with intuition, the scientific method with inspired fancy. He is challenged with facts by day and is the sport of notions by night.

Perhaps the secret of genius is to be possessed by an instinct that unconsciously knows when you should keep your feet on the ground and when you should take wings.

This dichotomy of behavior is the despair of the administrator. In my youth I received from the Director of the Imperial Cancer Institute in London advice that I have always cherished and sometimes followed. He said "If you have an idea, go into the laboratory and work for six months. Then you may enter the library and search the literature. If you find that someone has done the same thing before, and if you have obtained the same results as he did, you can pat yourself on the back as a good experimenter. If he obtained a different result—then, my boy, you have a problem."

I wonder if a project outlined in these terms would find favor with an advisory committee.

In my youth I held a great reverence for committees. With advancing years I have been drawn more and more into their orbits and I have found them to be composed of tired, conservative old men like myself.

Fancy free as these men may be in the conduct of their own investigations, when they come to Washington, or indeed when they operate on the editorial boards of our journals, they don a cloak of orthodoxy that is veritably sacerdotal.

These men who, in their laboratories, are our Discoverers become, in the committee room, the great defenders of the Discovered. They seem to feel a heavy responsibility to uphold the sanctity of that myth that has been called the scientific method. They demand plain answers to plain questions and no nonsense.

This is a judicial climate that encourages projects that have a foreseeable outcome, those that are neatly tied together with a rigid and narrow methodology. This is a climate that promotes the exhaustive documentation of a familiar idea that may already have become sterile —the timid project that always succeeds but never advances.

Administrators and committees can do much to promote the Art of the Possible. They are almost impotent to foster the Cultivation of the Improbable.

Somewhere I have read: "The best man to say how research should be done is the man doing it. The next best man is the head of his department. Here we leave the area of best men. The research director is wrong half the time, the research committee most of the time and the board of directors all of the time."

About all that we *can* do is to pick the men, provide the tools and keep open the lines of communication.

Ladies and Gentlemen, I promised you some reflections on matters of mutual concern. But I have spent most of my time on my own insecurities rather than yours. In your research you are not, I believe, much oppressed by administrative restraints. In its wisdom the Veterans Administration has adopted a policy of executive decentralization of the direction of research. Institutions, I understand, have a large measure of local autonomy.

I could wish that other agencies of government who are in the business of administering research would imitate your example. Then we might hope that the responsibility for the cultivation of knowledge will be returned to the academic institutions where it belongs.

This would put it up squarely to these institutions to maintain a climate of inquiry that encourages the mind that is not confined to a narrow methodology, the mind that is fancy free.

It has been said: "Man rose from the apes because he was always monkeying around." It seems to me that some monkeying around is essential to the soul of an institution for research.

Finally, I have a parting thought for the individual investigator.

If you should be tempted to try to keep up with the Jones who are churning out papers at a merrier rate than you can,

If you should be tempted for this reason to go after a larger share of the almost unlimited funds that appear to be available for medical research nowadays,

If you should be tempted to surround yourself with much equipment that records results automatically and many technicians that, as automatically, observe,

If you should be so tempted, pause to reflect that instruments and technicians remove you from immediate contact with the raw facts.

New ideas lie down the road of the Unexpected and an experiment that fails may be the beginning of understanding. But instruments and technicians are not wired to read the portent of the unexpected observation or the experiment that fails.

In brief, if you should be so tempted, remember the fate of the young lady of Kent:

> You recall the young lady of Kent
> Who said that she knew what it meant
> When men asked her to dine
> Gave her cocktails and wine
> She knew what it meant—but she went.

MEDICAL HISTORY
AND BIOGRAPHY

SOME LAY CONTRIBUTORS
TO MEDICINE

Medicine had its origin:

In the primal sympathy
Which having been must ever be;
In the soothing thoughts that spring
Out of human suffering.

Primitive man experienced the discomforts of his excesses, the pains of trauma, and the symptoms incident to disease and decay. His woman suffered the pangs of childbirth. The inherent urge of self-preservation and the protective device of the maternal instinct apparently dictated the first efforts directed toward the alleviation of human suffering. The evolution of modern medicine from these ill-formed and frequently misdirected beginnings has been uncertain and tedious. Perhaps the earliest advances were the outgrowth of observations of the habits of lower animals under conditions that appeared analogous to human disorders. Certain repetitious experiences led to the avoidance of offending causes or the application of remedial agents. The similarity of the leaf, flower, stem, or root of certain plants to human organs perpetuated a singular therapeutic practice in the use of these parts for the treatment of the suspected or recognized disease, the so-called doctrine of signatures.

Obviously the sum of human intelligence and knowledge was, and still is, limited. The ancients were inclined to relate the inexplicable to

Reprinted from *The Phi Kappa Phi Journal* 21 (December 1941): 167–72.

supernatural forces. Hence efforts were made to propitiate the kindly gods by votive offerings and to defend themselves against the forces of evil by the wearing of amulets. Lest we indulge ourselves in a false sense of superiority we should look to the hex doctor of Pennsylvania, the voodoo of the Negro population in the South (the Christian Scientist of the country at large), and the vast areas of the world where magic, charms, and incantations still constitute the sole defenses against disease.

Among uncultured people it is still customary to find the functions of priest, physician, and philosopher united in one person. This circumstance affords a clue to the original status of medicine in the earliest records of the profession. In Egypt and India medicine was subordinated to religion. Greek medicine, from which we take our lineal descent, had outgrown this relationship. The afflicted were, it is true, taken to the temples of Asclepius for the incubation sleep, but the priests were not practitioners of the healing art. Hippocrates, the father of medicine (460–370 B.C.), was a member of the Asclepiad family at Cos. Certain of the fundamental truths of physiology and medicine arose from Aristotle, another Asclepiad, who received medical training.

If the origin of medical practice insured the early attention of laymen, the ubiquitous order of medical phenomena, the multifaceted contacts of sciences with medicine, and the universal interest in affairs medical would suffice to explain the continued lay contributions to its growth through the centuries. The curiously minded layman was naturally attracted by the mysteries of human physiology. Our story may regularly begin with Galileo (1564–1642), brilliant but inattentive medical student, who was destined to desert medicine and gain immortality in astronomy and mathematics. Attendant upon the services in the cathedral at Pisa, his thoughts wandered and the swinging bronze lamp caught his attention. Galileo fixed its rate of swing by the rhythm of his own pulse. Thus arose the law of isochronism of the pendulum. He likewise constructed crude thermometers, a method of precision destined to lie fallow for three hundred years.

A contemporary fellow-countryman, Sanctorius (1561–1636), made further contributions to thermometry. His most interesting studies were upon insensible perspiration. A cut published posthumously shows Sanctorius seated on a steelyard before a table. Accurate weights of food intake and body wastes enabled him to estimate the insensible perspiration. These observations were the direct precursors of the modern basal metabolic determinations.

Interest in natural philosophy advanced to its highest degree in the seventeenth century in England. The Invisible College was founded by a group of kindred spirits in London who met for intellectual interchange in Gresham College (1645). Charles II granted its charter as the Royal Society of London in 1660. As usual a catalyst was active in the evolution and remarkable fruition of the plan. Robert Boyle (1627–91), an Irishman, who had studied at Eton, Geneva, and Florence (under Galileo), was the central force about whom all of the activities of the Royal Society centered. A tall, pale aesthete, Boyle was never endowed with great physical strength. Yet his native wit, social grace, and scientific insight like a lodestone attracted the finest minds in Britain about him. Boyle's most notable contribution to biological (and medical) knowledge was the demonstration of the dependence of life upon air.

Closely associated with Boyle as secretary of the Royal Society was Robert Hooke (1635–1703), who was as dissimilar from his patron as is humanly possible. Crooked in figure and in nature, Hooke suggested innumerable physiological facts but perfected little. He constructed the air pump with which Boyle made his revolutionary experiments. In a series of ingenious studies Hooke proved that the motion of the lungs was not necessary for life. Of him Samuel Pepys wrote, "Who is the most, and promises the least, of any man in the world that ever I saw."

Among the correspondents of these omnivorous members of the Royal Society was Antony van Leeuwenhoek (1632–1723). A draper in Delft, this amazing individual found time to grind 419 lenses and to construct 247 microscopes. In all he communicated 375 separate papers or observations to the Royal Society and twenty-seven to the French Academy of Sciences. Leeuwenhoek first described bacteria, red blood corpuscles, spermatozoa, voluntary muscle fibers, and many other tissues of the body.

The physiology of respiration continued to interest laymen. Joseph Priestley (1783–1804), the discoverer of oxygen, was beset by religious and political conflicts. His clerical profession occupied his time and energies only sporadically. When he might have anticipated the peace of a rural parish, his political sympathy with the French Revolution led to the burning of the chapel at Fairhill and the sacking of his home with the irreparable loss of many of his manuscripts. Priestley came to America in 1794 and declined invitations to the finest chairs of chemistry in the New World. The fate of his friend, Antoine-Laurent Lavoisier (1743–94), was most tragic. He discovered the true nature of the interchange of gases in the lung. He remarked the irony of the greatest requirement for food by those least able to pay. Lavoisier became a farmer-general and devoted a portion of his personal fortune to the common weal. He fell a victim to Madame Guillotine in 1794.

An English clergyman, Stephen Hales (1677–1761), was one of the first contributors to the physiology of the circulation. In 1733 he attached a long glass tube to the femoral artery of a horse by appropriate means. The blood rose eight feet three inches in the tube. This constitutes the first observation of arterial blood pressure, which has risen to plague patient and physician in recent years.

Smallpox was a pestilence of prime magnitude in the olden days. Rare was the adult without the disfiguring pock-marks. On March 18, 1718, Lady Mary Wortley Montagu, wife of the ambassador to Turkey, submitted her three-year-old son to inoculation. Three years later she introduced the procedure into England by having her daughter inoculated. Cotton Mather in New England and Benjamin Franklin in Pennsylvania fathered the movement in the Colonies. The medical profession was not always in the vanguard in this advance. Late in the eighteenth century Edward Jenner reported to his old teacher, John Hunter, the lay belief of the protection of cowpox against smallpox. Hunter replied: "Don't think, try; be patient, be accurate." The first boy thus vaccinated was James Phipps, from the arm of a milkmaid, Sarah Nelmes. Inertia and worse perpetuate smallpox, a disease that could be wiped from the face of the earth in a decade of universal vaccination.

The wife of the Viceroy of Peru, Countess of Chinchon, sickened of the intermittent fever in the palace at Lima (about 1630). The reputed virtue of the bark of a native tree was finally put to the clinical trial by her physician, Don Juan de Vego. The amazing cure effected led the Countess to carry a supply of the bark on her return to Europe. Here it was known as the Countess' bark until its importation by the priests, when it was termed the Jesuits' bark. Indeed, the latter circumstance caused Protestants to reject the remedy for many years. A charlatan, Robert Taylor, sold the open secret of the preparation of the bark to Louis XIV for 2000 louis d'or, a pension, and a title. So important was the introduction of this remedy that Ramazzini declared: "Cinchona did for medicine what gunpowder did for war."

In Shropshire, William Withering was practicing medicine with indifferent success. Becoming curious in the matter of the surprising results of a herb woman in the treatment of dropsy, he asked the composition of her remedy. From the twenty ingredients recited, Withering concluded that only foxglove (*digitalis purpurea*) could possibly possess any therapeutic virtue. After an extended clinical trial he finally published his epochal monograph on this drug in 1785. Its use revolutionized medical thought and practice in the treatment of heart failure.

The Pasteurs of Dôle and Arbois were a thrifty, hard-working family whose cultural background scarcely promised a world-renowned scientist among their offspring. The father of Louis Pasteur, a tanner, had been a soldier under Napoleon. His son (1822–95) found ample time for fishing in the Cuisance which ran behind the tannery. Furthermore, the young Pasteur's interests in chemistry and physics were far afield from the ultimate realm of his surpassing accomplishment.

Pasteur's acute powers of observation were reflected in his earliest studies in the crystallography of tartaric acid. The story of his life has been gloriously preserved by his nephew, Vallery-Radot. It is the recital of indomitable courage and singular tenacity in the approach to a series of problems that had baffled man from the beginning of time. Not even the tools of attack had been welded. To Pasteur was given the single-sighted vision to flout conventional philosophies and to penetrate into the mysteries of nature. Singularly, many of his contributions were highly materialistic and practical. His researches on the mechanism of spoiling wine and beer exploded the aging theory of spontaneous generation. The failure of the silk-worm industry initiated a five-year study with the discovery of the factors involved. Anthrax threatened the wool industry until his brilliant work, confirming the studies of Davaine, Klebs, and Koch, placed the responsibility upon a bacterial form. In the course of this work Pasteur isolated the first pathogenic anaerobe. The truism, "In the field of science chance favors only the prepared mind," was never better exemplified than in his discovery of a preventive vaccine for the chicken cholera. Cultures neglected in the laboratory during a vacation period proved very protective when injected upon his return. Most spectacular of all of Pasteur's great discoveries was the prophylactic treatment of rabies that bears his name.

Out of the layman Pasteur's studies came the science of bacteriology that has contributed so abundantly to medicine and human welfare. His name is perpetuated in the pasteurization of milk and the Pasteur treatment of individuals exposed to rabies. Every community in his native France has given his name to some street or place. Far beyond such recognition comes his responsibility for Joseph Lister's gift of antisepsis in surgery that has advanced regularly to modern asepsis. Without this boon the growth of surgery would have been greatly retarded. The world acclaims him as the greatest contributor to modern medicine.

A Dutch-German physicist, Wilhelm Konrad Roentgen (1845–1922), was working with a Crookes tube in a dark room in his laboratory at Wurzbürg in 1893 when the ability of the ray to penetrate the hand was demonstrated on a screen covered with barium platino-cyanide. The marvels of the x-ray have greatly lifted the horizon of scientific research.

At no other point of impingment has a measure of beneficence approached that attendant upon its application to medicine in diagnosis and treatment.

The picture changes and we find an expatriated Pole and her husband toiling in a damp shed in Paris. In honor of her native land the Curies named the first radioactive element isolated polonium. Later (1896) radium was discovered and the world acclaimed the Curies. The application of this lay contribution to the treatment of cancer could not have been predicted. Marie Curie has given the world an intimate word picture of her distinguished husband and Eve Curie has lent further luster to the fame of her brilliant mother in the finest biography of recent times.

Thus we pass to the dawn of a new century and into a civilization of increasing complexity. The lay interest in matters scientific has grown apace in recent years. Furthermore, the vast growth of knowledge in fields closely allied and related to medicine has insured an erasure of the sharp lines of demarcation that once separated medicine to its own detriment. Chemistry, physics, and biology now blend almost imperceptibly into medicine. Physiology, nutrition, and endocrinology particularly reflect this impact.

If we but take our local situation, you would be astounded to learn how well beaten the path is between the medical school and bacteriology and biochemistry in agriculture on one hand and physics, chemistry, and zoology on the other. The world would be poorer medically and materially without the contributions of Elvehjem, Guyer, Hart, Hastings, Hisaw, and Steenbock—all but one of whom are at work today at the University of Wisconsin. The Medical School proudly admits its subscription to this policy of cooperation in the chairmanship of four of its departments in the hands of nonmedical men.

Perhaps the time is ripe for the definition of a layman. In the earliest sense it connoted a distinction to the clergy; but more recently the term has designated one not of a particular profession. Medicine in its gratitude for the support of its growing allies is satisfied to consider them alien only in the application of their scientific knowledge, viz., the practice of medicine. Marie Curie touched the point when she said: "In science we should be interested in things, not persons." Medicine is essentially interested in people.

THE GOLDEN AGE
OF MEDICINE

Within sight of the Golden Gate only the warm hospitality and the indulgence of the citizens of the Golden State could afford a guest from the Middle West the temerity to speak of that precious metal. In the classical mood, Hesiod divided the history of mankind into five significant periods: the Golden Age in the reign of Cronus and the elder gods was an era of human contentment. Man was spared from heavy manual labor and from bodily handicaps. This period was succeeded by the Silver Age under Zeus and the younger gods, wherein innocence and reverence were forsaken. In the Bronze Age that followed, the contentious and violent peoples of the earth destroyed each other. Thereupon heroes and demigods vied in mortal combat at Troy and Thebes in the Heroic Age. Finally, in the Iron Age degenerate mankind was condemned to endless toil and strife to expiate their selfishness. In the modern usage Golden Age connotes a span of years marked by unusual happiness, prosperity, or progress. Hence the term, Golden Age of Medicine, must be used with careful discrimination.

Andrew Lang cautioned: "The little present must not be allowed wholly to elbow the great past out of view." For historical perspective let us turn back the pages of history 100 years. California was celebrating her first birthday as a state. Unselfishly, instead of receiving the traditional birthday tokens from her sister states, she was already opening her treasure trove to the world at large. With a decrease in her min-

Read before a meeting of the California Academy of Medicine, San Francisco, California, December 8, 1951. Reprinted from *The Western Journal of Surgery, Obstetrics and Gynecology* 60 (June 1952): 288–98.

eral wealth over the intervening years, California has found a diversity of channels through which to maintain her wide balance of credit in the national treasury. Eighteen hundred and fifty-one marked the beginning of one of the most momentous decades in American history. Material and cultural advances were to bless the land until the crisis of 1857. A remarkable coterie of writers, Longfellow, Whittier, Bryant, Lowell, Hawthorne, Holmes, and Emerson, brought a new brilliance to American letters. Yet, in sequence the Missouri Compromise (1820), the Wilmot Proviso (1846), the Omnibus (Compromise) Bill (1850), and the Fugitive Slave Law (1850) gave full warning of the evolving, sharp sectional division. Able statesmen, like Henry Clay, Daniel Webster, John C. Calhoun, and Jefferson Davis, dominated the national scene, but an indifferent president, Millard Fillmore, sat in the White House. Soon the Kansas-Nebraska Bill (1854), Dred Scott Decision (1857), Lecompton Constitution (1857), Lincoln-Douglas Debates (1858) and John Brown's Raid on Harper's Ferry (1859) were to bring the United States inexorably to the hour of decision.

While the witches' pot of war was seething to the boiling point in America, medical advance was by no means stayed a hundred years ago. Indeed, Garrison termed the decade from 1846 to 1855 "the most brilliant in the whole history of medicine." Well may he have extolled the surpassing contributions of Claude Bernard and Carl Ludwig to physiology. Louis Pasteur was then pulling the shrouds of skepticism from spontaneous generation and lending a scientific explanation for the etiology of infectious diseases. Joseph Lister had not yet applied these principles to surgical antisepsis, but he was laying the foundations for a sound career in surgery. Surgical anesthesia had been given impetus by Crawford W. Long (1842–43), Horace Wells (1844), and William Thomas Green Morton (1844–46) in the United States and James Young Simpson (1847) in Scotland. Rudolf Virchow was revolutionizing the pathological concepts of disease. The torch of clinical medicine, which had burned so brightly in France and Central Europe, was held high by the British clinicians, Richard Bright, Thomas Addison, and Thomas Hodgkin in this decade. The continental methods had been substantially transplanted to Dublin by William Stokes and Dominic Corrigan before this period; but Irish medicine reached its zenith in the middle of the nineteenth century. The infusion of French clinical methods into American medicine anticipated this decade; but the influence of Henry I. Bowditch, Oliver Wendell Holmes, Valentine Mott, William Wood Gerhard, Thomas D. Mütter, Alfred Stillé, and William Pepper (primus), all of whom studied in Paris, was still potent throughout the land. Perhaps one of the most significant medical contributions of the decade was Daniel Drake's publication of *A Systematic Treatise on . . . Diseases of the Interior Valley of North America* (1850–54), a classic in medical geography. In the surgical field, J. Marion Sims was establishing the feasibility of the repair of vesicovaginal fistula for the first time. In 1850, Samuel D. Gross, the greatest of American surgeons, was graduated from Jefferson Medical College. The American Medical Association was four years old in 1851; but the California Academy of Sciences had to await parturition three years later (1854).

As a barometer of professional interest and study, a survey of the programs of the scientific sessions of medical societies is most revealing. Let me caution you to avoid premature judgment. While the curves of interest as measured by presentations before representative medical groups and publications in recognized medical journals may follow a reasonably predictable trend, there is commonly an inverse relation between the quantitative and the qualitative values. A hundred years hence, the historian who attempts to relate progress in medicine to the textbooks, medical journals, and society proceedings of our generation, will be struck by the sudden flow and ebb of interest as reflected in the subject matter. Certainly this observation becomes evident when decennial samples are taken. In the program of one national medical society ten of forty-one papers were on infections and anti-infectious agents in 1941, while only three of twenty-seven were so related in 1951. Of the ten papers listed in 1941, four were on sulfonamides, four on gramicidin, and one on penicillin; and in 1951 not a single topic was directed to these agents. In three scientific groups, titles on endocrine subjects appeared on the programs in the following ratios to the total papers in 1941: ten of forty-one, eight of forty-one, and four of twenty-two, respectively. In 1951, for the same societies, the figures were three of twenty-seven, two of thirty, and one of thirty-six, respectively. Adrenocorticotropic hormone and cortisone came to their merited notice in 1951. In the programs of the three societies, five of twenty-seven, seven of thirty, and seven of thirty-six papers were devoted to this subject. Cardiovascular subjects showed an increase in each of the programs over the same period as follows: one to two, nine to twelve, and two to six, respectively. Hematological considerations showed a sustained interest in only one of the three groups, although a temporary upsurge in the reports of erythrocyte survival and blood plasma substitutes reflected the impending war in 1941. Involved technics and the almost universal recourse to biochemical support are interesting signs of the times. Radioisotopes attracted two places on the program of one society in 1941, and two, two, and three places, respectively, in the several programs in 1951. While such cursory studies are enlightening, detached from their chronologic precursors or successors they lose much of their potential weight. Obviously straddle surveys of two three- to five-year periods would constitute a more reasonable basis of comparison. Yet it is astounding how quickly an incompletely exploited area of medical research is to all intents and purposes deserted in favor of a newer and more promising field. Only fifty of the 3000 odd sulfonamides had been subjected to adequate study when the clinical value of penicillin was announced; yet over night the medical attention was almost completely diverted from sulfonamide research. Perhaps some future workers will glean untold harvests from this deserted field.

If one be not completely overwhelmed by the sheer mass and intricacy of modern medical advances, his first reaction must be amazement at the changing order of study and contribution in medical science. Certainly never has medical research pursued more closely the newer technics nor utilized more promptly the new tools of the physical and biological sciences than in the recent past. At a glance, the unusual advantages of such rapport to medical research must become apparent. The adaptation of electronic principles to the specific needs of basic medical research is a notable example. In electrocardiography the cathode oscillograph and vacuum tube amplifier have replaced the string galvanometer. Further applications of these principles have made electroencephalography a practical device in clinical neurology. No research laboratory in medicine can operate effectively without the spectrophotometer, photofluorometer, flame spectrophotometer, electrophoretic (Tisselius) apparatus, and oximeter. (I hasten to deny any profound knowledge of the manipulation of such equipment. I merely have a speaking acquaintance. As an administrator I validate the importunate requisitions from my associates.) The electron microscope promises ultimately to simplify certain basic principles. Its most recent contribution has been the visualization of the gene. Chromatography is a more humble newcomer for the characterization of serum proteins. Fascinating, indeed, are the potentialities for research in physical chemistry emanating from the use of the ultracentrifuge (Svedberg). This instrument at 50,000 to 60,000 revolutions per minute develops a force 200,000 times gravity. Applied to an isolated problem, each erythrocyte contains 300,000,000 molecules of hemoglobin. Each molecule of hemoglobin in turn holds four atoms of oxygen-binding iron and hundreds of electrically charged groups required in internal respiration. The internal environment of the mammalian body is indeed complex.

Enzyme chemistry is making itself felt with increasing force in medical research and practice. Clinicians speak freely of the competitive excretion of caronamide and penicillin from the renal tubule; but there is an interesting enzymatic activity involved in this important therapeutic device to increase blood levels of penicillin. Dimercaptopropanol (BAL) is an interesting adaptation of another aspect of this principle in the treatment of arsenical and certain other heavy metal poisonings. By combining with the tissue sulfhydryls, arsenic interrupts the vital pyruvate-oxidase system. In competition with the dithiol proteins of tissues, dimercaptopropanol has a greater affinity for arsenic and thus spares the sulfhydryls for their normal role in the pyruvate-oxidase chain. The pharmacologist has extended clinical insight into the action of certain drugs on the basis of their adrenergic or cholinergic functions. Acetylcholine and sympathin live in our therapeutic planning through their enzymatic activation and inactivation. The Coris have evolved a very significant theory of the action of insulin. From the evidence they have adduced, the diabetogenic hormone of the anterior lobe of the pituitary body inhibits the hexokinase reaction, whereas insulin accelerates it. In effect insulin is antidotal to the diabetogenic hormone. Now arises the neglected question of a bypassing of the bottleneck of the hexokinase reaction in the utilization of fructose through fructokinase. At least there are theoretical possibilities. Medical students of today have a sound working knowledge of decarboxylation, phosphorylation, and other essential enzymatic reactions and enzyme chemistry takes an increasingly important place in medical thinking and practice.

Not to be outdone, steroid chemistry has become a clamant newcomer in medical thought. Perhaps the spectacular introduction of cortisone has constituted one of the most revolutionary medical discoveries of our period (Kendall, Reichstein). The physiological interrelationship of the anterior lobe of the pituitary body and the adrenal cortex is even more impressive than the pituitary-thyroid interdependence. Important as was the initial clinical application of cortisone in the treatment of rheumatoid arthritis (Hench), even more significant have been the fundamental observations of resultant physiological changes. Profound influence upon endocrine function is noted. Steroid excretion and electrolyte balance are greatly affected.

The submergence of inflammatory and constitutional reactions upon its use in infections constitutes a revolutionary development (Finland; Smadel and Woodward). A sixty-nine-year-old white male in the State of Wisconsin General Hospital, receiving cortisone for the treatment of Felty's syndrome, experienced a sharp pain in the right flank. This pain was attended by local muscle spasm above the right iliac crest. Later, there developed increasing resistance and a mass in this region. The temperature remained normal, the leukocytes never rose above 3000 per cubic millimeter, and the erythrocyte sedimentation rate was unchanged. When the surgeons finally incised the area, 500 cc. of pus was evacuated from the retrocecal region. The beneficent cortisone had drawn a velvet curtain over the ordinary clinical guideposts to local suppuration. A similar situation exists in experimental syphilis and tuberculosis, with substantial clinical evidence to contraindicate the use of cortisone in these diseases. With the extending use of adrenocorticotropin and cortisone, their clinical indications and limitations are being more sharply drawn; yet the manner of their action in many respects remains an enigma. The clinic has outpaced the laboratory at a hazard. To consolidate our position we must proceed with the utmost caution. With the release of these agents for general use will come a wave of disastrous results. Fortunately most of these byeffects are reversible; but security will come only with an elucidation of their manner of action and medical expediency apparently will not await the inevitable scientific lag in this area. To date, we have merely cracked the shell of steroid chemistry in its relation to medicine.

In 1895, Wilhelm Konrad Roentgen announced the discovery of x-rays from his laboratory at Wurzbürg. Two years later a young American, Walter B. Cannon, made a significant contribution to the study of gastrointestinal mobility with this new tool. Using the goose because of its long esophagus, Cannon studied the progression of an opaque bolus through the upper gastrointestinal tract. (By a coincidence, Cannon was born in Prairie du Chien, Wisconsin, where at Fort Crawford, William Beaumont, pioneer physiologist, had performed approximately one-half of his experiments on Alexis St. Martin). In 1897, Henri Becquerel discovered that uranium emitted radiations that fogged the photographic plate. In 1900, the Curies isolated radium and ascertained the physical properties of radioactive substances. They listed these rays in the order of their penetrating properties, as alpha, beta, and gamma. Nuclear fission became the next logical objective of physicists. From their industry and brilliant perspicacity, a new field of fundamental science unfolded. Radioactive isotopes opened new vistas in medical research that are finding substantial applications in basic science and practice. Isotopes are substances of the same chemical formula, but different mass. They are divided into stable and unstable forms. The stable isotopes, which may be measured by the mass spectrograph, give no radiations. The radioactive forms radiate beta particles and gamma rays. The beta particles are high speed electrons which ionize more strongly but are less penetrating than the gamma rays. The latter resemble x-rays, but have shorter wave length. The millicurie, the unit of measurement, represents the disintegration of 37,000,000 atoms per second. The microcurie is 1/1000 of the millicurie. In biological experi-

mentation the "half-life," i.e., the time it takes for one-half of the radioactive atoms present to disintegrate, has an important bearing upon the
availability of a given radioisotope. A long "half-life" increases the
hazard of a given agent in the human subject. Among the instruments
for the detection of beta and gamma rays is the Geiger counter. A scientific wag has given some indication of the sensitivity of the method
by stating that a single radioactive penny could be detected in the
national debt!

World War II seriously interrupted the natural evolution of certain
phases of essential research in this area. By the same token the finest
scientific minds in western civilization lent every effort to the chaining
of atomic energy for destruction. The major dividends of their vast
expenditure were not gained in the military sphere, but are still being
won in the chemical, biological, physical, and medical advances through
this new medium. Geiling and others have utilized the ingenious device
of growing digitalis and tobacco in an atmosphere containing CO_2
tagged with C_{14} to trace the action of digitoxin and nicotine in subsequent pharmacologic experiments. Tagged elements have afforded
physiologists and allied scientists the means to establish incontrovertible
evidence of the channels of absorption and utilization of calcium, sodium, phosphorus, iron, and iodine. We are still hesitant to use C_{14} in
human studies, because of its very long "half-life," but radioactive iodine
(I_{131}) has lent itself most readily to physiological and clinical studies.
Indeed so sensitive are its determinations that one billionth of an ounce
can be determined in the human subject. The affinity of the thyroid
gland for iodine makes it an ideal area for research. If there be no com-
plicating factors, radioactive iodine uptake by the thyroid gland constitutes one of the most reliable tests of its activity. Furthermore, I_{131} has
found favor in the treatment of thyrotoxicosis and a limited group of
carcinomas of the thyroid gland. The use of radioautographs has afforded added information as to the activity of the several portions of the
thyroid gland upon excision after the administration of I_{131}.

Radioactive phosphorus (P_{32}) has also received wide medical attention. With its predilection for bone, research turned naturally to its
distribution and then its effects upon the marrow elements. A limited
therapeutic indication for its use in leukemia and lymphomas has
emerged. Lawrence and his fellows have established beyond a peradventure the supremacy of P_{32} in the treatment of polycythemia rubra
vera.

In recent years cardiologic research and practice have been engaged
largely in consolidating the advantages of electrocardiography, teleoroentgenography, and orthodiagraphy by refinements of technic and

minor exploratory forays. Heart sounds have been amplified by electronic means and adapted to clinical research. Largely through the work of Cournand, cardiac catheterization has become not only a technic for physiological study, but also for clinical evaluation of the cardiac patient. Cardioangiography has been developed apace. Both of these technics are now essential elements in every organized cardiac clinic. I say "organized" advisedly because these methods require technical skills and teamwork of a high order. Their performance is indicated in a small, well-selected group of patients, particularly the subjects with congenital heart lesions, for whom the boon of modern surgery is sought. Ballistocardiography and spatial vectorcardiography are currently experiencing well-deserved revivals of interest which promise sound contributions to the physiological and clinical understanding of cardiac disorders. In this relation let us heed S. Weir Mitchell's admonition to beware "dementalization" by gadgets.

In the hectic pace of modern medicine, may we pause to consider how truly great medical discoveries are made. Perhaps there is no royal road to scientific success. Pasteur once wrote: "In the fields of observation chance favors only the prepared mind." Not entirely opposed to this thesis is the principle of serendipity which presupposes the fortuitous discovery of a valuable or important object. Truly the two may overlap; but let us attempt to analyze certain surpassing contributions of our period on these grounds.

On the return from the San Francisco meeting of the American College of Physicians in 1932, the magic of the Bay loosed the bonds of conventional restraint and I asked Professor A. J. Carlson: "How did you miss insulin?" His classical experiments upon the pregnant bitch by which he showed that pancreatectomy in the later weeks of gestation was not succeeded by diabetes mellitus, but that this state promptly followed upon delivery of the litter, constitute one of the most notable "near misses" in this field. Professor Carlson answered, "Plain damn fool! Blind damn fool!" A trained physiologist had the revelation of the mystery of the internal secretion of the pancreas in easy reach; but he had closed his eyes and had missed this surpassing opportunity. Yet a general practitioner, Frederick G. Banting, recently returned from military duty in France, read an article by Moses Barron in which he cited the classical observations of von Mering and Minkowski on the atrophy of the pancreatic acini upon ligation of the pancreatic ducts. The rest of the story is familiar history and Macleod and Best share Banting's glory in the discovery of insulin. The Scots are a dour people. When the Nobel Prize had been awarded to the Toronto group and the world was acclaiming their epochal contribution, a worthy country practitioner, Dr. MacLachlan, came under my care. He was an uncle of Banting and

I commented warmly upon his nephew's attainment. Whereupon the doctor responded: "Yes, it is very fine; but Fred is the dumbest of the Bantings. Mark my words, he'll never discover another thing!"

When Whipple and Robscheit-Robbins announced the singular value of liver in the regeneration of hemoglobin in the standard anemia dog, many clinicians applied their observations to the anemic patient; but George R. Minot and William B. Murphy made the key contribution by noting its potency in the treatment of pernicious anemia. Minot had been a productive student of hematology for many years. His candid account of this basic discovery, while it raises the issue of serendipity, may be interpreted as an example of "chance [favoring] the prepared mind." Shortly after the announcement of the discovery of the usefulness of liver in pernicious anemia (1926), I visited Dr. Minot in Boston. Upon inquiring the steps of their approach to the problem, Dr. Minot countered: "You must have tried liver in treating your anemic patients after Whipple's report." When I assured him that I had, he continued: "Well, so did we; and among our early patients was one with pernicious anemia. He is a druggist nearby. Let me call him in and have him tell his own story." The subject proved to be a florid, well-nourished man who gave the following account: "Dr. Minot called me in with a group of other anemic patients. He told us of the unusual value of liver in restoring the blood in experimental animals and recommended its trial. I am very fond of liver, and ate it once or twice a day. When I returned for a check on my blood in a month, I had gained over a million red blood cells. Dr. Minot immediately inquired what I had done differently in the previous month." With the clue in hand, Minot and Murphy recalled their patients with pernicious anemia and instructed them to eat one-half pound of liver a day, with the results so familiar to the medical world. At that conference I had the temerity to tell Dr. Minot that I would predict much farther reaching results from the widened horizon of hematology than in the direct clinical application of this new therapeutic agent. With characteristic forthrightness, he agreed.

Graham and Cole had labored assiduously on the problem of the visualization of the gallbladder. The continued negativity of their results was most discouraging. Then came a perfectly visualized gallbladder in a dog whose protocol differed in no discernible detail from a score of others. Step by step they retraced the stages of the experiment without establishing a point of departure from the routine. Then, shamefacedly the diener came to them and confessed: "I notice you have been paying a lot of attention to the x-rays of that dog, and I'll have to tell you something about him. He was the only one I did *not* feed before you took the x-rays." So was born cholecystography!

The story of penicillin is too fresh in all of our minds to require its elaboration. Even the high school student in his general science course has learned that a British bacteriologist at St. Mary's Hospital, London, was fortunate enough to have a culture of staphylococci contaminated by airborne spores of the penicillium notatum. What the lad is not apt to learn at this stage of his education is the technical implications of such an overlay of fungi. To his elders there must be afforded the added background of the worker, for here, "chance [favored] the prepared mind." Alexander Fleming had long been interested in lytic agents. In 1922, he discovered lysozyme in the saliva and tears. Hence, any agent that would liquefy bacterial colonies immediately arrested his attention. The title of his paper "On the Antibacterial Action of Cultures of a Penicillium, With Special Reference to Their Use in the Isolation of B. Influenzae" (1929), indicates the direction of his primary interest. Although Fleming foresaw the clinical application of penicillin, the catalytic action of World War II and the energy of the Oxford group under Florey were required to exploit his discovery.

To the epochal discovery of penicillin a host of other antimicrobial agents has been added. Their beneficence in controlling infectious diseases is daily extended. Yet a more significant role awaits elucidation. Within the period of recorded history infections have undergone a tremendous change in their clinical mode. Allowing for the difficulties in reconciling certain Biblical accounts, leprosy has obviously decreased perceptibly in incidence and severity. Yellow fever devastated Atlantic ports as far north as Philadelphia until the end of the eighteenth century. Pandemics of Asiatic cholera swept this country until the middle of the nineteenth century. Indeed, miners from the lead fields of Wisconsin joined the '49'ers in the quest for gold and carried with them to Fort Leavenworth and Sacramento the cholera which had plagued their native state. Smallpox stalked every lumber camp and concentration point in the country down to the beginning of the present century. Two early personal recollections color this picture. Close to my boyhood home in Pennsylvania was an old fairground with a deserted pavilion. When smallpox appeared in our community, this building at the town limits became the pesthouse and we passed it at a distance with bated breath. In nearby Philadelphia, the sporadic occurrence of smallpox resulted in the roping off of a city block and the compulsory vaccination of all citizens within these confines. More impressive to the youthful was the posting of guards, armed with shotguns, at the front and the rear of the quarantined house. "Black" measles and "black" smallpox carried the connotation of gravity that struck terror to every heart. Scarlet fever has undergone a perceptible change in clinical expression. In general, the exanthematous diseases have shown qualitative as well as quantitative abatement. During my student and hospital training, typhoid fever was still rampant in Philadelphia. Its importance is attested by the fact that Professor James Tyson devoted ten to twelve hours of lecture to its consideration, while thirty-four pages of our edition of Osler dealt in meticulous detail with its manifestations. The hour now allotted to the discussion of typhoid fever in the third year of medicine is ample and the current textbooks devote an average of five pages to this topic. Despite protestations to the contrary, the common experience favors the opinion that pneumococcus lobar pneumonia is waning. Indeed, on the wards of teaching hospitals its occurrence has become so unusual as to constitute a signal for the general demonstration to medical students. Tuberculosis is also on the decline. Through prophylactic measures diphtheria and tetanus may one day become "deceased" diseases.

Replacing bacterial diseases in certain respects, viral and rickettsial infections have taken the ascendency. In the European Theatre of Operations in four years, there were 19,477 instances of viral (nonbacterial) pneumonia as contrasted to 12,046 with the bacterial pneumonia among the American troops. At first glance this transition might be attributed to the advent of the sulfonamides and antimicrobial agents; but the movement actually anticipated this revolutionary phase of therapy. In certain areas, sanitation and education must be given due credit for the amelioration of infectious diseases. In others, immunization programs had begun to exercise effects far beyond the immediately immunized subject. To the principle of spaced immunes, the augmentation of the initial objective can be ascribed. In essence this epidemiologic result is an unearned dividend.

Before the advent of the sulfonamides the treatment of pneumococcus lobar pneumonia constituted one of the most involved problems in clinical medicine. Indeed, its management taxed the resourcefulness of the most able physician and nurse. Shortly before his death, Sir William Osler said: "I hope to live to see the true treatment of lobar pneumonia." Initiated in South Africa and greatly extended in the Rockefeller Institute, bacteriologic studies were to make possible specific and effective antipneumococcus sera. Before this advance had been consolidated, Whitby announced the efficacy of sulfapyridine in the treatment of pneumococcus pneumonia. Dejectedly an official of one of our prominent pharmaceutical houses interested in the manufacture of biological products told me that their firm had just completed a plant to produce antipneumococcus sera, at the cost of $250,000, when this discovery was released. Such is the price of progress even in the world of science.

Scarcely had the miracle of the sulfonamides become a part of medical thinking and practice when penicillin was successfully used for systemic infections (1940). Although Fleming had discovered the bacteriostatic property of penicillium notatum in 1928 and described its action the following year, only the quest for bacteriolytic substances by Florey and his fellows at Oxford, impelled by the exigencies of war, rescued it from temporary oblivion. The new vista of the management of infectious diseases opened by penicillin has been vastly extended by the discovery of a number of other effective antimicrobial agents. Indeed, their efficacy has encompassed spirochaetal and rickettsial diseases. The viral disorders have only isolatedly fallen under their spell, but of singular significance is the susceptibility of pathogenic amebae to aureomycin and terramycin.

Amazing as are the potentialities of these antimicrobial agents derived from lowly fungi, even more arresting is the manner of their respective actions. In general their competition with bacteria for some essential foodstuff or an enzymatic interference with nutrition will explain the bacterial decline. Just as significant from a practical standpoint is the possibility of developing strains of bacteria resistant to these agents. Among the available antimicrobial agents, streptomycin has this propensity in the highest degree. In fact, it is the rule for bacteria sensitive to streptomycin to become resistant, a property that limits its usefulness. On the other hand, bacteria may develop an actual dependence upon the antimicrobial agent, literally an acquired taste. (In a collateral field, flies have developed a high resistance to DDT, to which they had been very susceptible upon earlier exposure.) The suppression of the bacterial flora has been attended by unanticipated fungus infections. Indeed, in certain instances the antimicrobial agent has appeared to sensitize the patient with resultant "id" reactions. In devious manners medicine has modified the biological balance in nature. The related changing modes of infectious diseases may unquestionably be traced in some measure to these imbalances. We must be alert to new and greater departures, which cannot be predicated.

The wave of interest in hematology initiated by Minot and Murphy's discovery of the liver therapy of pernicious anemia has continued in productive flood. Castle's enunciation of the extrinsic-intrinsic factors served as a good working hypothesis for many years. Meanwhile folic acid proved an effective agent in resolving the hematopoietic aspect of pernicious anemia; but its inadequacy in controlling or preventing neurologic complications established further knowledge of the mechanism of erythropoiesis. Vitamin B_{12} brought added light to the subject. From a practical standpoint, the physician had passed through phases of therapeutic doses of grams of liver to milligrams of folic acid to micrograms of B_{12}. As previously stated, radioactive phosphorus (P_{32}) has proved to be highly efficacious in polycythemia rubra vera. Nitrogen mustard has a limited usefulness in the treatment of polycythemia and certain leukemias, but an assured place in Hodgkin's disease. Urethane and P_{32} also have spheres of usefulness in leukemia. Cortisone and adrenocorticotropin are likewise under study in this area. Their especial therapeutic role appears to be in thrombocytopenic purpura and acquired hemolytic anemia. Antifolic acid substances, especially aminopterin, have received much attention. Although temporary remissions have been induced in a minority of younger patients with acute leukemia, their importance lies in the difference of approach. We may be on the verge of fundamental discoveries in this area.

Obviously I have taken you to only a few of the high mountains of medical advance and indicated the far horizons. To quote S. Weir Mitchell: "I must have told my story ill if to every physician who hears me, its illustrations have not the invigorating force of moral tonics." To each of us comes the challenge of a period of medical achievement unexcelled in history, truly a Golden Age of Medicine. And there are even brighter vistas ahead!

THE MEDICAL FRANKLIN

"and all diseases may by sure means be prevented or cured, not excepting even that of old age, and our lives lengthened at pleasure beyond even the antediluvian standard."

BENJAMIN FRANKLIN to JOSEPH PRIESTLEY

In an intellectual sense, Benjamin Franklin was singularly a man of his times. In few periods of history has intellectual curiosity been more encouraged. Never have men of inquiring minds delved into esoteric fields more productively. To consider Franklin's manifold interests without this background is to invite anachronistic dislocation and distortion.

Furthermore, Franklin was definitely a cosmopolite. Shaking the shackles of an unwelcome indenture in his brother's printing office, young Franklin fled to New York and thence to Philadelphia. Later he declared that he was born in Philadelphia at the age of seventeen. His urbanity and mental horizon were vastly extended by a period of residence in London, but he had a very limited formal education. He never attended college although he did receive honorary degrees from five different colleges and universities.

As a measure of his self-education abundant evidence may be adduced in an unquenchable thirst for knowledge, a splendid library, diversified experimental equipment, and his acceptance in learned circles and societies. When abroad he invited and attracted the company of seekers for knowledge and truth in natural philosophy. Accordingly, the organization and the functions of the Royal Society were carefully studied.

Returning to Philadelphia, Franklin drew kindred spirits about himself, first in the Junto, which had social and material advantages of association as a significant objective (1727). Then, for the intellectual

Reprinted from *The Pennsylvania Gazette* (November 1959; December 1959), pp. 14–18; 16–20.

outlet the American Society for Promoting and Propagating Useful Knowledge (later, 1769, the American Philosophical Society) was established under his leadership, in 1766.

THE IMPORTANCE OF DIET

To Franklin's inquiring mind, medicine offered an unusual opportunity for observation and study. In his *Autobiography* early attention is given to diet. Boarding at his brother's expense during the indenture, his vegetarian diet led to some discussion: "My refusing to eat flesh occasioned some inconveniency, and I was frequently chid for my singularity." Whereupon he struck a bargain with his brother to support himself on half the cost of his board.

Preparing his own food in the printing shop gave Franklin the following advantage: "dispatching presently my light repast, which often was no more than a bisket or a slice of bread, a handful of raisins or a tart from the pastry-cook's and a glass of water, [I] had the rest of the time till their return for study, in which I made the greater progress, from that greater clearness of head and quicker apprehension which usually attend temperance in eating and drinking." This dietetic foible persisted for some time and was broken under very interesting circumstances:

> I believe I have omitted mentioning that, in my first voyage from Boston, being becalmed off Block Island, our people set about catching cod, and hauled up a great many. Hitherto I had stuck to my resolution of not eating animal food, and on this occasion I considered, with my master Tryon, the taking every fish as a kind of unprovoked murder, since none of them had, or ever could do us any injury that might justify the slaughter. All this seemed very reasonable. But I had formerly been a great lover of fish and, when this came hot out of the frying-pan, it smelt admirably well. I balanc'd some time between principle and inclination, till I recollected that, when the fish were opened I saw smaller fish taken out of their stomachs; then thought I, "if you eat one another, I don't see why we mayn't eat you." So I din'd upon cod very heartily, and continued to eat with other people, returning only now and then occasionally to a vegetable diet. So convenient a thing is to be *a reasonable creature*, since it enables one to find or make a reason for every thing one has a mind to do.

Franklin's frugality persisted into his married life. He noted: "We kept no idle servants, our table was plain and simple, our furniture of the cheapest. For instance, my breakfast was a long time bread and milk (no tea), and I ate it out of a two-penny earthen porriger, with a pewter spoon." When his wife, Deborah, replaced these humble settings with china and silver, Franklin remonstrated with her.

In a more technical vein, he wrote a very significant letter that is reminiscent of William Heberden's classical notes on angina pectoris:

> In general, mankind, since the improvement of cooking, eats about twice as much as nature requires. Suppers are not bad, if we have not dined, but restless nights follow hearty suppers after full dinners. Indeed, as there is a difference in constitutions, some rest well after these meals; it costs them only a frightful dream and an apoplexy after which they sleep till doomsday. Nothing is more common in the newspapers than instances of people, who after eating a hearty supper, are found dead abed in the morning.

While working in Watts' printing house in Lincoln's Inn Fields, London, Franklin's abstemious habits led his beer guzzling fellow-workers to call him "Water American." Franklin noted that his associates drank six pints of beer a day:

> I thought it a detestable custom; but it was necessary, he supposed, to drink *strong* beer that he might be *strong* to labor. I endeavored to convince him that the bodily strength afforded by beer could only be in proportion to the grain or flour of the barley dissolved in the water of which it was made; that there was more flour in a pennyworth of bread, and therefore, if he would eat that with a pint of water, it would give him more strength than a quart of beer. He drank on, however, and had four or five shillings in pay out of his wages every Saturday night for that muddling liquor; an expense I was free from. And thus these poor devils keep themselves always under.

SEX AND ALCOHOL

From this account it should not be assumed that Franklin was a total abstainer from alcoholic beverages. He did attribute his long life to temperance in all things. Among thirteen virtues to which he aspired and against which he kept an inventory for a short time are listed the following of medical interest:

1. Temperance.
   Eat not to dullness; drink not to elevation.
9. Moderation.
   Avoid extreams; forbear resenting injuries so much as you think they deserve.
10. Cleanliness.
    Tolerate no uncleanliness in body, cloaths, or habitation.
11. Tranquillity.
    Be not disturbed at trifles, or at accidents common or unavoidable.
12. Chastity.
    Rarely use venery but for health or offspring, never to dullness, weakness, or the injury of your own, or another's peace or reputation.

To avoid a semblance of sanctimoniousness, Franklin admitted his difficulty in attaining these high objectives in perfection and his human frailty in falling from grace. As he wrote: "for something that pretended to be reason, was every now and then suggesting to me that such extream nicety as I exacted of myself might be a kind of foppery in morals, which, if it were known, would make me ridiculous; that a perfect character might be attended with the inconvenience of being envied and hated; and that a benevolent man should allow a few faults in himself, to keep his friends in countenance."

In the matter of continence, Franklin admitted the weakness of the flesh: "In the meantime, that hard-to-be governed passion of youth hurried me frequently into intrigues with low women that fell in my way, which were attended with some expense and great inconvenience, besides a continual risque to my health by a distemper which of all things I dreaded, though by great good luck I escaped it." In his oftquoted "Advice to a Young Man on the Choice of a Mistress," without condoning Franklin's earthy sentiments we must in charity translate them to the period of his communication.

ON PHYSICAL FITNESS

Franklin's reflections on general hygiene are most refreshing and certainly far in advance of his day. In 1773 he wrote to Jean Baptiste LeRoy: "but as this is heresy here, and perhaps may be so with you, I only whisper it, and expect you will keep my Secret. Our Physicians have begun to discover that fresh Air is good for People in the Small-Pox and other Fevers. I hope in time they will find out that it does no harm to People in Health."

Indeed, fresh air was a fetish with him and he claimed unusual relaxation from sitting naked after bathing, "a *bracing* or *tonic* Bath." Interestingly, Franklin remarked that perspiration was almost doubled in the naked state as compared with the clothed.

Manasseh Cutler, who deemed Franklin's acceptance of the Presidency of the Executive Council of Pennsylvania, "a sure sign of senility," described his bathing vessel: "It is copper in the form of a slipper. He sits in the Heel and his legs go under the Vamp; on the Instep he has a place to fix his book and here he sits and enjoys himself. . . . But would it not be a capital subject for an historical painting . . . the Doctor at the head of the Council Board in his bathing slipper?"

Benjamin Franklin advocated and maintained physical fitness in his youth and early adult life. Swimming was his favorite exercise. In this sport he apparently excelled, if his *Autobiography* be accepted as evidence. With his friend, Wygate, and others Franklin had gone to Chelsea to see the College and Saltero's curiosities:

> In our return, at the request of the company, whose curiosity Wygate had excited, I stripped and leaped into the river, and swam from near Chelsea to Blackfryar's performing on the way many feats of activity, both upon and under water, that surpris'd and pleas'd those to whom they were novelties.
>
> I had from a child been ever delighted with this exercise, had studied and practis'd all Thevenot's motions and positions, added some of my own, aiming at the graceful and easy as well as the useful. All those I took this occasion of exhibiting to the company and was much flatter'd by their admiration.

In a more physiologic mood, Franklin once wrote to Doctor Dubourg:

> The exercise of swimming is one of the most healthy and agreeable in the world. After having swam for an hour or two in the evening, one sleeps cooly the whole night, even during the most ardent heat of summer. Perhaps, the pores being cleansed, the insensible perspiration increases and occasions this coolness. It is certain that much swimming is the means of stopping a diarrhoea, and even of producing a constipation. With respect to those, who do not know how to swim, or who are affected with a diarrhoea at a season which does not permit them to use this exercise, a warm bath, by cleansing and purifying the skin, is found very salutary, and often effects a radical cure. I speak from my own experience, frequently repeated, and that of others to whom I have recommended this.

FRANKLIN'S MEDICAL ASSOCIATES

The Philadelphia scene of the eighteenth century found medicine in a preferred position. True, organized medical education was not established in Philadelphia until 1765 after the return of John Morgan and William Shippen from Edinburgh. Interesting in this relation is John Morgan's inscription in Franklin's complimentary copy of " 'Discourse on the Institution of Medical Schools in America,' which I shewed you in Ms."

Benjamin Franklin was ever active in furthering the interests of his compatriots seeking educational advantages in London and Edinburgh. He gave Morgan a letter of introduction to Professor Cullen. In the case of Benjamin Rush he welcomed him to his home, introduced him to his London friends and gave him letters to leading medical men in Edinburgh and Paris. Learning Rush's straitened financial status he afforded him a letter of credit for £200 for his continental trip.

Addressed to Dr. Thomas Bond of Philadelphia, a letter from Franklin (1772) evaluated the advantages of instruction in anatomy and surgery in London, but admitted the strength and prominence of the Edinburgh faculty. There follows a most enlightening passage:

> And to tell you frankly my Opinion, I suspect there is more valuable knowledge in Physic to be learned from the honest candid Observations of an Old Practitioner, who is past all desire of more Business, having made his Fortune, who has none of the Professional Interest in keeping up a Parade of Science to draw Pupils, and who by Experience has discovered the Inefficacy of most Remedies and Modes of Practice, than all the formal Lectures of all the Universities upon Earth. I like therefore a Physician's breeding his Son to Medicine, and wish the Art to be continued with the Race, as thinking that must be upon the whole most for the Public Welfare.

Through his wide circle of acquaintance, Franklin was on easy terms with the medical leaders of London, Edinburgh, and Paris. His close friendship with Sir John Pringle, physician to the Queen, is evinced by a continental tour they took together in 1766. Perhaps his most intimate English medical friend was Dr. John Fothergill, whose interest in American medicine was fostered, if not initiated, by Franklin. Some idea of their close relationship may be gathered from Franklin's letter (1765) to his friend urging more leisure and greater attention to the social amenities:

> To be hurried about perpetually from one sick chamber to another is not living. Do you please yourself with the fancy that you are doing good? You are mistaken. Half the lives you save are not worth saving, as being useless, and almost all the other half ought not to be saved, as being mischievous. Does your conscience never hint to you the impiety of being in constant warfare against the plans of Providence? Disease was intended as the punishment of intemperance, sloth, and other vices, and the example of that punishment was intended to promote and strengthen the opposite virtues. But here you step in officiously with your Art, disappoint those wise intentions of nature, and make men safe in their excesses, whereby you seem to me to be of just the same service to society as some favorite first minister who out of the great benevolence of his heart should procure pardons of all criminals that applied to him; only think of the consequences.

THE PENNSYLVANIA HOSPITAL

Benjamin Franklin's friendship with Dr. Thomas Bond led to one of his major contributions to Philadelphia medicine. In his *Autobiography* Franklin gives this account:

> In 1751, Dr. Thomas Bond, a particular friend of mine, conceived the idea of establishing a hospital in Philadelphia (a very beneficent design, which has been ascrib'd to me, but was originally his), for the reception and cure of poor sick persons, whether inhabitants or

strangers. He was zealous and active in endeavoring to procure subscriptions for it, but the proposal being a novelty in America, and at first not well understood, he met with but little success.

Discouraged, Dr. Bond turned to Franklin for assistance: "For I am often ask'd by those to whom I propose subscribing, 'Have you consulted Franklin upon this business? And what does he think of it?' And when I tell them that I have not (supposing it rather out of your line), they do not subscribe, but say they will consider of it."

Not only did Franklin subscribe to the good cause, but he actively solicited further financial support. When the subscribed sums fell short of the goal, he helped frame a petition to the General Assembly of the Province of Pennsylvania for "a small Provincial Hospital." Especial attention was herein directed to the lack of facilities to care for "Lunatics, or Persons distemper'd in Mind, and deprived of their rational Faculties" who endangered themselves, family and community.

The request for matching funds seemed destined to failure through the Assembly's fear that these monies would be completely absorbed by professional fees. Franklin undoubtedly was responsible for the decision of Drs. Lloyd Zachary, Thomas Bond, and Phineas Bond to serve without remuneration for three years. "I more easily excused myself for having made some use of cunning," Franklin reported. This position expedited the passage of the Bill (February 7, 1751), under whose terms the Province, duplicating the voluntary contributions, voted an appropriation of £2000.

The consummation of this plan was delayed by the failure of the nonresident Proprietors to accede to the request for a specific building site. Instead, through their agents a substitute area was offered for this purpose with an ominous reversion clause. In a letter to the agents, Thomas Hyam and Sylvanus Bevan, the Managers thus characterized the situation:

> It is contiguous to the Brick-Makers Grounds, from which the City hath been furnished with Brick above Forty Years past, so that their large Ponds being continually filled with standing Water, renders the Neighborhood unhealthy, and of course absolutely improper for our Purpose, which is to restore the Sick to Health; and the only proper Use of that Square will be for a Burying-ground to which Service some Part of it hath been applied by a Grant from the Proprietaries.

Further objection to the reversion clause was emphatically expressed.

Eventually the Pennsylvania Hospital was erected on an independent site in Eighth Street between Spruce and Pine Streets. The Cornerstone was laid May 28, 1755. The following inscription was written by Franklin:

In the year of Christ
MDCCLV
(For he sought the happiness of his people)
Philadelphia flourishing
(For its inhabitants were publick spirited)
This building
By the bounty of the Government,
And of many private persons
Was piously founded
For the relief of the sick and
miserable;
May the God of mercies
Bless the Undertaking

As Franklin and Thomas Bond were walking to the cornerstone laying, the latter expressed concern that the hospital would attract strangers to the city. With characteristic insight Franklin retorted: "Then our institution will be more useful than we intended it to be." As a manager Benjamin Franklin served as its first Clerk. *Some Account of the Pennsylvania Hospital; From its first Rise to the Beginning of the Fifth Month, called May, 1754* was printed by B. Franklin and D. Hall. Futhermore, Franklin solicited gifts of books and other medical materials from his British friends. Notable among these donations were the anatomic models and charts from Dr. John Fothergill. Hence the oldest general hospital in the United States takes justifiable pride in Franklin's important role in its foundation and early development.

INOCULATION AGAINST SMALLPOX

Smallpox was a pestilential scourge in the eighteenth century. His "afeckthone wife" Deborah wrote to Franklin in England (1773): "I shall tell you what concernes myself our yonegest Grandson is the finest child as alive he has had the small pox; and had it fine and got abrod agen." An earlier tragedy in his own family was recalled, since over his own signature in the *Pennsylvania Gazette* (December 13, 1736), Franklin had published the following note:

Understanding tis a current Report, that my Son Francis, who died lately of the Small Pox, had it by Inoculation; and being desired to satisfy the Publick in that Particular; in as much as some People are, by that Report (join'd with others of the like kind, and perhaps equally groundless) deter'd from having that Operation performed on their children, I do hereby sincerely declare that he was not inoculated but receiv'd the Distemper in the common way of Infection, and I suppose the Report could only arise from its being my known Opinion, that Inoculation was a safe and beneficial Practice; and from my having said among my Acquaintance, that I intended to have my child inoculated as soon as he should have recovered sufficient strength from a Flux with which he had been long afflicted.

In a letter to his sister, Mrs. Mecom (1731), Franklin had indicated the efficacy of inoculation against smallpox. His sustained interest in this prophylactic measure led him to enlist Dr. William Heberden's support in extending a knowledge of the method in the Colonies. Upon his representations this distinguished English physician wrote "Plain Instructions" and had a large number printed for free distribution in America.

This small pamphlet, with an introduction by Franklin, "Some Account of the Success of Inoculation for the Small Pox in England and America Together With Plain Instructions, By Which Any Person May be Enabled to Perform the Operation, and Conduct the Patient through the Distemper," was published in London in 1759 and played an important role in the acceptance and the extension of this procedure in America.

THE COMMON COLD

The common cold was a familiar ailment in Colonial days and Franklin had advanced ideas on its etiology and pathogenesis. He vigorously resisted the prevalent theories of a causal relationship in moisture and cold. His natural reference to the freedom of sailors and others in exposed occupations from such disorders was stoutly held. He formulated an outline of a logical approach to a consideration of the subject but did not write the proposed paper. In this outline Franklin remarked on *"Taking Cold.* The Disorder only called so in English and in no other Language . . . Every Pain or Disorder now ascrib'd to a Cold. It is the Covering Excuse of all Intemperance."

In article four of the outline he made a portentous observation: "By particular Effluvia in the Air, from some unknown Cause, General Colds thro'-out a County. By being in a Coach close, or small Room with a Person having a Cold."

In a particularly cogent letter, Franklin expounded his theory of the common cold to Dr. Benjamin Rush:

> I hope that after having discovered the benefit of fresh and cool air applied to the sick, people will began to suspect that possibly it may do no harm to the well. I have not seen Dr. Cullen's book, but am glad to hear that he speaks of catarrhs or cold by contagion. I have been long satisfied from observation, that besides the general colds now termed *influenzas,* (which may possibly spread by contagion, as well as by a particular quality of the air), people often catch cold from

one another when shut up together in close rooms, coaches, etc., and when sitting near and conversing so as to breathe in each others transpiration; the disorder being in a certain state. I think, too, that it is the frouzy, corrupt air from animal substances, and the perspired matter from our bodies, which being long confined in beds, not lately used, and clothes not lately worn, and books long shut up in closed rooms, obtains the kind of putridity, which occasions the colds observed upon sleeping in, wearing, and turning over such bedclothes or books, and not their coldness or dampness. From these causes, but more from too full living, with too little exercise, proceed in my opinion most of the disorders which for about one hundred and fifty years past the English have called *colds*.

Franklin took particular exception to Professor Cullen's subscription to "cold or catarrah *a frigore*": "Dampness may indeed assist in producing putridity and these miasmata which infect us with the disorder we call a cold; but of itself can never by a little addition of moisture hurt a body filled with watery fluids from head to foot."

A passage of Franklin's letter to Thomas Percival is especially pungent:

Thus, tho' it is generally allowed that taking the Air is a good thing, yet what Caution against Air, what stopping of crevices, what wrapping up in warm clothes, what shutting the doors and windows! Even in the midst of Summer! Many London families go out once a Day to take the Air; three or four Persons in a Coach, one perhaps Sick; these go three or four miles, or as many turns in Hide Park, with the Glasses both up close, all breathing over and over again the same Air they brought out of Town with them in the Coach with the least change possible, and render's worse every moment. And this they call taking the Air. From many years' observation on myself and others, I am persuaded we are on the wrong Scent in supposing moist or cold Air the cause of that Disorder we call a Cold. Some unknown quality in the Air may perhaps produce colds as in the Influenza, but generally I apprehend they are the effects of too full living in proportion to our exercise.

John Adams's *Autobiography* affords an amusing episode in this connection. Franklin and Adams were travelling together (1776):

At Brunswick, but one bed could be procured for Dr. Franklin and me, in a chamber little larger than the bed, without a chimney and with only one small window. The window was open, and I who was an invalid and afraid of the air at night, shut it close. "Oh," says Franklin, "don't shut the window, we shall be suffocated." I answered I was afraid of the evening air. Dr. Franklin replied, "The air within this chamber will soon be, and indeed is now, worse than that without doors. Come open the window and come to bed, and I will convince you. I believe you are not acquainted with my theory of colds?"

The window was opened and Adams fell asleep while Franklin expatiated on his theory.

THE BIFOCALS

Of wide application was Franklin's invention of bifocal lenses. As was his habit, Franklin made a study of his personal difficulty and the construction of spectacles of divided lenses, with the upper and the lower halves of different convexities, resulted. Their widespread use bears testimony to the sound quality of Franklin's ingenuity. His own description affords a clear picture of his logical approach to the problem:

> By Mr. Dolland's saying, that my double Spectacles can only serve particular eyes, I doubt he has not been rightly informed of their Construction. I imagine it will be found pretty generally true, that the same Convexity of Glass through which Man sees clearest and best at the Distance proper for Reading is not the best for greater Distances. I therefore had formerly two Pair of Spectacles, which I shifted occasionally as in travelling I sometimes read and often wanted to regard the Prospects. Finding this Change troublesome and not always sufficiently ready, I had the Glasses cut, and half of each kind associated in the same Circle.
>
> By this means, as I wear my Spectacles constantly, I have only to move my Eyes up or down, as I want to see distinctly far or near, the proper Glasses being always ready. This I find more particularly convenient since my being in France, the Glasses that serve me best at Table to see what I eat, not being the best to see the Faces of those on the other Side of the Table who speak to me; and when one's Ears are not well accustomed to the sounds of a Language, a sight of the movements in the Features of him that speaks helps to explain, so that I understand French better by the help of my Spectacles.

As a rule Benjamin Franklin eschewed the role and the responsibilities of a medical counsellor. In a letter to his parents he wrote: "I apprehend I am too busy in prescribing and meddling in the doctor's sphere, when any of you complain of ails in your letter. But as I always employ a physician myself, when any disorder arises in my family, and submit implicitly to his orders in everything, so I hope you consider my advice, when I give any, only as a mark of my good will, and put no more of it in practice than happens to agree with what your doctor directs."

Yet Franklin's ubiquitous interests found absorption in reflections on the use of wormwood for cancer of the breast and pokeweed for cancer in general. When "fixed air" (nitrogen) was recommended for the treatment of cancerous ulcers, he advised the following procedure to

Dr. John Hawkesworth: "I would first syringe the sore strongly with warm water impregnated with Fix'd Air so as to cleanse well the part. Then I would apply to it a succession of Glasses filled with Fix'd Air, each glass to remain till the sore had absorbed the Fix'd Air contained in it." Nor was Franklin above friendly advice as to specific therapy as witnesses his letter to Rev. Samuel Jackson (September 1750) regarding the treatment of "fever and ague":

> Don't imagine yourself thoroughly cured, and so omit the use of the bark too soon. Remember to take the preventing dose faithfully. If you were to continue taking a dose or two every day for two or three weeks after the fits have left you, 'twould not be amiss. If you take the powder mixed quick in a tea-cup of milk, 'tis no way disagreeable, but looks and even tastes like chocolate. 'Tis an old saying, that an ounce of prevention is worth a pound of cure, and certainly a true one, with regard to the bark; a little of which will do more in preventing the fits than a great deal in removing them.

HISTORY AND THE GOUT

Gouty attacks were to plague Franklin during the latter part of his life. Not only did they bring great personal suffering but at times they interfered with the interests of his country. After the failure of the Canadian invasion by the Continental Army, Franklin was named on a commission to negotiate with the British. After a strenuous journey by boat and wagon, "enfeebled and dispirited" he interrupted his journey to rest and recuperate at the home of General Schuyler in Saratoga.

His years and gout were taking their toll. On June 21, 1776, he wrote to George Washington: "I am just recovering from a severe fit of the gout, which has kept me from Congress and Company ever since you left us, so that I know little of what has pass'd there except that a Declaration of Independence is preparing." He neglected to add that his own infirmity had deferred the drafting of this historic document to Thomas Jefferson.

In Paris, Madame Brillon thus settled Franklin's pragmatic argument: "There would be many little things, in truth, to criticize in your logic, which you fortify so well, my dear papa. 'When I was a young man' you say, 'and enjoyed the favors of the sex more freely than at present, I had no gout.' Therefore, one might reply to this, when I threw myself out of the window, I didn't break my leg. Therefore, you could have the gout without having deserved it, and you could well have deserved it, as I believe, and not have had it."

For some time Franklin manifested a philosophical air toward the

recurrences of gout. To Jean-Baptiste LeRoy, he made the following
light suggestion: "I had sometimes wished I had brought with me from
France a balloon sufficiently large to raise me from the ground. In my
malady it would have been the most easy carriage for me, being led
by a string held by a man walking on the ground."

As many gouty sufferers have observed, he spoke of the unusual
well-being of mind and body that succeeded the acute bouts. From
personal observation he found cold more comforting than local heat
in the acute episodes. By some he is credited with the introduction of
colchicum for the treatment of gout into America. However this has
not been confirmed. His "Dialogue between Franklin and the Gout"
is a classic (October 22, 1780). In this whimsy Madame Gout gives
him recurrent twinges of pain. Certain passages are particularly cogent:

> Franklin—I repeat; my enemy; for you would not only torment my
> body to death, but ruin my good name; and reproach me as a glutton
> and a tippler; now all the world, that knows me, will allow that I am
> neither the one or the other.
> Gout—The world may think as it pleases, it is always very complaisant
> to itself and sometimes to its friends; but I very well know that the
> quantities of meat and drink proper for a man, who takes a reasonable
> amount of exercise, would be too much for another, who never takes
> any.
> Gout—Well, then to my office; it should not be forgotten that I am
> your physician. There!
> Franklin—Oh-h-h! What a devil of a physician.
> Gout—How ungrateful you are to say so! Is it not I who, in the char-
> acter of your physician, have saved you from the palsy, dropsy, and
> apoplexy, one or other of which would have done for you long ago
> but for me?
> Franklin—I submit and thank you for the past, but entreat the dis-
> continuance of your visits for the future; for in my mind one had bet-
> ter die than be cured so dolefully. Permit me just to hint that I have
> also not been unfriendly to you. I never feed a physician or quack of
> any kind to enter the list against you; if, thus, you do not leave such
> my repose, it may be said you are ungrateful too.
> Gout—I can scarcely acknowledge that as an objection. As to quacks,
> I despise them; they may kill you, indeed, but cannot injure me. And
> as to regular physicians, they are at least convinced that the gout, in
> such a subject as you are, is no disease, but a remedy; and wherefore
> cure a remedy? But to our business; there!
> Franklin—Oh! Oh! for heaven's sake leave me, and I promise faith-
> fully nevermore to play at chess, but to take exercise daily and live
> temperately.
> Gout—I know you too well. You promise fair, but after a few months
> of good health you will return to your old habits; your fine promises
> will be forgotten like the forms of the last year's clouds. Let us, then,
> finish the account, and I will go. But I leave you with an assurance of

visiting you again at a proper time and place; for my object is your good, and you are sensible now that I am your real friend.

ANOTHER PROBLEM—URINARY STONE

Added to the growing handicap of gout Franklin suffered from urinary tract stone. Ironically he reflected on the fate that contradicted the terms of the wishing song:

> May I govern my Passions with an absolute sway,
> Grow wiser and better as my strength wears away,
> Without Gout or Stone, by a gentle Decay.

From widespread sources he sought relief from his painful disorder. At an earlier age he had suggested to his parents the probable efficacy of honey and molasses in holding in suspension particles that might otherwise form gravel. Benjamin Rush quoted Franklin's benefit from blackberry jam. However, the latter concluded that its sugar content was probably the active ingredient, since one-half pint of syrup (brown sugar in water) gave as much relief as opium at night.

In a letter to John Jay (1784), Franklin expressed the hope that abstemious living and gentle exercise might prevent the growth of urinary stone. He added: "I am cheerful, enjoy the company of my Friends, sleep well, have sufficient appetite and my Stomach performs well its Functions. The latter is very material to the preservation of Health. I therefore take no Drugs, lest I should disorder it. You may judge that my Disease is not very grievous, since I am more afraid of the Medicines than of the Malady."

To Dr. Jan Ingenhousz he wrote: "I have taken therefore, and am now again taking the Remedy you mention which is called *Blackrie's Solvent*. It is the Soap Lie, with Lime Water, and I believe it may have some Effect in diminishing the Symptoms, and preventing the Growth of the Stone, which is all I expect from it. It does not hurt my appetite; I sleep well, and enjoy my Friends in cheerful Conversation as usual. But, as I cannot use much Exercise, I eat more sparingly than formerly and I drink no Wine."

Interestingly, the following month Franklin instructed his nephew, Jonathan Williams, to purchase "Blackrie's Disquisition on Medicines that dissolve the Stone," from Wilkie's No. 71, St. Paul's Churchyard, London.

THE CUP OF LIFE

In 1787 Franklin wrote to M. LeVeillard: "People who live long, who will drink of the cup of life to the very bottom, must expect to meet with some of the dregs, and when I reflect on the number of terrible maladies human nature is subject to, I think myself favoured in having to share only the stone and the gout." Yet in another letter he referred to "near eighty-three, the age of commencing decrepitude."

The tenor of Franklin's letters changed perceptibly in 1789. To M. LeVeillard he wrote: "I have a long time been afflicted with almost constant and grievous Pain, to combat which I have been obliged to have recourse to Opium, which indeed has afforded me some Ease from time to time, but then it has taken away my Appetite and so impeded my Digestion that I am become totally emaciated, and little remains of me but a Skeleton covered with a Skin."

In a similar vein he addressed Benjamin Vaughan: "I thank you very much for your intimations of the virtues of hemlock, but I have tried so many things with so little effect, that I am quite discouraged, and have no longer any faith in remedies for the stone. The palliating system is what I am now fixed in. Opium gives me ease when I am attacked by pain, and by the use of it I still make life at least tolerable. Not being able, however, to bear sitting to write, I now make use of the hand of one of my grandsons, dictating to him from my bed."

Mary Hewson, Franklin's protégée, who had spent the winter of 1784–85 with him at Passy, came to Philadelphia to be with him in his failing days. Her intimate picture of the fallen lion constitutes a most human story. In spite of his suffering he rallied to enjoy the company of his books and his friends whenever the pain relented.

Resigned to his fate, he remained mentally clear until just before the end, which came at eleven o'clock on the evening of April 17, 1790. His attending physician, Dr. John Jones, has left a detailed clinical account of this illness. The sequence of pleuritic pain, fever, cough, and dyspnoea with the explosive expectoration of a large amount of pus led to the conclusion of a pulmonary abscess (or empyema).

EPITAPH AND WHIMSY

Thus passed one of the truly great Americans. The conventional epitaph of Franklin, written in 1728, reads:

The Body
of
Benjamin Franklin
Printer
(Like the cover of an old book, its
contents torn out and stript of its
lettering and gilding)

Lies here, food for worms,
For it will (as he believed) appear
once more
In a new and more elegant edition
Revised and corrected
by
The Author

A more characteristic reaction on Franklin's part stemmed from two reported observations, namely the survival of toads long buried in sand and of flies drowned in wine. On this score he wrote in a whimsical mood, "I wish it were possible . . . to invent a method of embalming drowned persons, in such a manner that they may be recalled to life at any period, however distant; for having a very ardent desire to see and observe the State of America a hundred years hence, I should prefer to any ordinary death, the being immersed in a cask of Madeira wine, with a few friends, till that time, to be then recalled to life by the solar warmth of my dear country!"

Were Benjamin Franklin to return to Philadelphia today, 169 years after his death, he would be quite overwhelmed by the changes wrought by science and time. Even in his beloved adopted city he would be hard put to find his physical bearings. Unquestionably Christ Church, Friends Meeting, and St. Peter's Church would prove helpful landmarks. The emergence of Independence Hall, Carpenters' Hall, and other familiar haunts in the splendidly conceived historic shrine of Independence Mall would give him deep satisfaction.

The submergence of the Library Company, to which he lent such impetus, would be understood as a measure of growth. The strength and the stature of the American Philosophical Society would be a source of great personal gratification. Assuredly he would glory in the good name and works of Pennsylvania Hospital, which has indeed proved "more useful than we intended it to be."

In all probability his greatest reward would be found in the growth and development of the tiny, struggling Charity School and Academy into the University of Pennsylvania. Truly the spirit of Benjamin Franklin prevails in her academic halls and works, even though his whimsical return in the flesh is denied.

TURNER'S LANE HOSPITAL

The medical life of Philadelphia was greatly disrupted by the Civil War. Not only were the University of Pennsylvania School of Medicine and Jefferson Medical College favored institutions for Southern medical students, but at that time their faculties included a number of members of Southern origin. The withdrawal of the Southern students and the increasing exactions of military service seriously depleted the enrollment in the Philadelphia schools. Nor was the public sentiment of the community wholly behind the Federal administration at the outset of hostilities. S. Weir Mitchell puts words to Mrs. Alice Westerley's reaction: "I wish, for my part, we could tow Massachusetts and South Carolina out to sea, and anchor them together and let them settle their difficulties."[1]

From its geographic and strategic position Philadelphia was destined to play an increasingly important role in provisioning and supporting the Union forces, both on land and sea. Its medical resources made it one of the most important hospital centers for the sick and wounded soldiers and sailors of the North. The Christian Street Hospital between Ninth and Tenth Streets admitted its first patient on May 6, 1861, in Moyamensing Hall.[2] Eventually the Department of

Presented at the thirty-eighth annual meeting of the American Association for the History of Medicine, Philadelphia, April 30, 1965. Reprinted from *Bulletin of the History of Medicine* 60, no. 1 (January-February, 1966): 14–42. Grateful acknowledgment of sustained assistance from Dr. W. B. McDaniel 2nd and the staff of the Library of the College of Physicians of Philadelphia is herewith rendered.

1. S. W. Mitchell, *In War Time* (Boston: Houghton, Mifflin, 1885).

2. F. P. Henry, *Standard History of the Medical Profession of Philadelphia* (Chicago: Goodspeed, 1897), pp. 263, 270–71.

Pennsylvania was responsible for 18,709 beds, of which 14,508 were in the environs of Philadelphia. Only Washington with 21,426 beds cared for a greater segment of the total Union hospital bed capacity (118,057 in sixteen departments). On January 1, 1866, the United States Sanitary Commission reported that 157,000 soldiers and sailors had been treated in general hospitals in Philadelphia during the war.[3]

Among these military installations the Turner's Lane Hospital occupies a unique position that merits careful exploration and scrutiny. With some reservations imposed by family obligations and traditional Southern attachments, S. Weir Mitchell first entered military service as Acting Assistant Surgeon at the Filbert Street Hospital. Here the magnitude of the problem of peripheral nerve injuries impressed him. As these patients overflowed the Filbert Street Hospital, they were transferred to the Christian Street Hospital, where George Reed Morehouse and William Williams Keen joined Mitchell to form a remarkable team that was destined to leave its permanent imprint on the field of organic neurology.

The Surgeon General of the United States Army, William A. Hammond, happened to be a close friend of Mitchell. They had collaborated before the war in the study of the poisons, corroval and vao, and of the toxicological effects of sassy bark. They planned the investigation of snake venom.[4] Obviously the proposal of a special hospital for nerve injuries and disorders emanated from Mitchell. In 1872 he clearly stated their respective positions in the matter:

> In May 1863, Dr. William A. Hammond, then Surgeon-General of the United States Army, requested me to share with Dr. George Morehouse the material charge of an Army hospital for nervous diseases, the foundation of which I had suggested to the medical bureau, over which at that time Dr. Hammond presided with such ability as has caused his name to be inseparably associated with the medical and surgical history of the late Civil War.[5]

Especial commendation was accorded Surgeon General Hammond for the "watchful care with which he fostered the interests of scientific medicine, while organizing and perfecting that vast system of hospitals for which the country owes a debt of gratitude to a genius alike enterprizing, intelligent, and laborious."[6]

3. F. H. Taylor, *Philadelphia in the Civil War* (Philadelphia: The City, 1913), p. 226.
4. N. Mumey, *S. Weir Mitchell. The Versatile Physician (1829–1914). A Sketch of his Life and his Literary Contributions* (Denver: Range Press, 1934), p. 34.
5. S. W. Mitchell, *Injuries of Nerves and Their Consequences* (Philadelphia: Lippincott, 1872), p. 9.
6. S. W. Mitchell, G. R. Morehouse, and W. W. Keen, *Gunshot Wounds and*

Clearly then, S. Weir Mitchell (1829–1914) was the catalyst who formed the team and lent his brilliance and boundless energies to the exploration of the singularly fallow field of peripheral nerve injuries. Upon the opening of the Turner's Lane Hospital, Mitchell was thirty-three years old (Pl. 1). After his acadamic preparation at the University of Pennsylvania he entered Jefferson Medical College over the protest of his father, Dr. John K. Mitchell, who said, "You are wanting in nearly all the qualities that go to make a success in medicine. You have brains, but no industry."[7] Graduating in 1850, he spent the following two years in Paris where he came under the spell of Claude Bernard.[8] On one occasion Mitchell said: "I think so and so must be the case." "Why think," Bernard said, "when you can experiment? Exhaust experiment, and then think." Illness interrupted Mitchell's European interlude, and he returned to Philadelphia to find his father in failing health. In spite of the exactions of competitive practice and the responsibilities of supporting the family, Weir Mitchell kept the spirit of inquiry alive. His later associate, William Williams Keen, gave one of the most perceptive analyses of his basic attributes:

> Never have I known so original, suggestive, and fertile a mind. I often called him a "yeasty" man. His mind was ever fermenting, speculating, alert, and overflowing with ideas. With these he leavened the minds of his fellows and set their ideas fermenting. He was always desirous of putting everything to the test of experiment, and never satisfied until he had exhausted all possibilities. Almost every research but opened a vista of other and still more interesting problems to be solved. An hour in his office set my own mind in a turmoil so that I could hardly sleep. His was indeed an elevating, stimulating friendship. Ideas scintillated, plans were formed, and almost always took concrete shape.[9]

George Reed Morehouse (1829–1905) (Pl. 2) is by all means the most elusive of the team; yet the warm biographic sketch by S. Weir Mitchell[10] leaves no question as to his superior qualities of personality, intellect, and character. Classmates at Jefferson, they maintained a communion of the spirit in an anatomicophysiological study of the respira-

---

Other Injuries of Nerves, (Philadelphia: Lippincott, 1864), pp. iii–iv.

7. Mumey, S. *Weir Mitchell*, p. 53.

8. A. J. Carlson 1938, "Silas Weir Mitchell, 1829-1914," *Science*, 87:474–78.

9. W. W. Keen 1914, "Tribute to S. Weir Mitchell," *Tr. Coll. Physicians, Philadelphia*, 3rd s. 36:347.

10. S. W. Mitchell, "George Reed Morehouse (1829-1905)," in H. A. Kelly and W. L. Burrage, eds., *American Medical Biographies* (Baltimore: Norman, Remington, 1920).

tion of the chelonia.[11] Their observations first disclosed a nerve chiasm outside the cranium. Skillful and self-possessed, Morehouse worked quietly and effectively under pressure. Mitchell specifically asked for his transfer from the Filbert Street Hospital to Turner's Lane on its activation.

William Williams Keen (1837–1932) was the youngest of the group (Pl. 3). Furthermore, he was the only one of the trio who had seen active military service in the field. He had completed the literary course at Brown University. The account of his first encounter with Mitchell merits repetition:

> I had just begun the study of bones, Gray's Anatomy—then quite a new book—lay before me and in my hands was a skull. The window was open and the hot September sun was shut out by Venetian blinds, as in the early afternoon I sat in my preceptor's office where now the Jefferson Medical College building stands. Suddenly I heard the blinds move and turning around I saw a pair of eyes looking between the now horizontal slats, while a voice outside said, "Doctor, don't you want to help me on some experiments on snakes?"[12]

Flattery of the fledgling medical student or whatever may have been the primary impelling force, Mitchell was to remain "master" to the end. Meanwhile Keen's medical course was interrupted by military service. Sworn as Assistant Surgeon, July 4, 1861, in Washington, he was assigned to the Fifth Massachusetts Regiment and participated in the disaster at Bull Run, July 21, 1861. His vivid account of that battle emphasized the lack of preparedness, supplies, and logistical support.[13] In his official report, he took his appropriate share of the blame: "It is proper to state, in extenuation of the faults observed, that they were mostly, in my opinion, due to the utter lack of experience on the part of medical officers, and I would by no means exclude myself, of both the mode of obtaining supplies and the proper persons to apply to."[14] Returning to Philadelphia, he completed his medical course at Jefferson, March 1862, and two months later was again in uniform. After further field experience in medical units supporting the troops engaged in the second Battle of Bull Run and Antietam, Keen was assigned to the Satterlee Hospital, West Philadelphia. On the request of Mitchell

11. S. W. Mitchell and G. R. Morehouse, *Researches upon the Anatomy and Physiology of Respiration in the Chelonia* (Washington, D.C.: Smithsonian Institution, 1863).

12. Keen 1914, "Tribute to Mitchell," p. 345.

13. Keen, "Surgical Reminiscences of the Civil War," in *Addresses and Other Papers* (Philadelphia and London: Saunders, 1905), pp. 420–41.

14. Keen, in *Medical and Surgical History of the War of the Rebellion* (Washington, 1870–1883), Part I, Medical Volume, Appendix, p. 9.

and Morehouse, he was transferred to the Christian Street Hospital (1863) and thence to the Turner's Lane Hospital. Keen was twenty-seven years old at that time. In later years he maintained that Mitchell had asked for him, because "he never could kill me with hard work." In addition to their duties in successive military hospitals, Mitchell and Morehouse maintained their private practices in Philadelphia. As resident surgeon Keen lived in the hospital.

The Turner's Lane site has been variously described; evidently it was a country estate of that period. Keen told of the Hospital, "which then stood in the midst of a large farm near Twenty-second Street and Columbia Avenue."[15] In *The Case of George Dedlow*, Mitchell thus pictured the hospital: "It was a pleasant old-fashioned country-seat, its gardens surrounded by a circle of wooden, one story wards, shaded by pine trees."[16] Although contemporary accounts are limited, several excellent photographs afford a clear image of the Turner's Lane Hospital and its surroundings (Pl. 4).

The vision of Surgeon General Hammond, ably seconded by Surgeon General Barnes and Inspector of the Pennsylvania Department, Lieutenant Colonel Le Conte, vastly enhanced the scope and the depth of the studies at the Turner's Lane Hospital. Mitchell wrote: "When this hospital was organized, I urged upon the Surgeon General the necessity of freeing its medical staff from the usual administrative duties which take up so much of the time of our military hospital surgeon. Arrangements were therefore made which permitted us to devote to our cases all available time, and left the government of the house in charge of a competent surgeon-in-chief."[17]

In a later novel, Mitchell referred to "the awful harvest of Gettysburg."[18] In retrospect he wrote: "Never has such an opportunity for the study of nerve lesions and their results presented itself. A multitude of cases, representing almost every conceivable type of obscure nervous disease was sent to us from this department and that of Washington, by surgeons who felt conscious that these forms of disease were rarely amenable to treatment in wards crowded with grave wounds, constantly demanding all the time and care of overworked attendants."[19]

In an earlier publication this group stated that the range of nerve injuries was wide. "Among them were representatives of every con-

15. Keen 1914, "Tribute to Mitchell," p. 436.
16. S. W. Mitchell, *The Case of George Dedlow* (New York: Century, 1900), p. 134.
17. Mitchell, *Injuries of Nerves*, p. 9.
18. Mitchell, *In War Time*, p. 8.
19. Mitchell, *Injuries of Nerves*, p. 10.

ceivable form of nerve injury,—from shot and shell, from sabre cuts, contusions and dislocations. . . . Whatever may be wanting in this essay is, therefore, due alone to its authors, since never before in medical history has there been collected for study and treatment so remarkable a series of nerve injuries." Due credit was given the soldiers for the accuracy of their descriptions. "The large mass of our patients being Americans, they were usually possessed of at least some education, and often of considerable intelligence and power of observation, which was certainly not dulled by the interest with which such men regarded their own cases."[20]

The routine day of the special team, Mitchell, Morehouse, and Keen, at the Turner's Lane Hospital has been preserved by Mitchell.[21] As stated, Keen lived in the hospital. Mitchell and Morehouse would pay a cursory visit at 7:00 o'clock in the morning. Then, after their professional rounds of private practice, both would return to Turner's Lane in the late afternoon to complete detailed examinations and note-taking until midnight or early morning hours, at least several nights each week. There were no clerks or stenographers. All records were kept by members of the team. The night work completed, exhilarated by the exciting observations of the day, Mitchell and Morehouse would walk several miles to their homes. Mitchell wrote: "I have worked with many men since, but never with any who took more delight in repaying opportunity by labor. The opportunity was indeed unique and we knew it. . . . I sometimes wonder how we stood it. If urgent calls took us back into town, we returned to the hospital as if drawn by a magnet. In fact it was exciting in its constancy of novel interest. Thousands of notes were taken."[22]

Fortunately for posterity, their manuscript notes are preserved in the Library of the College of Physicians of Philadelphia. Moreover, their works were published in monograph form and were received with warm approval by the medical profession. The pamphlet on reflex paralysis (1864)[23] related primarily the experiences at the Christian Street Hospital. The authors averred, "so far as we are aware, the Medical Histories, which we are about to record, stand alone as the first reports of sudden reflex paralysis from mechanical injuries." Two

20. Mitchell, Morehouse, Keen, *Gunshot Wounds*, pp. 9–10, 20.
21. S. W. Mitchell 1914, "The Medical Department in the Civil War," *J.A.M.A.*, 62:1445–1450.
22. Ibid., p. 1449.
23. S. W. Mitchell, G. R. Morehouse, and W. W. Keen, Jr., *Reflex Paralysis* (Circular 6, U. S. General Hospital, Christian St., Philadelphia, Penna., Feb. 15, 1864).

monumental monographs, *Gunshot Wounds and Other Injuries of Nerves* (1864) and *Injuries of Nerves and Their Consequences* (1872), comprehensively covered the field and marked a new epoch in the advancement of organic neurology. Armed with the manuscript notes, one may trace certain of the casualties through three sources. The meticulous care and the accuracy of their observations become apparent. While duplication and overlapping are inevitable, in the formal treatises appropriate references are given to afford guidance. Vigorous exception to Duchenne's weakness in this area[24] was expressed. They declared: "his book is a model of confusion in the arrangement of subjects, and is without an index, so that it is not easy to be sure as to what is and what is not in it."[25] With the perspective of years, lesser importance has been assigned certain other contributions from the Turner's Lane Hospital. The study of the antagonistic actions of morphine and atropine[26] attracted more than passing notice at a period when these drugs were in great demand and use. Undoubtedly the touch of the masters gave their paper on malingering lasting value.[27] Particularly was the suggestion of a "malingerer's brigade" cogent from the psychological standpoint. As they argued, "add dishonour to hard labour and lose all hope of a discharge, malingerers would be rarely seen." Mitchell stated that at one time there were as many as eighty epileptics in the Turner's Lane Hospital.[28] The group's meticulous notes with certain original observations were destroyed by fire in Morehouse's home.[29]

Apparently guided by a knowledge of basic anatomy and fundamental ballistics, these workers made careful notes of the position and activity of the soldiers at the time of the wounding. They endeavored to trace the course of the missile from the point of entrance to its exit. Singularly, in later years Mitchell remarked that he had never seen a bayonet wound.[30] To illustrate the attention to the course of the missile, let the record speak: David Schiveley, 17 years old, 114th Pennsylvania Volunteers:

> At Gettysburg, July 2, 1863, while aiming, a ball entered one inch to

24. G. B. A. Duchenne, *De l'électrisation localisée* (Paris: Baillière, 1855).

25. Mitchell, Morehouse, and Keen, *Gunshot Wounds*, p. 74.

26. S. W. Mitchell, W. W. Keen, and G. R. Morehouse 1865, "On the antagonism of atropia and morphia," *Am. J. M. Sc.*, 50:67–76.

27. W. W. Keen, S. W. Mitchell, and G. R. Morehouse 1864, "On malingering, especially in regard to simulation of diseases of the nervous system," *Am. J. M. Sc.*, 48:367–94.

28. Mitchell 1914, "The Medical Department in the Civil War."

29. Mitchell 1906, "Memoir of George Reed Morehouse, M.D.," *Tr. Coll. Physicians, Philadelphia*, 3rd s. 28:lix–lxiii.

30. Mitchell 1914, "The Medical Department in the Civil War."

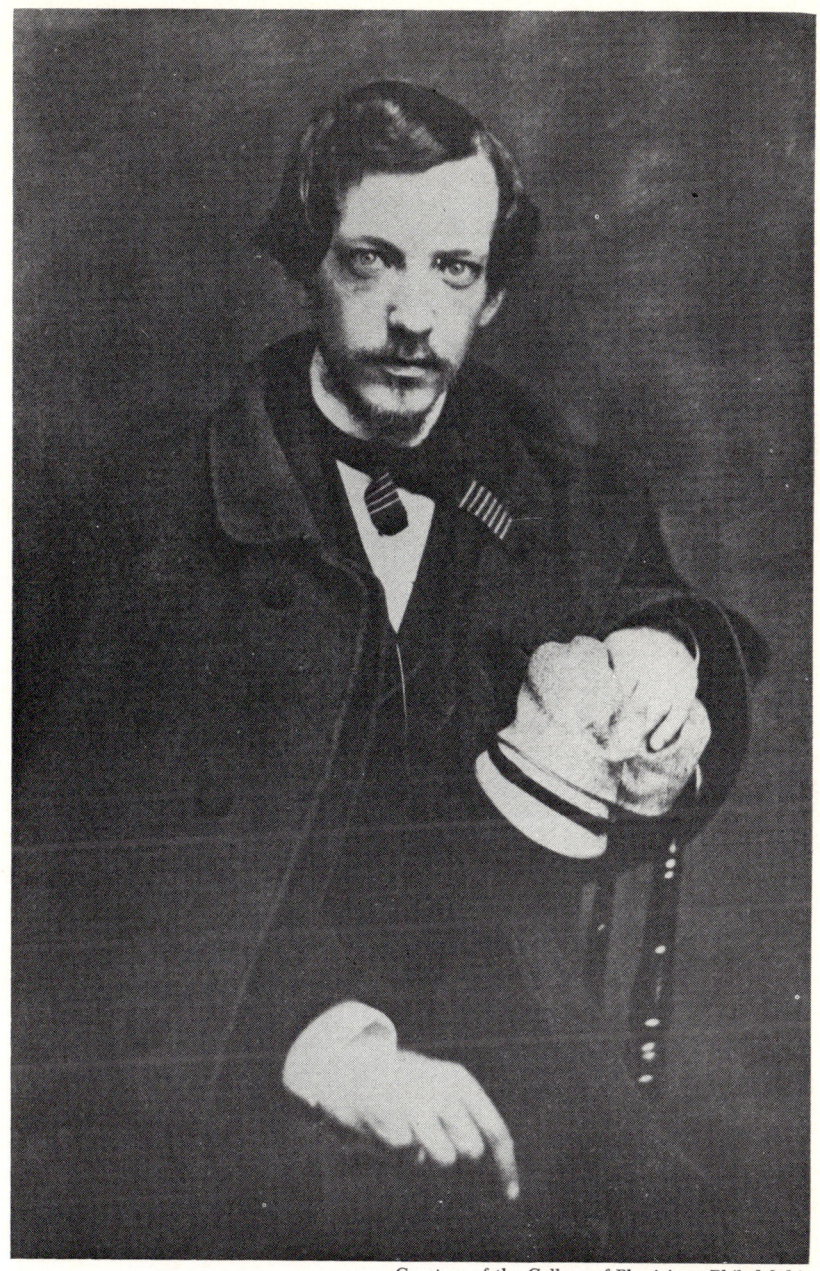

Courtesy of the College of Physicians, Philadelphia

Plate 1   S. Weir Mitchell.

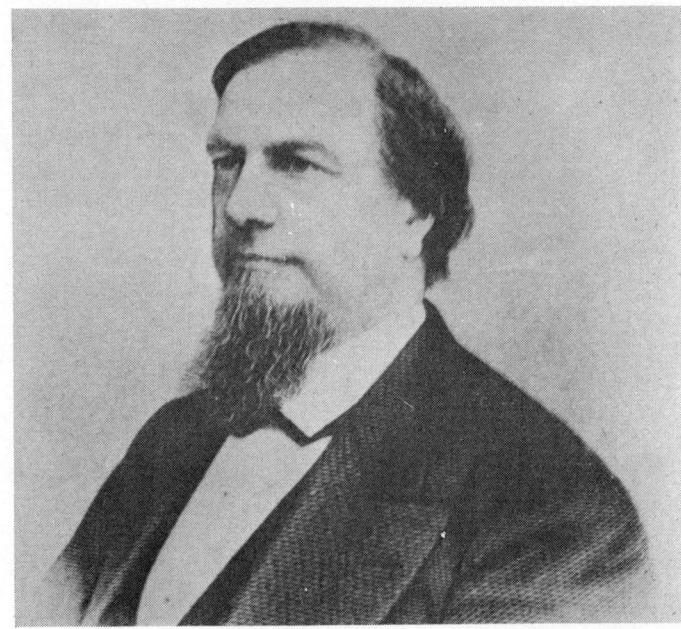

Plate 2   George Reed Morehouse.

Plate 3   William Williams Keen.

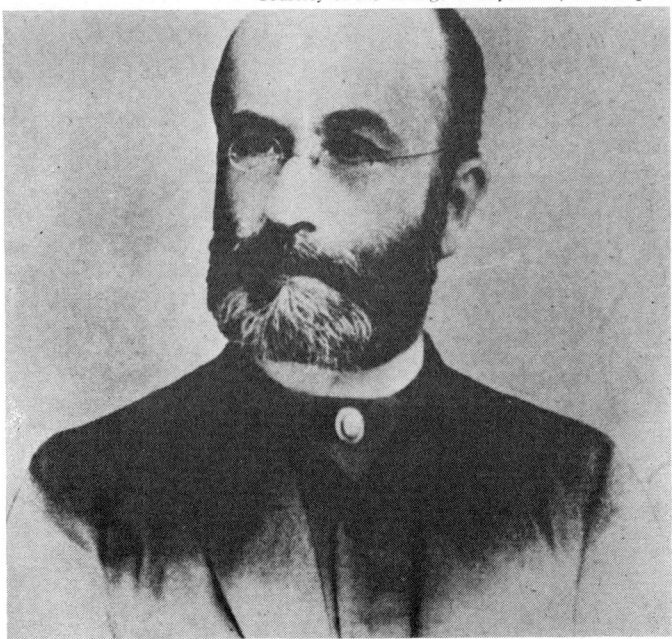

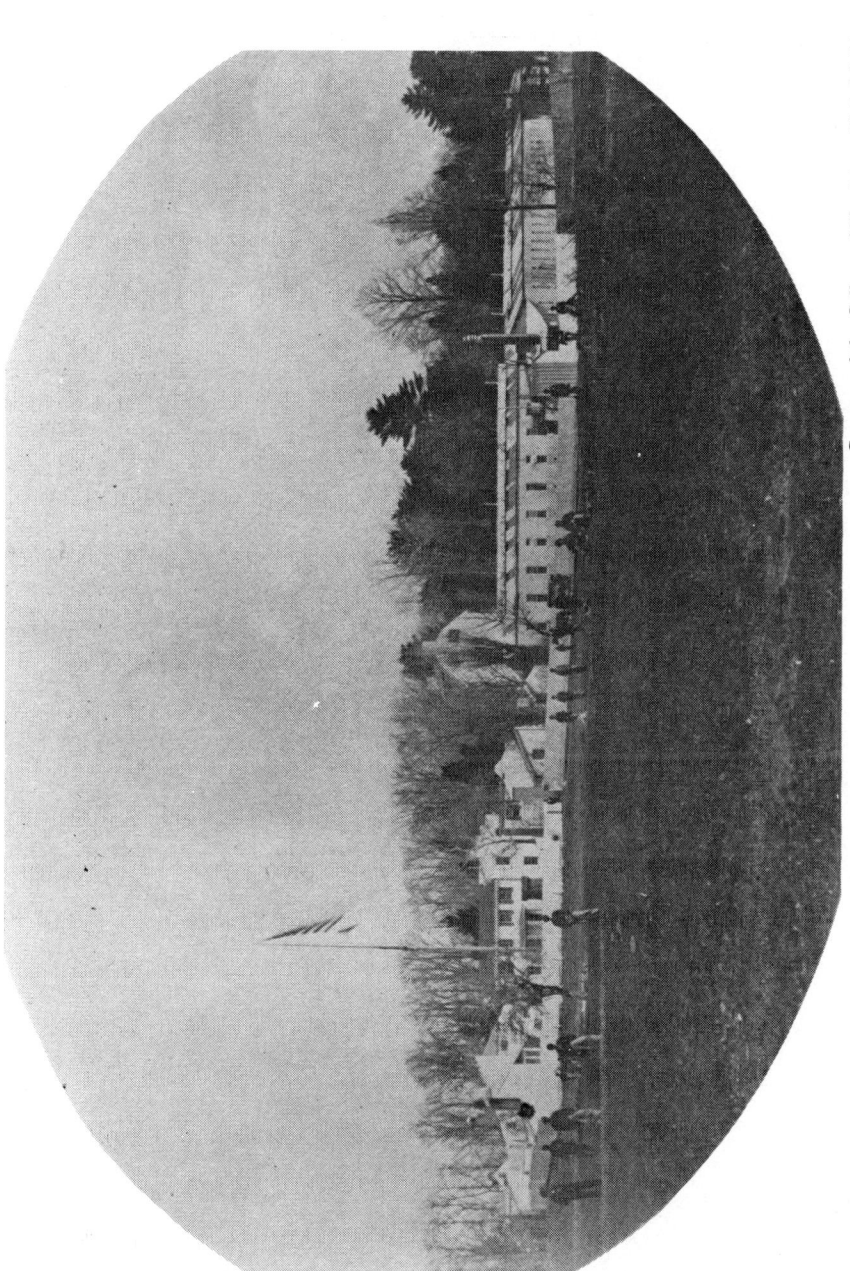

Plate 4   Turner's Lane Hospital.

GEORGE R. MOREHOUSE M.D.
2033 WALNUT STREET
PHILADELPHIA

My dear Dr Mitchell

I thank You for the copy of "Remote Consequences" you kindly sent me. And I feel personally indebted to you for putting before me the after history of some of those old inmates of Christian St + Turners Lane whose cases were so familiar to me thirty odd years ago. I think your work is very creditable. The facts you have judiciously collected, will stand for future reference. Facts are permanent, their interpretation changes color from the knowledge of the time.

With kindest regard I am sincerely yours

Geo R Morehouse

June 5ᵗʰ 95

Plate 5   Letter from Dr. G. R.
Morehouse to Dr. J. K. Mitchell.

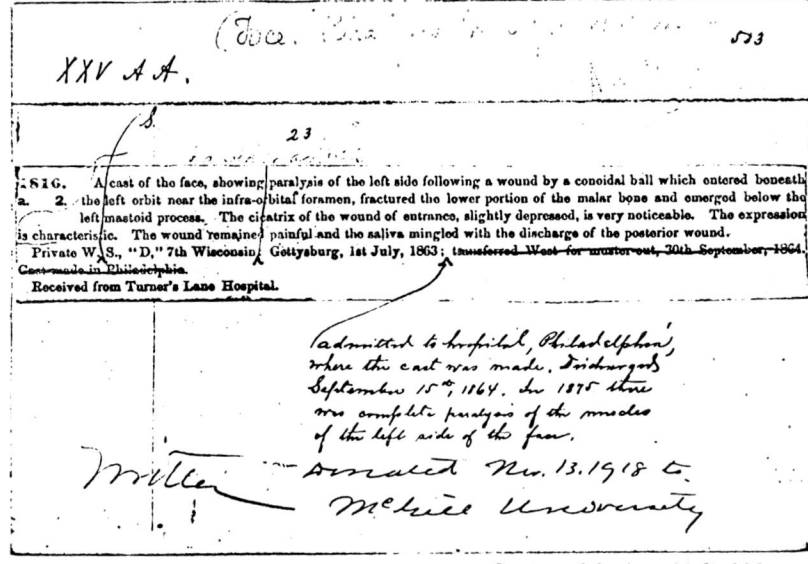

Plate 6   Turner's Lane
Hospital Accession Form.

Plate 7   Stethoscopes: Laennec, vintage
1819, below; Bowles, vintage 1908, above.

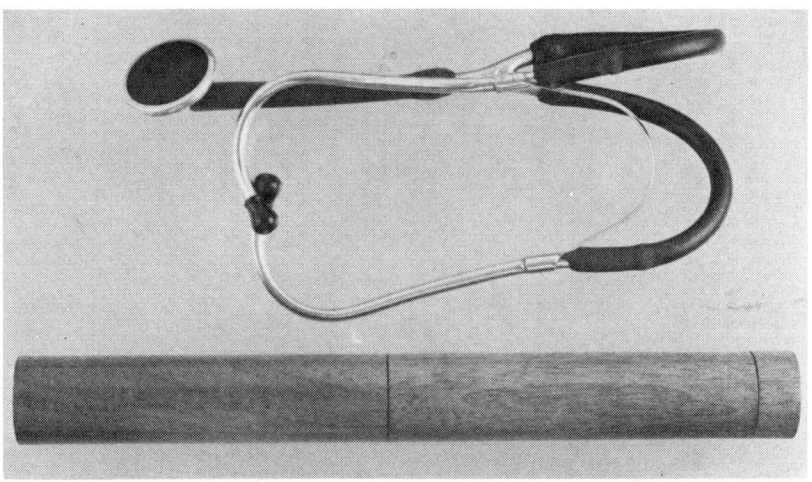

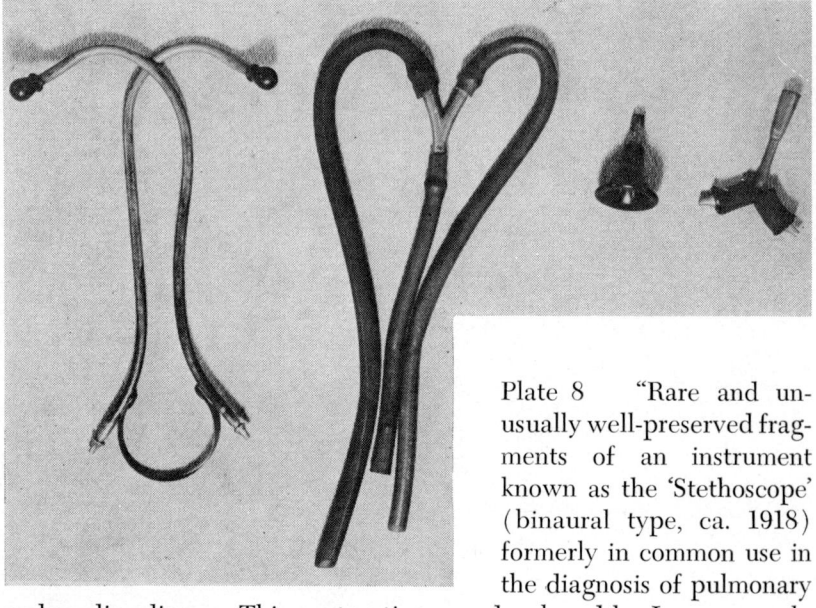

Plate 8   "Rare and unusually well-preserved fragments of an instrument known as the 'Stethoscope' (binaural type, ca. 1918) formerly in common use in the diagnosis of pulmonary and cardiac disease. This contraption was developed by Laennec early in the nineteenth century and was actually in general use until the Roentgen era." From the Sosman Exhibit, Peter Bent Brigham Hospital, Boston, Massachusetts.

Plate 9   The maximal physician-patient distance for a proper examination.

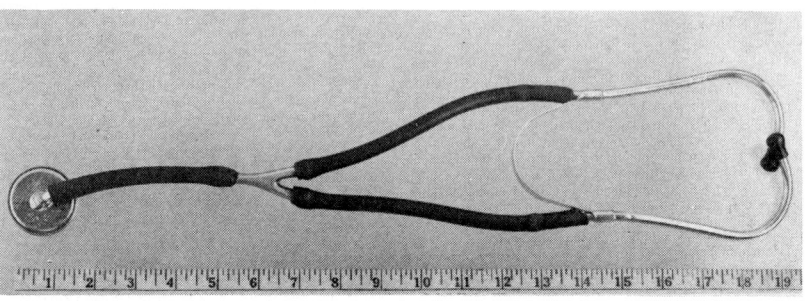

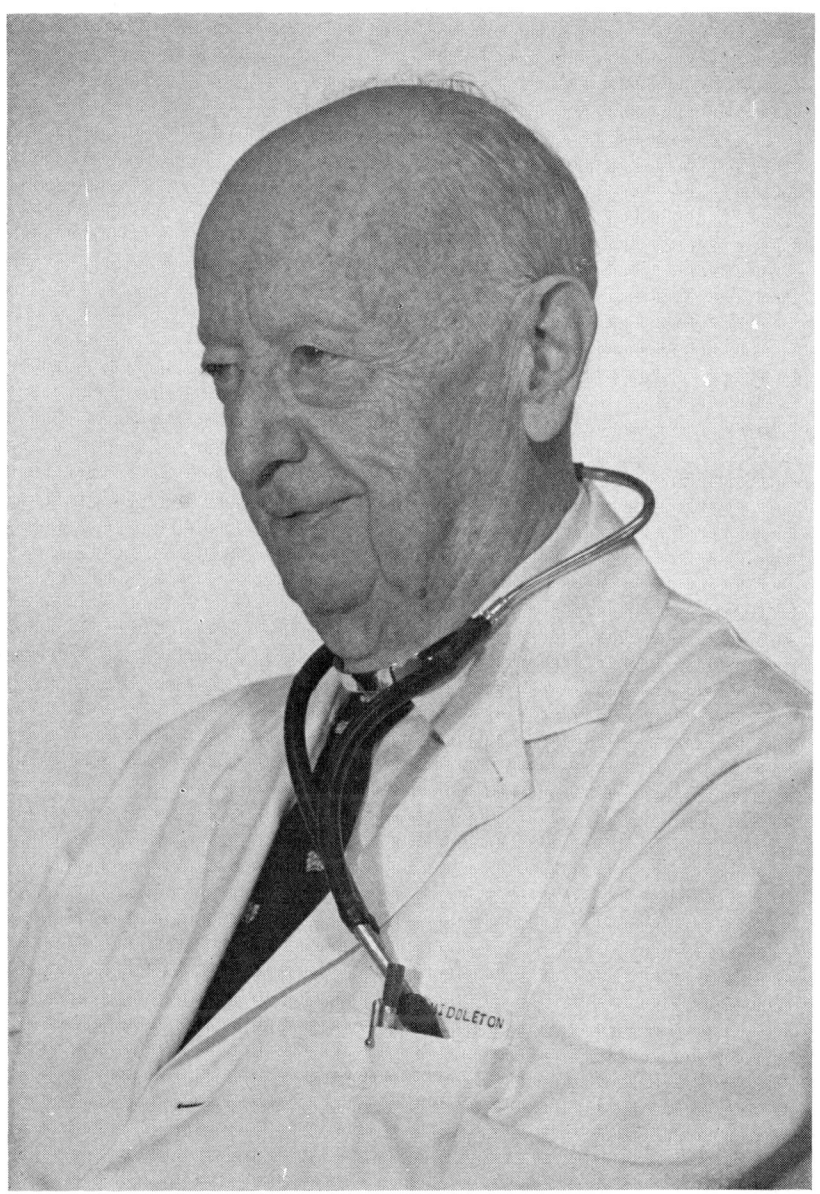

Plate 10   Dr. William Shainline Middleton.

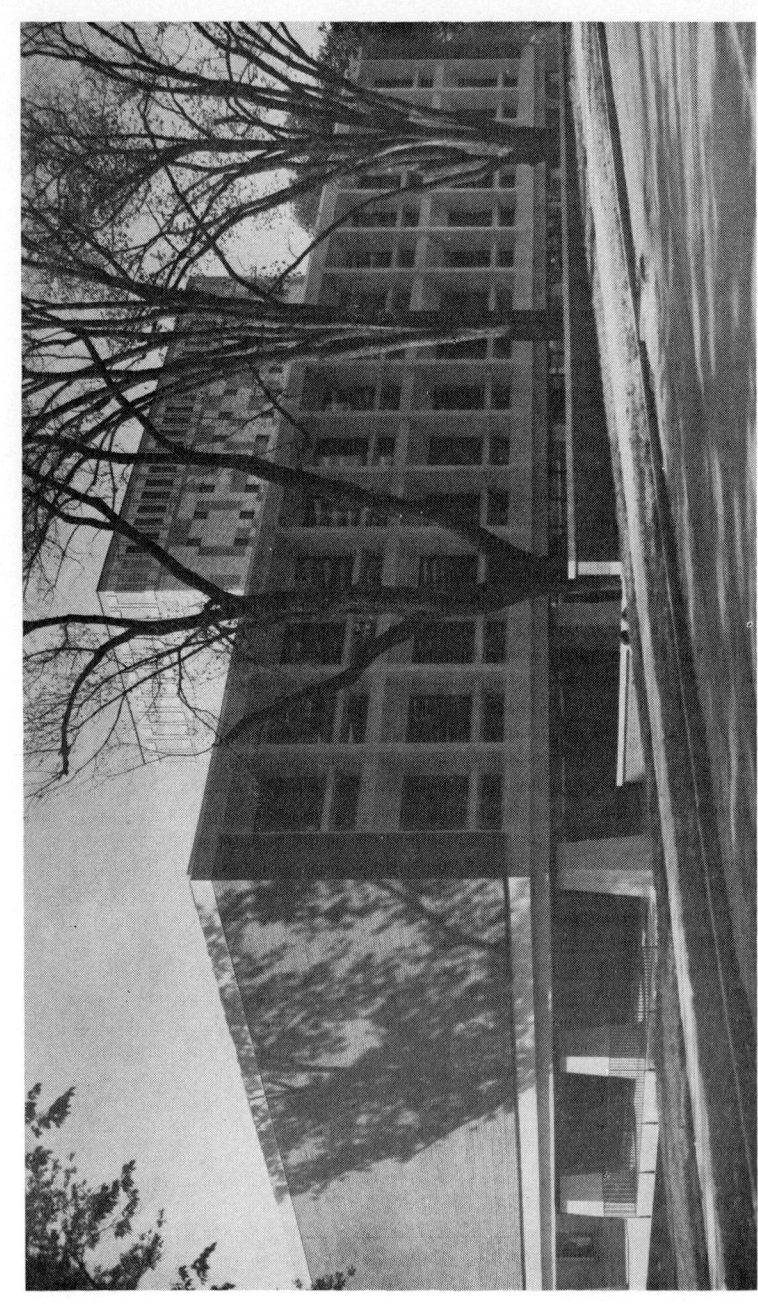

Plate 11   The Middleton Medical Library, University of Wisconsin—Madison.

the left of the middle line, and one inch above the sternal end of the clavicle. Exit on the posterior part of the right arm, at the middle line, two inches below the axilla. The ball passed in front of the trachea, broke the inner half of the right clavicle, went in front of the vessels of the neck and the subclavian artery, in front of the axillary artery and below the humerus, speaking of that bone as raised and abducted at the time. When hit, he thought his arm was shot off. It dropped, the gun fell, and, screaming that he was murdered, he staggered, bleeding freely, and soon fell unconscious.[31]

Of William Seymour, Mitchell gave an even more vivid account:

On May 5, 1865, in the Wilderness, while ramming a load, he was shot from the branches of a tree on his left. The ball entered one and a half inches immediately below the left auditory meatus, touching the lower lobe of the ear; it slightly splintered the posterior angle of the lower jaw-bone, and passed across the throat much below the level of the tongue, though as to its exact path little is known. It made exit in the right side of the neck at a level with lower edge of the thyroid cartilage, through the sternocleido-mastoid muscle about one and a half inches above the clavicle and two and a quarter inches from the middle line. He fell senseless, lay thus about an hour, and then awakening, crept half a mile, as he thinks, both wounds bleeding in jets. He now filled the wounds with dust and so checked the bleeding. He thinks both arms were at this time equally strong. The third night his wounds were dressed. Up to this time he had taken no food, and most of the water which he drank ran out of the right wound of the neck.[32]

Graphically the attitudes and reactions of the wounded were depicted.[33] Commonly the soldier felt as though he had been struck with a stick and turned to accuse a comrade of the attack. A few spoke of the sting of a whip, whereas on rare occasions the sharpness of the pain was likened to a knife thrust. At Chancellorsville Austin Lawton, 4th Ohio Volunteers, when struck by a shell fragment on the inside of the arm just below the axilla, had the following experience: "His fingers clutched the ramrod which he was using and required force to unlock the grip." Mitchell cited a soldier at Antietam with spasm of the hand and arm so severe that force had to be used to release the musket.[34] In a survey of ninety-one wounded soldiers, a third experienced no pain.[35]

The skin manifested a series of changes after wounds of the peripheral nerves and nerve plexuses. Mitchell remarked, "The tendency is

31. Mitchell, Morehouse, and Keen, *Gunshot Wounds*, p. 87.
32. Mitchell, *Injuries of Nerves*, pp. 216–17.
33. Mitchell, Morehouse, and Keen, *Gunshot Wounds*, pp. 13, 94.
34. Mitchell, *Injuries of Nerves*, p. 138.
35. Ibid., p. 136.

toward atrophy, and the thinned and shining skin, constantly fretted with tiny ulcers, seems at last to fail to shelter sufficiently its included nerve ends. Finally, the centers become over-sensitive, and radiate their state of sensitive wakefulness far and wide."[36] In another connection they described the changes thus: "Thence to the finger tips the skin is tense, shining, hairless, mottled red and blue, abraded in spots; the nails curved, and joints swollen and very tender. Palmar surface normal to wrist. The whole palmar face of the hand and fingers is polished, deep scarlet, abraded in points and eczematous all over to a remarkable degree. The eruption followed the burning in about six weeks. The palm of the left hand is nearly equally eczematous. It began to be so nearly a month before any eczema appeared in the wounded member."[37]

The first mention of alteration in the sweat to a sour quality is encountered in Clark, who suffered a gunshot wound of the median nerve.[38] John Fiting's ulnar nerve injury was succeeded by "vinegar" sweat. Particularly was this change apparent in patients with causalgia. Mitchell noted that: "the sweat was not abundant, but intensely acid, so that when some of these patients passed me in the wards I was aware of their presence because of the disagreeable odor, like vinegar, which their hands exhaled, despite the constant use of water, to which they resorted for relief. In one man the smell was disgustingly heavy, and resembled that which comes from a bad drain."[39] The claw hand was repeatedly observed. Their explanation invoked the lack of opposition to the major flexors through paralysis of the interossei (second and third phalanges).[40]

In the discussion of reflex paralysis the team advanced a theory of shock that merited the favorable notice of Fulton some seventy-six years later.[41] They wrote:

> The majority of physicians will no doubt be disposed to attribute the chief share in the phenomena of shock in its various forms to the indirect influence exerted upon and through the heart. There are, however, certain facts, which duly considered, will, we think, lead us to suppose that in many cases the phenomena in question may be due to a temporary paralysis of the whole range of nerve centers, and that

36. Ibid., p. 181.

37. Mitchell, Morehouse, and Keen, *Gunshot Wounds*, p. 88.

38. S. W. Mitchell, G. R. Morehouse, and W. W. Keen, Manuscript notes in the Library of the College of Physicians of Philadelphia.

39. Mitchell, *Injuries of Nerves*, p. 173.

40. Mitchell, Morehouse, and Keen, *Gunshot Wounds*, pp. 132–33.

41. J. F. Fulton 1940, "Neurology and war," *Tr. & Stud., Coll. Physicians, Philadelphia*, 4th s. 8:157.

among these phenomena the cardiac feebleness may play a large part, and be itself induced by the state of the regulatory nerve centers of the great circulatory organ.[42]

Still in the philosophic area, Mitchell pursued the issue:

> Shock, then, is a reflex disturbance, or, in some cases, paralysis of centers. Why in one case the cerebrum should suffer, another the heart, or in a third, the motor centers of the leg, or arm, is as yet inscrutable. A ball crushes a nerve, and the tremendous shock instantly propagated to the spine falls ruinously upon some one of the numerous ganglia through which it travels. Is this because it finds a weak point or is it that conduction checked somewhere causes at the spot destruction from the dangerous accumulation of nerve force?[43]

By most students of the disturbances of peripheral nerves the definition of causalgia is ascribed to Mitchell, Morehouse, and Keen. Certainly their manuscript notes and monographs are replete with graphic descriptions of this singular burning sensation incident to nerve injury. However, Garrison cited the description of cubitodigital neuralgia by Antonio Scarpa (1832) as the counterpart of the Civil War observations.[44] If so, the later workers were not cognizant of this report, for they wrote: "It is a form of suffering as yet undescribed, and so frequent and terrible as to demand from us the fullest description." Certainly they afforded the generally accepted designation, causalgia. The sensation was variously described as "Burning," "mustard red hot," "a red hot file rasping the skin" and in malnourished patients "almost unendurable anguish." One sufferer described the pain thus, "It is as if a rough bar of iron were thrust to and fro through the knuckles, a red-hot iron placed at the junction of the palm and the thenar eminence, with a heavy weight on it, and the skin was being rasped off his finger ends." Rarely was this sensation experienced immediately upon the injury and complete severance of the nerve or nerve trunk was never so attended. "The seat of burning pain is very various; but it never attacks the trunk, rarely the arm or thigh, and not often the forearm or leg. Its favorite site is the foot or hand." Certain significant contributions to the augmentation or relief of causalgia were regularly, if not consistently, observed. "Exposure to the air is avoided by the patient with a care which seems absurd, and most of the bad cases keep the hand constantly wet, finding relief in moisture rather than in the coolness of the application. Two of these sufferers carried a bottle of water

42. Mitchell, Morehouse, and Keen, *Reflex Paralysis.*
43. Mitchell, *Injuries of Nerves*, p. 142.
44. F. H. Garrison, *An Introduction to the History of Medicine* (4th ed.; Philadelphia and London: Saunders, 1929), p. 337.

and a sponge, and never permitted the part to become dry for a moment." Such minor incidents as the rustle of paper, drafts of air, footfall of marching steps, and band music apparently aggravated the causalgia. "He walks carefully, carries the limb tenderly with the sound hand, is tremulous, nervous, and has all kinds of expedients for lessening pain." In fact at times such patients refused to submit to an examination until the surgeon moistened his hands. The psychologic impact of the constant burning with attendant insomnia was terrific.[45]

The occurrence of motor weakness and actual paralysis without direct neural involvement in the trauma early arrested the attention of these workers. Obviously certain of these patients had hysterical paralysis; but recurring experiences in the Civil War and all subsequent wars afford ample documentation for reflex paralysis. Indeed, death may occur from proximity to an explosion (shell, bomb, or other missile) without demonstrable external wound. (The classical experiments of Zuckerman[46] have assigned the primary responsibility for such devastating results to the physical effect of the pressure wave of the high explosive missiles.) Continuing their interest in this aspect of neurologic injuries, repeated observations were incorporated in the two monographs that followed the transfer from the Christian Street Hospital to the Turner's Lane Hospital. Seven case reports were made in Circular 6.[47] By reason of overlapping and duplication it is impossible to cite comparable figures from the later notes and monograph. Again, the authors themselves question certain instances.[48] For example, Henry H. Burrows had suffered a wound of the brachial plexus. Three weeks later he was unable to hold a pen. Insensible for twenty minutes, when he regained consciousness his right arm was paralyzed. The following day he could write and electrical tests for motor function were normal. In the manuscript notes[49] the case of Morgan Emory was carefully documented and reappeared in Circular 6[50] and the monograph.[51] Sustaining a through and through wound of the neck without manifest bony or neural involvement, he experienced a quadriplegia. Motor power was promptly restored to all extremities, except the right arm. With faradization the strength in the

45. Mitchell, Morehouse, and Keen, *Gunshot Wounds,* pp. 101–111.

46. S. Zuckerman 1940, "Experimental study of blast injuries to the lungs," *Lancet,* 2:219–24.

47. Mitchell, Morehouse, and Keen, *Reflex Paralysis.*

48. Mitchell, Morehouse, and Keen, Manuscript notes.

49. Ibid.

50. Mitchell, Morehouse, and Keen, *Reflex Paralysis.*

51. Mitchell, Morehouse, and Keen, *Gunshot Wounds,* p. 31.

right arm was regained, and there remained only irregular areas of hyperesthesia that might have represented a commotion of the cervical cord from the proximate transit of the missile. The case of John Schultze was likewise reported in several media. The account in the monograph[52] related his clinical course from the Minié ball wound at Gettysburg until his discharge from the Turner's Lane Hospital. The missile entered the left cheek at the lower edge of the malar prominence and coursed across the ramus of the jaw to the anterior margin of the trapezius. He was unconscious for one half hour. There was no pain, but on the second day there was a sudden recurrence of sensation, especially in the distribution of the left mental nerve. When he regained consciousness the left arm was powerless. The fingers could be moved but he could not flex his arm at the elbow. The right arm was less involved. Lesser sensory changes were observed. Power returned to the right arm in one week. The left arm responded much more gradually.

The group's discussions of the mechanisms of the various neurological manifestations were supported by citations from the literature, personal observations, and experimentation. Compression and commotion received appropriate attention. Painstakingly Mitchell analyzed the periods and stages of nerve injury and repair.[53] Certainly his experimental work to delineate the pressure factor postdated the war period and the activity of the Turner's Lane Hospital.[54] Of the patient with a neural lesion the team left a vivid word picture that should be preserved: "A more wretched spectacle than this man presents can hardly be imagined. He lies in bed, motionless, emaciated to the last degree, and with bed-sores on both elbows and both hips. His hands lie crossed on his chest, perfectly rigid; the fingers extended; the skin congested and thin; the nails curved; false anchylosis of all the joints of the upper limbs; the head and neck rigid, with acute pain in these parts on movement."[55]

Singularly there are relatively few observations and notes of cranial nerve injuries. Upon reflection, several circumstances would explain this situation. In the first place, wounds of the head are usually grave and commonly fatal. Then, too, the period of the Civil War would practically assure infection. In addition, the mission of the Turner's Lane Hospital as a convalescent center for specially screened patients with neurological injury or disease would almost arbitrarily eliminate

52. Ibid., pp. 45–47.
53. Mitchell, *Injuries of Nerves,* pp. 108–110.
54. Ibid., p. 112.
55. Mitchell, Morehouse, and Keen, *Gunshot Wounds,* p. 23.

this group of the wounded. An exception was cited in the person of William S. Sylvester of the 7th Wisconsin Volunteers, who was wounded by a Minié ball at Gettysburg, July 1, 1863. From its point of entrance one inch below the outer angle of the left eye the missile travelled backward and outward across the external auditory meatus with fracture of the ramus of the jaw to emerge behind the fractured lower half of the mastoid process. All muscles of expression on the left side of the face were paralyzed, and taste was lost on the left side of the tongue. "He was long annoyed by the inability to cover his eye with the lid; but has now learned to roll his eye upward, so as to cover the iris. He then supposes he has closed the lid." No response to electrical stimulation could be demonstrated in the muscles supplied by the left seventh cranial nerve (portia dura).[56]

Edward Mooney was first encountered in the manuscript notes. His wound had involved the right superior cervical sympathetic ganglion. Their observations included flushed cheek, ptosis, altered line of the lid, and contracted pupil on the affected side. Unsuccessful attempts to record differences in the surface temperature were noted.[57] Later Keen afforded certain missing links. While serving at the Satterlee U. S. General Hospital, Keen had had a soldier presented to him. He proceeded: "On looking up at him I said to myself: 'You are Dalton's cat.'" Upon inquiry the patient stated that he had been shot in the neck. Thereupon he was transferred to the Christian Street Hospital, where he was attended by Keen and undoubtedly again moved to the Turner's Lane Hospital when it was opened. When Keen went to Paris after the war, he related the situation to Claude Bernard. The master was greatly excited to have the first confirmation of his research observation in man. Mooney had completed the scientific circle.[58]

Taking advantage of their excellent opportunity to observe the widest range of injuries of peripheral nerves, nerve trunks, and plexuses, with infinite patience these workers noted every subjective and objective detail that their studies disclosed.[59] Motor and sensory deficits were carefully evaluated for prognostic as well as diagnostic purposes. The dangers of the improper use of splints and crutches were emphasized. For example, John Fiting of the 27th Wisconsin sustained a wound of the forearm involving branches of the ulnar nerve. An improper splint and disuse led to extreme atrophy and paresis that re-

56. Ibid., pp. 52–54; also Fig. 6.

57. Mitchell, Morehouse, and Keen, Manuscript notes; Mitchell, *Injuries of Nerves*, pp. 319–22.

58. Keen, "Surgical Reminiscences of the Civil War," p. 437.

59. Mitchell, Morehouse, and Keen, Manuscript notes.

sponded to appropriate therapy. Richard McCabe had a similar experience after a wound of the forearm involving the ulnar nerve. Loss of extensor power with contracture of the flexors greatly increased his problems and protracted his rehabilitation. James C. Meaning fractured his tibia and fibula in a fall. After two months of walking with the aid of crutches, he complained of numbness in the right arm. He admitted that he leaned more heavily on this arm. From paraesthesia his disability advanced to complete inability to move the right arm.

The phenomenon of the phantom limb had been recognized from the time of Ambroise Paré. To the Turner's Lane group came an unusual opportunity to study its physiologic and psychophysiological parameters. In Philadelphia the South Street Hospital had been established at Twenty-fourth and South Streets. Its function soon gravitated to the care of amputees, and within the Army it came to be known as "Stump Hospital." The soldiers spoke lightly of being "limbed." Mitchell delved deeply into many aspects of this problem.[60] Neuritis, neuralgia, neurofibroma, and chorea are sequelae that have concerned medicine for many years. Hence Mitchell studied the influence of environmental temperature on the sensitivity of stumps. About one-half of fifty amputees professed to some ability to predict a change in weather. Mitchell found no answer to this traditional claim. Turning to the phantom limb, he remarked: "Nearly every man who loses a limb carries about with him a constant or inconstant phantom of the missing member, a sensory ghost of that much of himself, and sometimes a most inconvenient presence, faintly felt at times, but ready to be called up to his perception by a blow, a touch, or a change of wind." The onset of this phenomenon may be immediate or delayed. There was cited an instance of a virtual absence of sensation on amputation of the foot; but with a reamputation above the knee there appeared a permanent phantom.

Mitchell's enlargement of the subject stated:

> Even in those who are least conscious of the missing part, I have amazed them by suddenly recalling it with the aid of a faradic current applied to the nerves of the stump. It is not easy to forget the astonishment with which some of these persons reawaken to a perception of the long lost leg or arm.
>
> I recently faradised a case of disarticulated shoulder without warning my patient of the possible result. For two years he had altogether ceased to feel the limb. As the current affected the brachial plexus of nerves, he suddenly cried aloud, "Oh, the hand, the hand!" and attempted to seize the missing member. The phantom I had conjured up

60. Mitchell, *Injuries of Nerves*, pp. 345–360.

swiftly disappeared, but no spirit could have more amazed the man, so real did it seem.

Singularly, the patient with a phantom limb experienced no sense of the intervening arm or leg when the absent hand or foot seemed so real. Then, too, there was a feeling of an approximation of the phantom part to the stump. In elucidating certain of these psychopathologic reactions Mitchell offered this explanation:

> It would appear, then, that when we will a movement, there arise coincidently, or from the spinal ganglia through which it is carried out, impressions as to the force of the act and the position of the parts which we will to move; so that given the volition, there springs up in the mind a consciousness as to the act and its qualities, which is too generally believed to originate altogether from the external parts disturbed. On the other hand, the second series of experiments proves, or makes probable, that certain nerves carry centrally, during motion, impressions which, with those nascent in the centres when the act is willed, go to complete the general knowledge as to motor activities.

One of the most famous literary hoaxes with a medical background is *The Case of George Dedlow*.[61] Mitchell had always had a literary flair. Indeed, he had taken counsel of Oliver Wendell Holmes, who advised him to submerge such aspirations until he had passed fifty years. His fantasy took form in the psychologic reaction of a soldier who was a quadruple amputee. At a circle of spiritualists the tale reached its climax in the collapse of the victim, who had trusted himself to the support of his phantom legs. Several incidents leading to its publication are noteworthy. Presumably, when Weir Mitchell entrusted his manuscript to Mrs. Caspar Wistar, daughter of Dr. William Henry Furness, he had no plan for publication. His first knowledge of its submittal was a check for eighty dollars from the *Atlantic Monthly*, with the page proof. Aside from his first financial return for his literary effort, other unexpected reactions were encountered. His account of George Dedlow's unhappy state loosened the sympathetic purse strings of a number of people, who sent monies for his comfort. Others called in person at Stump Hospital to visit Dedlow. Even spiritualists found some solace in Dedlow's short-lived support on the nonexisting legs.[62] Mitchell concluded this fantastic story thus: "It is needless to add that I am not a happy fraction of a man, and that I am eager for the day when I shall rejoin the lost members of my corporeal family in another and a happier world."

61. Mitchell, *The Case of George Dedlow*.
62. C. W. Burr 1919, "S. Weir Mitchell, physician, man of science, man of letters, man of affairs," *Tr. Coll. Physicians, Philadelphia*, 3rd s. *41*:227–49.

Malingering is the *bête noire* of medical men at all times, in war or peace. Since mutual respect and understanding are so essential to the practice of medicine, any breach in the cooperative pattern is disruptive to the best interests of all concerned. In a military setting the epidemiology of this psychologic plague is traditional. Without careful study and fair discipline it may spread like a prairie fire and irreparably impair the morale of a unit or command. Purposeful misrepresentation can mislead and may defy detection by even skilled attendants. Such evasion or actual malingering becomes increasingly difficult of discovery if the evidence is subjective. The Turner's Lane Hospital team was primarily concerned with the "simulation of diseases of the nervous system."[63] According to their observations, malingering was more common in the Regular Army. "The older soldiers are fast learning deceit, and if we be not mistaken, the attempts to malinger are now much more frequent, and far more clever, than they were two years ago." The evils and temptations of the bounty system were cited. Discharge and reenlistment under the premium of a mounting bounty proved a profitable transaction. The cited "malingerer's brigade" was too radical a remedy for adoption by the Army. Other basic principles were enunciated. Inhalation of ether to uncover feigned contractures and ankylosis was an expedient of wide usefulness. At times limping and lameness disappeared on recovery from a general anesthetic. Presumed aphonia and deafness stood revealed as false on appropriate anesthesia. Convulsive attacks were rarely spurious. If the attacks did not occur more than once a month, the patient was transferred to the Veterans Reserve Corps but not discharged. Attention was directed to an important point in the differential diagnosis of epilepsy. By general consent, dilated, unresponsive pupils at the height of a seizure were deemed diagnostic of true epilepsy. However, these workers reproduced the pupillary changes by violent effort against the restraint of broad bands across the shoulders and girdles about the waist. In addition to the close surveillance of malingerers in the hospital, the discharge to the command unit included a statement of the alleged handicap, so that the responsible officer would be in a position to make independent observations.

An atmosphere of study was continuously abroad at the Turner's Lane Hospital. One of the thoughtful projects of the group was the effort to study the skin temperature of wounded extremities.[64] Having

63. Keen, Mitchell, and Morehouse 1864, "On malingering."
64. Mitchell, Morehouse, and Keen, *Gunshot Wounds*, pp. 134–35; Mitchell, *Injuries of Nerves*, p. 174.

failed with a bulb thermometer, the workers were supplied with Becquerel thermoelectric disks by Professor Rand of Central High School, Philadelphia. Apparently this device was too sensitive for the purpose, since the needle flew to the limit in nearly every case. On direct observation with a small thermometer (one half of the circumference of the bulb being covered by a cork), there were determined declines in temperature of 2 to 5° F if nerve section were complete and 2 to 3° F if incomplete. If there were causalgia or a glossy skin, the temperature was found to be normal or slightly elevated. The affected muscles were invariably tested electrically. "Of this we are distinctly sure that there is no test of the restoration of nerve supply except the electric current."[65] As the notes and texts are studied their strict adherence to this rule emphasizes their dependence on this measure in diagnosis and prognosis. In Mitchell's monograph a number of anatomic and physiologic experiments were outlined. Furthermore, attention was directed to the use of the metronome in timing the transmission of nerve impulses and of the sphygmogram in defining muscle activity. Since these observations postdated the Turner's Lane period, they are not herein considered, with one exception. Mitchell concluded that: "we are without absolute proof of the existence of true trophic nerves, devoted solely to regulating nutrition, and are equally without just reasons for asserting that the nerves of sense and motion may not be largely concerned in propagating to the tissues irritative and other influences quite competent to occasion disease."[66] The apt expression catches the eye and holds the attention. In describing the confusion of the proprioceptive sense that attends the interlocking of fingers behind the back Mitchell and his colleagues referred to the "tactile squint."[67]

The prognosis of the injuries of peripheral nerves is one of the most elusive and difficult aspects of the problem. They remarked: "among the injuries which fail to palsy a limb at once and completely, those which bruise a nerve have seemed to us to be the most likely in the end to cause atrophies."[68] Repeated reference was made to the confusion of contractures with primary paralysis. Mitchell noted: "The future of any case of long continued subacute neuritis is rather a dark one, and is grave in proportion to the length of nerve involved, and the extent to which it has traveled in a central direction; since if it has passed up as far as the parent plexus, so as to be beyond surgical reach, the case may usually be regarded as one to be relieved, but rarely

65. Mitchell, Morehouse, and Keen, Gunshot Wounds, p. 71.
66. Mitchell, Injuries of Nerves, p. 16.
67. Mitchell, Morehouse, and Keen, Gunshot Wounds, p. 118.
68. Ibid., p. 71.

cured."[69] Many of the obvious failures in their experience related to delay and neglect in adequate treatment. As their records are reviewed, ample justification is found for their optimism, thus expressed: "No class of cases with which we have been called to deal seemed to us, at one time, so sadly hopeless as injuries of the nerves; none has better rewarded enduring and steady efforts to afford relief. We look back with unfeigned pleasure upon the great number who came to us, despairing cripples, and left us eased of pain, and either entirely well or so far aided as to enable them to employ their limbs in useful occupations."[70]

In general, the therapy of these injuries was conventional and reflected the practice of the times. Wet dressings were supplemented by poultices and blisters in certain patients with neuritis. Actual cautery was occasionally resorted to. Leeching was apparently effective in some instances; but cold applications proved helpful both objectively and subjectively in severe neuritis. "The relief afforded is often remarkable, and the loss of the nerves in size, hardness and tenderness most gratifying."[71] Counterirritation and faradisation were employed upon subsidence of the acute manifestations. Vesicants were not applied directly over the involved nerves. Morphine and other sedatives were extensively employed. Mechanical devices, as bandages and splints, afforded necessary support. On occasions tenotomy was performed to overcome disabling contractures.[72] Due attention was directed to the general hygiene and nutrition of these patients.

Of especial interest is the detailed hydrotherapy and physiotherapy of the neurological patients at the Turner's Lane Hospital. Repeated reference was made to "douching" and "shampooing" of the wounded. The massage consisted of deep kneading short of pain. Mitchell continued: "the results, which I have seen obtained by practiced rubbers were certainly to be gained by no other equally rapid treatment." In another relation, he added that the "manipulation must be not only tender and gentle, but also strong and enduring."[73] Most noteworthy was his further statement: "New modes of treatment were devised, and gymnastic classes instituted, under the care of intelligent sergeants of the invalid corps; electricity was constantly employed, and hypodermic medication—at that time somewhat novel—was habitually re-

69. Mitchell, *Injuries of Nerves*, p. 68.
70. Mitchell, Morehouse, and Keen, *Gunshot Wounds*, pp. 156–57.
71. Mitchell, *Injuries of Nerves*, p. 73.
72. Ibid., pp. 205–6.
73. Ibid., pp. 249–53.

sorted to, and its effects carefully studied."[74] As to the electrical modality employed, Mitchell concluded: "Whatever current is the readiest excitor is the one to be preferred, and galvanism in traumatic, as in infantile palsies, is active where induced currents fail us. It is, however, very largely a question of time and patience."[75] As noted, morphine was regularly used, but the hypodermic route was an innovation, and Mitchell noted that sixty to eighty injections were given daily and perhaps 40,000 in a year without incident at the Turner's Lane Hospital. The experiences with conia, hyoscyamus, daturia, and atropia did not warrant their replacement of morphine.[76]

Hostilities ceasing and the need for military hospitals decreasing, the smaller, and particularly the specialized, institutions were consolidated or closed. "On the same day (8 May 1865) the Army hospitals at Broad and Cherry . . . Turner's Lane, . . . were finally closed, and the remaining patients transferred to other hospitals."[77] The actual duties at the Turner's Lane Hospital were concluded in June 1865. The Surgeon General ordered the relinquishment of all records. These invaluable data were copied in a month and the original notes consigned to the oblivion of the official files in Washington.[78] Through the Bureau of Pensions and the National Home for Disabled Veterans and by personal correspondence, efforts were made to maintain contact with the wounded who had come under the care of the staff at the Turner's Lane Hospital. Unfortunately, the returns were desultory and the dividends did not justify the expenditure of time and effort. Finally, S. Weir Mitchell's son, John K. Mitchell, with commendable zeal and tenacity of purpose and with the added influence of Hon. J. W. Noble, Secretary of the Interior, and Dr. Ingram of the Bureau of Pensions, established among other conclusions the status of some fifteen of the Turner's Lane Hospital patients.[79] His observations, published thirty years after the Civil War, constituted a material contribution to the knowledge of the ultimate results of peripheral nerve injuries. While certain familiar names and situations are missing, there is still a continuity that bridges a generation and emphasizes the youth of the soldiers in that

74. Ibid., pp. 10–11.
75. Ibid., p. 247.
76. Ibid., pp. 269–70.
77. J. T. Scharf and T. Westcott, *History of Philadelphia*, 3 vols. (Philadelphia: Everts, 1884), 1:825.
78. Mitchell 1914, "The Medical Department in the Civil War"; Mitchell 1906, "Memoir of Morehouse."
79. J. K. Mitchell, *Remote Consequences of Injuries of Nerves and Their Treatment* (Philadelphia: Lea, 1895).

terrible conflict. Morehouse wrote a letter of appreciation to John K. Mitchell on receipt of *Remote Consequences* (Pl. 5).[80]

Somewhat more intimate has been the experience in attempting to locate certain specimens and models of that period. Alonzo A. Lambert, nineteen years old, Private, Company H, 7th Wisconsin Volunteers, was wounded in the Battle of the Wilderness. His left arm was amputated and sent to the College of Physicians of Philadelphia. Many years ago, a zealous Curator of the Mutter Museum discarded all specimens without appropriate identification.[81] Apparently this was the fate of the Lambert arm. Recurrent through the manuscript notes and monographs are references to masks of the face and casts of the extremities. A majority of these notes indicated the Army Medical Museum as their repository. General Joe M. Blumberg traced accession forms for fifteen of these specimens.[82] A few of them were lost; but on November 13, 1918, the majority found their way to McGill University (Pl. 6). Professor McMillan has diligently pursued this clue, without disclosing any trace of the masks or casts.[83]

Both in his literary and in his medical publications after the Civil War, Mitchell spoke most highly of the contributions of medicine to the common cause and deprecated the apparent lack of civic appreciation. In *In War Time* he wrote: "Vast hospitals were planned and admirably built, without the advice of architects, by physicians who had to learn as they went along the special constructive needs of different climates, and to settle novel and frequent hygienic questions as they arose."[84] Shortly before his death, Mitchell said: "I propose to deal briefly with the place our great profession held morally and technically in the war of the sixties. It is a record to be proud of, or I should not so willingly revert to it. . . . We gain nowhere a sense of the immensity of the task which as a profession we dealt with. We hear little or nothing of the unequaled capacity with which we met the call on energy and intelligence, or of the extraordinary power of the trained American to deal with the unusual." In a similar vein he decried the lack of recognition in life, or of a memorial in death, for the medical officers who served their country in the Civil War. Yet posterity has granted its accolade to the team that worked so assiduously and achieved so vastly at the Turner's Lane Hospital. Not only has their contribution had a

80. Letter, G. R. Morehouse to J. K. Mitchell.
81. Personal correspondence of the author with Dr. W. B. McDaniel 2nd.
82. Personal correspondence of the author with Brigadier General J. M. Blumberg.
83. Personal correspondence of the author with Professor G. C. McMillan.
84. Mitchell, *In War Time*, p. 44.

lasting influence on American medicine; but to its fundamental roots may clearly be traced the origin of organic neurology in this country.

The dramatic story of medical achievement in the Turner's Lane Hospital, which Fulton characterized as "one of the great milestones in the history of American neurology and American clinical medicine,"[85] has been related. There remains a natural curiosity as to the subsequent careers of its principals. George Reed Morehouse, a product of Princeton and Jefferson, proved to be the worker in the vineyard. A highly respected family counselor, he had a large private practice, and his services were widely sought in consultation after the war. A most congenial companion, he eschewed public appearance and discussion. Weir Mitchell bore repeated testimony to his surgical skill. Although intellectually endowed for great attainment, Morehouse purposefully directed his superior talents to the care of patients, in which he found the greatest personal satisfaction. Princeton granted him the honorary degree of Ph.D. *honoris causa* (1892). In his memorial notice, Mitchell referred to Morehouse's dilatory habit of deferring writing assignments on joint projects. "I have never yet been able to determine wherein lay a man's difficulty in putting on paper what seemed to be clear and definite and of which he could talk so lucidly. What this remarkably able man was competent to do, and did do, I have here recorded. What he did not go on to do is still to me a matter of wonder, interest, and friendly regret."[86] Warm in the devotion of his patients and friends, Morehouse died November 12, 1905.

After the Civil War, William Williams Keen[87] was destined for a long and distinguished career in surgery. He first spent two years in the clinics of Paris and Berlin. In the latter center he came under the influence of Rudolph Virchow. An early proponent of Lister's revolutionary technique, he steadily advanced in academic circles to become in turn professor of surgery at Woman's Medical College and at Jefferson Medical College. "Although fragile in frame and almost diminutive in stature, his intellect coupled with an extraordinary capacity for hard work brought him well merited leadership." A master surgeon, he assisted Dr. Joseph D. Bryant in the clandestine surgery on President Cleveland aboard a yacht in the East River. At the First International Congress of American Physicians and Surgeons (1888), Keen reported the successful removal of three brain tumors that marked him among the pioneers in this area. Active in organized medicine, he was hon-

---

85. Fulton 1940, "Neurology and war."
86. Mitchell 1906, "Memoir of Morehouse."
87. W. Pickles 1927, "William Williams Keen," *Rhode Island M. J.,* 10:1; Obituary notice, *J.A.M.A.* 1932, 98:2228.

ored by the presidency of the American Medical Association (1900–1901), the American Surgical Association (1899), and the International Congress of Surgery, Paris (1920). A crusader at heart, Keen valiantly contested the efforts of ill-advised zealots to curtail vivisection. Keen had the unusual distinction of being the only medical officer serving in both the Civil War and World War I. Although he had volunteered in the Spanish-American War, hostilities ceased before he was called to active duty. His commission as Major in World War I was essentially an honorary one. At this time he published a monograph, *The Treatment of War Wounds,* the popular appeal of which was evinced by an early (1918) second edition. Anachronistic license affords mild amusement in the emergence of the Carrel-Dakin treatment to supplant acriflavine, proflavine, brilliant green, and mercurophen between the two editions. Perhaps no American surgeon to his day was so showered with honors as Keen, who died at ninety-five years, mourned as a noble exemplar of the highest ideals of the medical profession.

By breeding, instinct, and personality, Silas Weir Mitchell was the leader of this remarkable cast. His postwar career was marked by a steady advancement in medical proficiency and recognition. Yet his highest ambition, a University professorship, eluded him. The occasion when such an objective might have been realized was thus related: "He was a teacher of those who taught, although he was never a professor in any medical school except for five minutes during the time that he was a trustee at the University of Pennsylvania. At a board meeting he was asked to retire, and during his absence was elected Professor of Physiology. He immediately resigned after being informed of his appointment."[88] His boyhood zeal for investigation never waned; but in later life it found expression largely in the stimulation and support of younger workers. He contributed approximately 250 articles or books to the medical literature, a majority of which dealt with neurological, physiological, pharmacological, and toxicological subjects. His flair for writing made him one of this country's conspicuous medical litterateurs. Although the psychological quirks of his characters colored some of his novels, unusual merit attaches to *The Red City,* an account of the yellow fever epidemic of 1793 in Philadelphia, and to *Hugh Wynne, Free Quaker,* a remarkable historical novel of Philadelphia life in the Revolutionary period. Of Mitchell's manifold interests, none approached his dedicated efforts in behalf of the College of Physicians of Philadelphia and its Library. Widely honored in this country and abroad for his literary and medical achievements, Mitchell died in his

88. Mumey, S. *Weir Mitchell,* p. 47.

eighty-fifth year. Among the many tributes paid his memory, none more fully measured the man than the eloquent words of William H. Welch:

> However the verdict of history may modify contemporary judgments of the achievements of men, it cannot change the place which Dr. Mitchell holds in our affection and esteem. He was a great physician; our leader, endeared, admired; our friend and counselor, generous, wise, inspiring; a man of singular graces and accomplishments, active in advancing knowledge, and in good works, a poet and a man of letters, a sweetener of life to both sick and well. Happy such a life and happy the memories thereof which we shall ever cherish! As he said of Harvey, we may say of him—Weir Mitchell represented all that is best in the physician and the gentleman.[89]

Turner's Lane Hospital, the scene of this medical drama, has suffered the vicissitudes of time and material deterioration. It falls in an area designed for urban renewal. There is no historical marker of its site. Yet here, following the precepts of Hippocrates and Sydenham, there was written a chapter in medical history during the Civil War that has affected clinical thought and practice to the present day.

89. W. H. Welch, "S. Weir Mitchell. Physician and Man of Science," in S. *Weir Mitchell, M.D., LL.D., F.R.S., 1829–1914. Memorial Addresses and Resolutions* (Philadelphia, 1914).

MEDICAL BRIDGES

"Doctors are a social cement."

LORD SALISBURY

Singularly through the centuries of recorded history, medicine has ignored national boundaries.While chauvinism may prevail in art and the humanities on many occasions and nationalism reign in policy and diplomacy almost as a rule, to the everlasting credit of medicine its limits are not sectional, national, religious, or ethnic. The origin of medicine does not concern us in the present relation. Modern clinical medicine had its roots in the clinics of Boerhaave of Leyden (1668–1738). Although his stature has assumed reduced proportions in later years, his revival of the Hippocratic methods of observation and deduction merited the contemporary attraction of progressive young men from Western Europe and Great Britain. As a measure of his influence, his pupils promulgated his philosophy in many centers. In turn, the medical schools of London and Edinburgh under such masters as the Hunters, Baillie, Cullen, and the Monros drew eager youths not only from their own countries, but from the English-speaking colonies across the Atlantic ocean.

So it came to pass that two young Philadelphians, William Shippen, Jr., and John Morgan, drank from the fountainhead in Edinburgh. As they pursued their doctoral curricula, they planned a new medical school in their native land. Graduating before Morgan, Shippen initiated private lectures in anatomy on his return to Philadelphia (1762). Whatever may have been the understanding between these young men, Morgan gave the Commencement Address before the College of Philadelphia (May 30 and 31, 1765), that actually launched this proj-

Presented at the Medical College of South Carolina, March, 1966. Reprinted from *The Pharos of Alpha Omega Alpha* 29 (October 1966): 116–21.

ect. His "Discourse Upon the Institution of Medical Schools in America" is a classical exposition of an involved subject. His vision and perspicacity bespoke a profound insight into this field. To cite an isolated instance, Morgan foresaw the need for specialized practice at that early day and limited his own services to medicine. Generations of Americans were destined to pass before his standards were approximated. Immediately after his address, he was made Professor of the Practice of Medicine. In the Fall (1765), Shippen was elected Professor of Anatomy and Surgery. They constituted the first faculty of the first medical school in North America. To them later were joined Thomas Bond, London, Paris, and Rheims (Clinical Medicine); Benjamin Rush, Edinburgh (Chemistry); Adam Kuhn, Upsala (Materia Medica and Botany). Thus, clearly the stamp of Edinburgh was deeply impressed on the young school in Philadelphia and its students. In fact, one of the professors was accused of reading his lecture from the Edinburgh notes unchanged through his long career as a teacher!

In a felicitous vein, Leon Israel has dealt with the medical ties between Charleston and Philadelphia, South Carolina and Pennsylvania in "A Medical Tale of Two Cities." Quite logically, David Ramsey explained the perceptible shifting of medical students from Edinburgh to Philadelphia. Added to the strength of the latter's faculty, he wrote: "The convenience of attending medical lectures in a neighboring city for some time past, and at the present draws three in four of the Charlestown medical students to Philadelphia in preference to Edinburgh at the distance of 3,000 miles and in a climate often too cold for young Carolinians." The official files of the University of Pennsylvania medical graduates afford inadequate data as to their origin. For example, in the 1812 Class of seventy-two, only James Moultrie is listed from South Carolina. Yet six men of this class came from that State. However, such surnames as Huger, Mazyck, Mitchell, North, Prioleau, Waring, and Waterhouse that recur among Pennsylvania graduates, require no confirmation of their origin.

By fortuitous circumstances, several theses of Pennsylvania graduates of an early period have come to hand. Two of these discourses prepared by young men from Charleston have more than passing interest. Philip Gendron Prioleau presented his "An Inaugural Dissertation on the Use of Nitric and Oxiginated Muriatic Acids in Some Diseases," May 22, 1798. He inscribed his thesis to Caspar Wistar, Adjunct Professor of Anatomy, Surgery, and Midwifery, for the "unceasing endeavors to give one every opportunity of improvement, which your extensive practice afforded, and the invaluable precepts, which you have with so much pleasure delivered to your pupils." Surgeon William

Scott of the East India Company had reported striking results from the administration of well diluted nitric acid in diabetes, intermittent fever, and syphilis. Paralleling the reaction to mercury, he noted salivation, redness and swelling of the gums, and pain in the occiput after nitric acid. First published in the *Bombay Courier,* April 30, 1796, this paper was reprinted in *Duncan's Medical Annals* and the *New York Repository.*

Fostered by Drs. William Boys, John Church, Samuel Duffield, and Thomas James, physicians of the Philadelphia Almshouse and House of Employment, young Prioleau pursued his clinical studies with commendable zeal. From the vantage point of removed analysis, the diagnosis of syphilis in fourteen patients must be questioned. A majority presented multiple genital lesions and bubos; but other aspects of his studies merit serious consideration.

Prioleau's prescription was:

Rx:
Gum. Arab. IV drach: IV
Aquae Menth: VI drach: VI
Acid: Nit: II drach II F.m.

A tablespoonful of this mixture with sweetened water was taken hourly through a glass "funnel" if necessary, to avoid contact with the teeth.

Enlarging on the action of nitric acid, Prioleau stated that:

It produces a soreness of the gums, looseness of the teeth, ptyalism, increased heat of body, and in every respect increases the combustion of life. This increased heat and action in the arterial system does not arise to such an height, as to wear down the system and bring an indirect debility. On the contrary, it appears to give strength and vigour to the body. . . . I shall not, I hope, be considered as chimerical, nor as giving virtues to medicines which they do not possess, when I say that I have no doubt but that Nitric Acid will hereafter be acknowledged to possess these two properties . . . i.e. restoring tone and strength to every part of the system, justifies the opinion of its being an universal tonic . . . and if given long enough durable effects.

Convinced that oxygen was the essential factor in the action of nitric acid, Prioleau sought a greater source of this beneficent element. Muriatic acid appeared to be the logical choice. "The Oxiginated Muriatic Acid . . . contained the largest possible quantity of *Vital Air.* I made it by distilling the common Muriatic Acid on Manganese." The product, hydrochlorous acid, was used in the same manner as nitric acid with comparable results. One notable therapeutic effect has apparently escaped subsequent notice. Without exception, the patients receiving "oxiginated muriatic acid" experienced marked diuresis. One patient "complained that in the night she could not remain long enough in bed to get warm, on account of the frequent calls to evacuate her urine. . . . On an average she discharges three large potfuls of urine a day." The case report of E.S., a pauper in the Almshouse, is also most interesting. She experienced "an anxiety about her breast, a difficulty of breathing, which was increased when she attempted to walk fast and more especially when she ascended the stairs, she had also with these symptoms oedematous legs, and scantiness of urine." Under "oxiginated muriatic acid" therapy, diuresis began on the third day and became extreme the following day. Progressive and sustained improvement with complete disappearance of the edema and increased exercise tolerance attended the continuance of this treatment. In fact, Prioleau compared the response to "oxiginated muriatic acid" favorably with digitalis. Many years passed before the mechanism of diuresis on lowering of the pH of the body fluids was elucidated.

In 1805, Daniel Legare of Charleston prepared his inaugural thesis at Pennsylvania on "An Experimental Inquiry Into the Effects of Tobacco Fumes on the System: and Their Use in Suspended Animation From Submersion." He dedicated his thesis to his preceptor, Thomas Harrison McCalla of Charleston, in appreciation of his example and friendship, and to Caspar Wistar for his "polite attention and valuable instruction." As early as 1667 tobacco fumes had been recommended by the Humane Society of Amsterdam for resuscitation of the drowned. Since this procedure had fallen into disuse, Legare set up a logical experimental approach. He, personally, submitted to a series of injections of tobacco fumes "*per anum.*" After the third injection at 25 minutes, he recorded, "I experienced much uneasiness and heat, in the region of the abdomen; in 30, a nauseated stomach and vertigo of the head came on. These effects, however, did not continue longer than twenty-five or thirty minutes. The pulse, throughout the experiment, was not perceived to be the least increased in fulness." There followed a series of experiments on dogs, in which, along with the pulse rate, the intestinal mobility was observed directly. Upon anal injections of tobacco fumes, the quiescent gut resumed active peristalsis, the lacteals were distended, and "the mesenteric arteries pulsated with preternatural force and frequency." Repetition of the experiment in the same dogs was attended by a decrease to absence of these responses. To establish the possible influence of heat in the recorded changes, Legare lowered the temperature of the fumes from 90° F to 65° F. When there was still a rise in the pulse rate, he resorted to enemata of water at varying temperatures without consistent changes. Finally, tobacco fumes were completely ineffective in resuscitating any of eight drowned dogs. His concluding deduction is reflective of the medical period: "In my opinion, they prove prejudicial, not by diminishing action (as the term, *sedative*, is intended to imply), but, on the contrary, by producing, through means of their stimulating power, an excitement disproportionate to the excitability of the system, thereby extinguishing the remaining sparks of life."

An interesting observation relative to medicine in colonial America is encountered: "The Carolinas, with Charleston as the center, had according to some historians, a larger percentage of European-trained practitioners than any other colony. But the urge to return home was strong among the university-trained physicians, and after staying a short time in the colonies, many returned to a safer and easier existence." The establishment of four medical schools in the American colonies and early United States, i.e., College of Philadelphia, 1765, King's College, 1768, Harvard, 1782, and Dartmouth, 1796, in some measure stemmed the outgoing tide of foreign medical training. Yet, the total graduates from these medical schools numbered only 250 out of a total estimate of 4000 practitioners in the country at the end of the eighteenth century. Naturally, Charleston, a progressive medical community, sought its place in the sun. Founded in 1789, the Medical Society of South Carolina early interested itself in medical education. President Thomas Cooper of South Carolina College took the initiative in proposing the establishment of a medical college to the Medical Licensing Board and the Medical Society of South Carolina (1822). In the Summer of 1823, Henry Dickson and James Ramsey gave a series of lectures to medical students. In January 1824, upon the authorization of the Legislature, the Medical College was organized in Charleston without requisite financial support. A disagreement within the faculty led to the foundation of a second medical school, the Medical College of South Carolina, chartered in 1832. With one notable exception, the faculties of the two schools were identical. This school perpetuated the dubious policy of combining licensure with education. The reconciliation of the two medical schools (1839) as the Medical College of the State of South Carolina, marked the beginning of a most successful period in the history of the school that was to be interrupted by the calamitous Civil War.

Of the architects of South Carolina medicine, much has been recorded. It is carrying palmetto to Charleston to attempt an adequate account of their individual lives and contributions. The efforts of three graduates of the University of Pennsylvania, Samuel Henry Dickson,

Henry Rutledge Frost, and James Ramsey, gave form and substance to the teaching and the practice of medicine in South Carolina at a critical period in her history (1823–32). The fourth of these staunch pioneers, James Moultrie, was also a Pennsylvania graduate; but he declined to join the first faculty because of inadequate State support. His later acceptance of the professorship of physiology in the Medical College of South Carolina (1832) and his forthright position on major issues mark him as a leader. Essential as were the roles played by this group of outstanding men, it is to two remarkable addresses that attention is drawn in the present relation. On December 5, 1835, before the South Carolina Society for the Advancement of Learning in Representative Hall, James Moultrie delivered his notable "Memorial on the State of Medical Education in South Carolina." After outlining the curriculum, physical facilities, and manifest gains in enrollment and support, with perceptive insight, he analyzed the weaknesses and deficiencies of the young school. In his judgment, the lectures were too few and too short. The lack of an orderly approach was condemned. "There is a mental running here, and there, and everywhere—no preliminary acquaintance with the elements of general knowledge, none with fundamental principles of the plainest and best understood department of philosophy." With reference to the actual system of lectures, he observed that "It is addressed exclusively to the ear, and not sufficiently to the eye." In his amazing analysis, Moultrie recommended the graded, sequential approach in this passage: "Let the period of lecturing be extended to six or eight months and let each student be compelled to attend three or four courses." He, moreover, urged searching examinations to assure the graduate's competence to practice. He noted "the nurture of a generation which, in the main, have conferred little honor either on themselves or their Alma Mater. The diplomated quacks far outnumber the legitimately initiated." Fearlessly, he attacked the existing methods of faculty appointments. Instead of its "hit or miss" procedure, he recommended the following: "Let there be a substitute provided for the concours, or the concours itself be established, in which each applicant for a professorship shall give a *practical* or *demonstrative* proof of his abilities and competence to fill the situation."

At a period when two medical schools existed in Charleston (1835), James Moultrie took a statesmanly and practical position in urging the Legislature to support a single project. Rivalry and the dispersion of appropriated monies spelled hardship for both schools. As he expressed the broad principles, "Let the Legislature take the *whole subject* of education under its paternal care; and let the system be so regulated in accordance with the views and principles which have been exposed. Let the medical department be made a branch of that system, and a college be established by its authority; and let all other grants be abrogated, or expire naturally, at the end of the term for which they were given." By European standards, the medical facilities in Charleston were woefully inadequate. The Marine Hospital with fifty beds and the Poor House without fixed hospital beds afforded the only clinical outlets. Moultrie said: "Obstetricy wants the appendage of a suitable hospital." Furthermore: "The chimical department is not very deficient. It needs, however, replenishment from year to year." On the other hand, there was no deficiency in anatomical material. In his judgment, Charleston did not suffer by comparison with other American medical centers.

This astounding pronouncement of Moultrie arouses a great respect and admiration for the man, when the place and the time of its delivery are considered. As indicated, the medical profession of Charleston was divided and it took a high degree of moral fortitude to assume a position of judicial detachment. To afford perspective relative to his curricular recommendations, existing conditions of medical education of that period must be examined. With few exceptions, three years of preceptorship were required for admission to a medical school. Thereafter, two courses of fourteen to sixteen weeks each were pursued befor the candidate was eligible for admission to the doctoral examination. To compound the weakness of the curriculum, the lectures of the second course frequently duplicated the first. Supplementary subjects were offered in private lectures and seminars. Not until 1859 through the efforts of Nathan S. Davis did the Chicago Medical College (Lind, later Northwestern, University), offer the first systematic graded course of three years of medicine in the United States. Harvard and Syracuse followed twelve years later (1871).

In his "Introductory Lecture read at the Commencement of the Course," November 9, 1846, Samuel Henry Dickson bespoke more stringent entrance requirements for admission to the medical school or more searching final examinations for the doctoral degree. Since the diploma was tantamount to licensure to practice, the examination of all candidates devolved upon the Trustees and the Faculty. "This apparent privilege is a real burden and a very embarrassing one—not only is the seeming benefit shared in fact with the patent right, which opens the door to every ignorant pretender and mountebank; but our diploma, with its pretty seal, its fine motto and its learned and high-sounding phrases—the insignia of the highest professional rank is thus brought practically into competition and contrast with the mere certificate of license; the latter being obtainable by a brief exhibition of retentive memory." To the ease or lack of licensure, Dickson attributed much of the deterioration and low estate of American medicine. By his criteria, the individual states would determine the fitness or unfitness of the individual candidate: "Let the diploma of no college weigh with them, except so far as it is proved by experience to be conferred exclusively upon diligence, character, and merit. Let no patent right to play upon the credulity of the miserable be in any manner recognized; no miraculous pretensions considered." Commending the tributes to notable individuals in other spheres of human endeavor, he closed on a lugubrious note: "But no wreath is turned for the brow of the physician; his silent labors go unheeded and unrecorded; confounded by the neglect of the law with the empiric and the vender of nostrums, neither honor nor advancement in any shape are attainable by him, nor place nor pension render less wretched the decline of life or the incapacity of old age."

While Moultrie and Dickson were distinct pioneers in medical thought, and as such well merit their place in the historical linkage with later advances, they were by no means isolated "prophets crying in the wilderness." Physicians of vision through the country were increasingly aware of the degraded state of American medicine and the factors contributing thereto. In 1847, under the presidency of Nathaniel Chapman, the American Medical Association convened in Philadelphia for the first time. Singularly, its proceedings might have followed the trail blazed by James Moultrie twelve years earlier. Although its recommendations were much more conservative, through its corporate body, the medical profession took official cognizance of the problems and the initial steps toward their correction. Quite appropriately, when the American Medical Association met in Charleston, in 1850, the stature of James Moultrie as a medical statesman was recognized in his election to its presidency. General acceptance of Dickson's radical position and proposals was delayed; but his vision is indubitable.

Professional communication is perhaps best exemplified in medical research, in which there can be no national boundaries. In this season of material abundance in the United States, the mere whisper of the word is open sesame in the legislative halls. Naively the laity cherishes the belief that money will purchase the answer to all the secrets of nature and the shibboleth has loosened the pursestrings of the nation. As might be anticipated, qualitative results have not regularly attended quantitative effort. The call to research is not confined to the men with outstanding ability and restless, inquiring minds. Instead, too frequently we find "research puppets, whose intellectual processes are responsive only to the strings of expediency." Then, too, there is a singular group of earnest workers engaged in trivial studies that hinge upon some more or less involved gadget. Whatever the shortcomings of the individual or the system, medical research offers the most fruitful examples of cross-fertilization. Perhaps the most involved example concerns the evolution of the sulfanilamides. An English lad, William Henry Perkin, in an effort to synthesize quinine isolated mauve, the first of the anilin dyes (1856). Gelmo, a German, synthesized sulfanilamide (1908). In 1919, Heidelberger and Jacobs established the bactericidal action of combined sulfanilamide and ethylhydrocupreine in this country. They overlooked the independent potency of the former. Prontosil was developed by the Germans Meitsch and Klarer (1932). Its protective action against streptococcemia in mice was established by the German Domagk (1935)—an epochal discovery. Interestingly, the German patents on prontosil covered only the azo dye. In 1936, the French workers, Tréfouël, Tréfouël, Nith, and Bovet, proved that prontosil was reduced to free sulfanilamide in the body and this element is the active antibacterial factor. The British team, Colebrook and Kenny (1936), discovered its efficiency in the septicemia of man.

The international flavor of the antimicrobial agents is not as broad as the evolution of the sulfonamides, yet a beginning was made in Belgium by Gratia and Dath (1924) in the destruction of staphylococci and gas bacilli by strains of streptothrix and penicillium. A Scotsman, Fleming, working in the laboratory of St. Mary's Hospital, London, discovered penicillin (1928)—a landmark in medicine. The catalytic action of war and the perceptive tenacity of Florey, an Australian domiciled in England, and his team at Oxford gave this neglected agent the impetus that has revolutionized the treatment of many infectious diseases. Nor is the story of penicillin completed until mass production became the American contribution under the pressure of the O.S.R.D. So the list might be extended in and beyond the field of pharmacology, whenever men work with a consuming enthusiasm for truth—and national bounds are obliterated.

With modern communication and transportation, many economic, ecologic, and demographic problems obtrude themselves in medical situations. Medicine is vitally interested in the population explosion. Experts predict that the world population, which was 1.5 billion in 1900, will increase to 6 billion by 2000. The birth rate is maintained, while the death rate from major diseases, as malaria and tuberculosis, is markedly reduced through modern measures of control and treatment. In the United States, 1 million acres of farmland are annually retired from cropping by highways and industry. At the present time, there are approximately twelve acres of land for each person in this country. In 2200 A.D., at the present rate of increasing population, each American will have one square yard. With the current accumulation of surplus grain, there is a hue and cry to feed the hungry of other lands. Were such an effort effectively implemented, each famished person in the underprivileged countries would receive a cupful of cereal every fortnight. Yet with added attention to the vegetation of the sea and by conversion of solar and nuclear energy to human needs, the worldwide gap in nutrition could be completely effaced.

In the changing world of the twentieth century, the practice of medicine has undergone radical adaptations. Rugged individualism prevailed until the scientific and technical advances in medicine made specialization inevitable and interdependence imperative. In the interest of the patient, group and associated practice have evolved on a comprehensive scale in this period. Among other factors, the requirement of diagnostic and therapeutic procedures has evolved complicated techniques and apparatus beyond the means of the individual practitioner. Hence the hospital has become the logical center of professional activity. With hospitalization insurance, and now Medicare, this trend is inescapable. The physician owes it to himself and the community to contain this tide of institutional care within justifiable bounds. By careful judgment, an appreciable proportion of the eligible patients can and should be cared for in the office and home. The bridges between medicine and society are increasing in number and utilization. Medicine has come to the realization that health is not the exclusive prerogative of our profession. As a member of the modern health team, the physician will maintain leadership. From his vantage point, he will encourage the intelligent participation of and give guidance to the host of fellow-workers, professional and voluntary, in the health arts and sciences.

In a materialistic world, it is vital to the future of medicine as a professional and a social unit that we do not burn important bridges behind us. With the burgeoning weight of scientific advance comes an interesting and commendable deference to objectivity in procedure and deduction. However, the intrusion of impersonality threatens a traditional bulwark of medical strength. Not only is the mutual understanding in the patient-physician relationship of inestimable value to the latter in his analysis of the clinical status; but such reciprocal respect plays an appreciable part in that intangible but potent element termed cooperative therapy. No thoughtful physician would impede or deny the advances of automation and kindred esoteric skills in medicine. By the same token, John Brown's characterization has a currency that must not be overlooked in the whirlwind of progress that is apt to divert our attention to less fundamental principles: "that gentleness and compassion for his suffering fellow-men, without which no man— be his intellect ever so transcendent, his learning ever so vast, his industry ever so accurate and inappeasable—need hope to be a great physician, much less a virtuous and honest man."

THE EVOLUTION OF MODERN CARDIOLOGY, BEING IN SOME MEASURE THE EXPERIENCE OF A STETHOSCOPE (1908-1968)

In 1908, my Bowles model stethoscope was purchased from Edward P. Dolbey on Woodland Avenue, Philadelphia, for $4.50. It has served me faithfully and has witnessed great advances in cardiology through the span of sixty years. Such errors as have risen from its use must be laid to faulty reception or interpretation on my part and not to defects inherent in the instrument.

This binaural stethoscope is the natural offspring of the monaural form devised by Laennec in 1816 (Pl. 7). His naive account of its discovery, as translated, reads:

> In 1816, I was consulted by a young woman labouring under general symptoms of diseased heart, and in whose case percussion and the application of the hand were of little avail on account of the great degree of fatness. The other method just mentioned (immediate auscultation) being rendered inadmissable by the age and sex of the patient, I happened to recollect a simple and well known fact in acoustics, and fancied it might be turned to some use on the present occasion. The fact I allude to is the great distinctness with which we hear the scratch of a pin at one end of a piece of wood, on applying our ear to the

Presented before the second general scientific session of the 101st Annual Meeting of the West Virginia State Medical Association at the Greenbrier in White Sulphur Springs, August 22–24, 1968. Reprinted from *The West Virginia Medical Journal* 65 (February 1969): 31–38.

other. Immediately, on the suggestion, I rolled a quire of paper into a kind of cylinder and applied one end of it to the region of the heart and the other to my ear, and was not a little surprised and pleased to find that I could thereby perceive the action of the heart in a manner much more clear and distinct than I had ever been able to do by the immediate application of the ear.

The impetus of Laennec's discovery to examination of the patient in general and the heart in particular cannot be overemphasized. Inspection and palpation were well established before his period. Percussion that had been neglected after Auenbrugger's enunciation of its principles (1761), had been restored to its appropriate place by Corvisart (1808). Mediate auscultation, however, was to forge the strongest link in the advancement of knowledge of the cardiovascular system at the beginning of the nineteenth century. Singularly, Laennec manifested a restricted grasp of the significance of cardiac signs, while his comprehensive interpretation of pulmonary phenomena has stood the test of time.

The early observations of Stephen Hales on the arterial blood pressure of the horse (1711) lay fallow for many years. Actually his own studies were not published until 1733. Finally, in 1896, the several experimental models to determine the blood pressure gave way to a clinically practical sphygmomanometer (Riva Rocci) that vastly improved the earlier instruments of Marey and Potain. The anaeroid blood pressure apparatus gradually replaced the mercury manometer by reason of its more compact and convenient form. Korotkoff, in 1905, described the auscultatory phases, determined by the altered pressure of the cuff over the artery, as an accurate method of sphygmomanometry. This method is still employed. *The* stethoscope bears witness to the excesses that early attended the overenthusiastic deference to these determinations.

Studies of the venous pressure were never as widely accepted for clinical purposes as those of the arterial blood pressure. Employing the indirect method with the instrument devised by Hooker and Eyster (1908), invaluable information of the capacity of the right heart to receive the returning blood may be derived. Direct readings of the venous pressure by venipuncture largely replaced the indirect method. In turn, central venous pressure determinations in the superior vena cava have superseded studies of the pressure in peripheral veins. Clearly such approaches bring Starling's curve of cardiac strain and overstrain into clinical focus.

For many years, medicine sought graphic methods of studying and recording the phenomena of movement of the blood in the heart and blood vessels. Marey (1860) had devised a polygraphic apparatus that would simultaneously record pulse waves and precordial activity. From his absorbing interest in cardiac arrhythmias (from 1880), Mackenzie evolved an ink polygraph. Although his monumental studies anticipate our Odyssey, they contribute a landmark in cardiology. From them, he was enabled to diagnose and prognosticate the simple from the grave arrhythmias—a detail that requires later attention.

In a lighter vein, as an intern in the Philadelphia General Hospital, I was interested in the observations of Dr. William Pepper, later Dean of the University of Pennsylvania School of Medicine, with the ink polygraph (1911). In response to my inquiry relative to its usefulness, with characteristic candor he declared: "Middleton, it is the most useless waste of time in which I have ever indulged." Scarcely an invitation to my personal participation.

Meanwhile, a new development arose to eclipse polygraphy. Although Matteuci, Weller, and others had appreciated the electrical potentials of muscle, including myocardial, contraction, Einthoven resolved the matter to a practical model for experimental and clinical investigation in the invention of a string galvanometer (1902). He termed the resultant procedure "electrocardiography," which gave a new dimension of accuracy to the clinical appraisal of cardiac conduction and myocardial disturbances. By this token, it truly revolutionized cardiology. When I came to Madison (1912), by a turn of fortune, a group of able physiologists (Eyster, Meek, and Gasser) was engaged in fundamental studies of neuromyocardial conduction. In 1911, an Edelman electrocardiographic apparatus had been purchased for the Department of Physiology at a cost of $6050.98—a stupendous sum at that time. It paid splendid dividends, however, in the scholarly contributions of its users. An unusual departmental technician, James Hipple, by his native ingenuity duplicated this apparatus for paired physiological experiments. The duplicate was shortly (1913–14) tranferred to the Student Infirmary (Raymer House) for clinical application. Here under primitive conditions, I was initiated to the Einthoven triangle and the conventional limb leads for the orderly study of changing electrical potentials under various clinical conditions.

Two circumstances in relation to those exciting days are recalled. The electrodes, imported from Germany, were finely drawn glass threads coated with silver. With the onset of World War I, this source of supply was interrupted. Mr. Hipple's substitutes, while useful, never attained the delicacy of the original German product and the resultant electrocardiograms were quite coarse. The apparatus was housed in the basement and the wires for the leads were brought through the floor to a room above, where the patient rested on a cot. The electrocardiograms were developed in a dark room in the unheated basement. The less hardy observers required topcoats if they wished to read the tracings before they were dry.

The year 1924 brought the distinguished Professor Willem Einthoven to Madison. Pains were taken to show him first our meager best. Having exhausted this prospect, he was taken to the Laboratories of Physiology in the basement of Science Hall. Thereupon he first removed his coat, then his waistcoat and finally his dickey. With a sigh of relief, he exclaimed: "Ah, now dis is home!"

With vast improvements both in the basic apparatus and in the techniques of electrocardiography, medicine today is infinitely better served in the evaluation of certain aspects of cardiac physiology and disease than a half century ago. Pipberger and Freis have evolved an interesting innovation in the computer field for mass interpretation of electrocardiograms. They have transferred electrocardiographic signals in analog form to the magnetic tape. The signals are then converted to digital form for automatic analysis by the electronic computer with an accuracy approximating 95 percent. Telephone telemetry is an early prospect in this field. Retracing our steps, certain early differences have been reconciled; yet, to the traditionalst, Mackenzie's suggestion of "auricular paralysis" has a more distinctive physiological connotation than the atrial fibrillation of current acceptance (Lewis). James Heard related an interesting observation from Mackenzie: "I don't mind telling you, Doctor, I hae taen all the cream off it. Tomas can hae the rest." The note of caution, sounded by Frank N. Wilson, should always be borne in mind: "Electrocardiography is one of the most exact of diagnostic methods. Its potential value is great, but it is not being used to the best advantage. Electrocardiographic abnormalities are not diseases. They have no important bearing upon the life expectancy of the patient, or the extent to which his mode of life should be altered when there is a reasonable doubt as to the nature of the factor or factors responsible for them in that particular case."

Meanwhile, as the role of electrocardiography was increasing apace in clinical medicine, radiology afforded an added parameter of objectivity in the study of the heart and great vessels. The Wisconsin group, Bardeen, Eyster, Hodges, et al., directed attention to determination of cardiac size by teleoroentgenography. Accepting the technical limitations of the period (1912–20), they clearly discredited the cardiothoracic ratio in this relation and proved that the cardiac silhouette (teleoroentgenogram) in the postero-anterior projection, as measured by planimetry, is a function of body area and not of the height or of the weight alone. Their charts, however, based on this correlation, never gained wide favor. Eventually, Eyster and Kurtz utilized orthodiascopy for the more precise definition of the cardiac size (Kurtz 1937).

Meanwhile *the* stethoscope had traveled far and had had one disquieting experience. In the Spring of 1918, I was Battalion Medical Officer with the First Battalion, King's Own Royal Lancaster Regiment, Fourth Division of the British Expeditionary Forces. The Division was in reserve when the German attack of Good Friday was launched to broaden their front between Amiens and Arras. Details of the military action only indirectly concern the whereabouts of *the* stethoscope. With the German advance south of the Scarpe River, our flank became more exposed and my aid post in a shack behind the railroad bank was untenable. At the same time, the third wave of the German advance overran the Essex positions and the King's Own held the British front line of defense. To maintain contact with our Battalion, I moved forward and established communications.

In this movement, Sergeant Stanley, a stout North County man, overlooked or mislaid *the* stethoscope. I was forced to use a British issue instrument. In about a week, I was transferred to the American Expeditionary Forces. My dismay in leaving my British associates without *the* stethoscope obviously deeply impressed Sergeant Stanley. My surprise and relief knew no bounds when, after a few weeks, the military dispatch delivered this precious companion to me at the Central Medical Laboratory, Dijon, France. The accompanying letter from the Sergeant told of his discovery of *the* stethoscope in the possession of one of the stretcher bearers, who on sick call was listening to another British Tommy's chest with it.

Certain sophisticated physical refinements have added materially to the advancement of cardiology. As an example, phonocardiography has afforded a definition to cardiac sounds, normal and abnormal, beyond the range of the unaided human ear; but no clinician worthy of the name has substituted this elegant apparatus for his stethoscope. Under certain circumstances, it becomes a welcome ally in the more complete elucidation of an involved problem. Interesting is the healthy renaissance in the basic interpretation of cardiac auscultation that at times is so involved as to recall Justice Cardozo's characterization: "There is an accuracy that defeats itself by overemphasis of details." Ballistocardiography offers specific information, viz, the ejection thrust, that can be established by no other method. Still it has never captured the measure of clinical attention it deserves. Vector-cardiography also is a technical approach that has not gained wide clinical acceptance.

Just on the horizon is the prospect of the application of the ultrasonic Doppler principle to auscultation. The signals registered by the Doppler cardiophone bid fair to open a new acoustical world in the auscultation of the heart. The conventionalist may perhaps change his basic concepts, if this occurs.

The physical potentiality of radiology could not rest upon mere morphology. By kymography, movements of the heart borders were recorded (Moore), and invaluable information as to pathological changes in the myocardium and pericardium gained. The revolutionary movement, however, awaited cardiac catheterization, which brought factors that previously had been implied or measured indirectly, under more or less precise control. As early as 1905, Bleichroeder had passed a catheter into the arteries and veins of a dog and into his own veins; but these cursory observations were not actively pursued. These studies were not controlled by x-ray; but no adverse result attended the intravenous manipulations of catheterization. With Unger (1912), Bleichroeder utilized the femoral artery approach for injection of Collargol into the lower abdominal aorta for the treatment of puerperal sepsis. Without knowledge of these earlier studies, Forssmann, in 1929, passed a catheter via the veins of his own forearm into the right atrium under the fluoroscope with a nurse holding a mirror for his guidance. Experiencing no discomfort, he then walked from the operating room to the x-ray department. In 1931, he opacified the heart chambers of a dog by injection of radiopaque material into the femoral vein. He could not, however, duplicate the result on himself. By intravenous injection of diodrast, Robb and Steinberg (1938) first visualized all chambers of the human heart.

The bridgehead had been established and the expansion of basic information of the structural and hemodynamic processes of the heart has been monumental. A generation past, we were satisfied to classify congenital heart lesions as cyanotic, delayed cyanotic, and acyanotic. Certain specific abnormalities were recognized; but, by and large, since there was no method of correction, the deficiency was not magnified by our ignorance. Now with the ability to enter any heart chamber or great vessel with an assurance (or abandon) undreamed of in an earlier period, not only are pressure readings momentarily available, but pressure gradients across valves give invaluable diagnostic data. Samples of blood taken from the several heart chambers and great vessels may be studied for oxygen content or pressure. Indicator dilution curves afford important information. The hemodynamics of the circulation may be directly measured. To cap these several parameters, cineangiocardiography has been developed to such a degree of technical excellence as to give definition to coronary as well as cardiac pathological lesions. Recently, other sophisticated physical principles have been adapted to clinical practice. Photoscanning with sodium pertechnetate, Tc99m, offers a ready method for the diagnosis of pericardial effusion. A halo surrounds the radioactive filled heart. In addition, the concentration of pertechnetate in the stomach affords a confirmatory detail in its abnormal separation from the similarly marked heart by the interposition of pericardial fluid. In some centers, injection of C_3131 has found favor in the definition of myocardial infarction.

With the support of these methods of precision from the chemical, physical, and physiological laboratories, there should be a conscious effort to maintain those proved bedside methods that have stood the test of time. Confirmation of the clinical diagnosis of coronary arterial compromise by chemical, electrocardiographic, and cineangiographic evidence is reassuring. On the other hand, a patient may die of coronary artery insufficiency without conclusive evidence from these sources. Conversely, severe grades of atherosclerosis may be demonstrated on cineangiography or at necropsy in patients who have no record of coronary artery insufficiency. These instances are exceptions to the rule. Enzyme studies on the blood have extended the earlier observations of leucocytosis and increased erythrocyte sedimentation rate in myocardial infarction. Without an iota of iconoclasm, each and every element of the newer cardiology is welcomed as a boon to the patient through the physician's clearer understanding of the problems involved.

Despite the vaunted progress in the knowledge of the physiology and pathology of the heart, diseases of the cardiovascular system still account for more deaths in the United States than those from all other causes. The partial containment of cardiopathic infections, as syphilis and rheumatic fever, has appreciably reduced the incidence of their crippling sequelae. Other infections, viz, viruses and fungi, have emerged as occasional etiologic threats. Overwhelming, of course, is the ascendency of the degenerative factors in cardiac pathology. Toward the prophylaxis and control of their contributing backgrounds with the common denominator of atherosclerosis, great efforts are being extended.

In the advance, the therapy of cardiovascular diseases has been almost as profoundly affected as their diagnosis. Whenever cardiac problems present, digitalis is the sheet anchor of treatment. Its administration should be reserved primarily for the patient in failure or threatened failure. Certainly the distinction between right and left heart failure has no place in this decision. Digitalis is indicated in both. Much wasted effort has gone into discussion of the relative merits of the Galenical preparations and the glycosides of digitalis. My admonition is to learn and to gain confidence in two forms of digitalis, i.e., a promptly acting form for intravenous use and a slow actor for continuous or maintenance oral administration. Of one thing be assured, in spite of the representations of the detail man and the advertisements, if it be a potent digitalis product, there will be the inherent hazard of byeffects. In recent years, a high incidence of gynecomastia apparently has attended the use of glycosides of digitalis that had not been recorded with the leaf. Significantly, the levels of serum calcium and potassium are now receiving merited attention in patients receiving digitalis. The inotropic and chronotropic action of catecholamines are being weighed in the use of adrenergic drugs. The control of cardiac arrhythmias has been subjected to clearer pharmacological rules. Quinidine sulfate, although much maligned, still is an effective drug in our hands. Reserved for the control of atrial fibrillation or more serious ectopic arrhythmia, its prompt action (ten to fifteen minutes by mouth) and its short duration of action (one and one-half to two hours) should govern its administration. In practice, doses of 200–400 mg. are given every two hours around the clock for thirty-six hours, or until normal sinus rhythm is restored. If there is no improvement in thirty-six hours, the drug is discontinued. If normal sinus rhythm has supervened, the dosage is first reduced and then the interval lengthened (by doubling the time), until it may be possible to eliminate the quinidine—or to fix a maintenance schedule. Procaine amide (pronestyl) is favored for the control of ectopic beats and ventricular tachycardia (250–500 mg. dose every four to six hours). Neosynephrine 0.5–1 mg. intravenously (Youmans) may have a dramatic role in the control of supraventricular tachycardia. Upon its administration, the sharp rise in blood pressure stimulates the carotid sinus with slowing of the heart. Lidocaine (Xylocaine) has earned an assured position in critical ventricular arrhythmias. The recommended loading dose is one mg. per kilo of body weight intravenously. Thereafter with careful monitoring, an intravenous drip is maintained at a rate not to exceed one mg./minute. Propanolol and diphenylhydantin (dilantin) are receiving extended study for the treatment of arrhythmia.

Cardiac edema to the point of anasarca ever has been a therapeutic target for physicians. My introduction to its control was by mechanical relief. Thoracentesis, paracentesis, Southey tubes, and scarification of the scrotum and legs were commonplace. Within the last generation, the ground shifted, so that the verdict arose that the physician's care and ability are in reverse ratio to the frequency of his recourse to these devices. Sound physiological principles dictate his correction of such variable contributors to the cardiac edema as are amenable to his management. Rest, low sodium intake, and digitalis usually suffice to turn the tide. Interesting has been the displacement of time-honored mercurial diuretics by hydrochlorothiazide (hydrodiuril), which latterly is being challenged by furosemide (Lasix) and ethacrynic acid. In the use of these diuretics, the electrolyte balance must be closely guarded.

Recent studies, largely by Lillehei and his associates at Minnesota, have seriously challenged the accepted management of shock. Reinforced by some basic observations of the response of the capitance vessels and the resistance arterioles to the increased sympathetic tone and increased levels of circulating catecholamines, they subjected a large series of dogs to controlled experimental myocardial infarction. Their results showed an advantage of phenoxybenzamine (dibenzyline), an adrenergic blocker, and corticosteroids, supplemented by sodium bicarbonate intravenously, over the vasopressor agents. In their hands, isuprel has a definite place in this situation. They subscribe to the long-held physiologic principle of a decrease in the *effective* circulating blood volume in shock (Meek). By central venous pressure studies, they differentiate peripheral vascular stagnation from central cardiac failure. Assuredly, their results merit careful reassessment of the entire question. Recently, some doubt has been cast on their basic premises. Meanwhile, from personal observation, the vasopressor drugs, metaraminol (aramine) and levarterenol (levophed) by slow intravenous infusion have been life-saving in isolated instances.

Physical measures have increasingly found expression not only in diagnostic but in therapeutic aspects of cardiology. Electrical shock (D.C.) is now widely employed in the conversion of arrhythmias. In the more dangerous atrial fibrillation and other potentially serious arrhythmias, cardioversion has an accepted place in treatment. Recently, electrical stimulation of the carotid sinus nerve has been used to control angina. Defibrillators are an essential element of every resuscitation unit. In addition to electrical stimulation, free airway, mouth to mouth insufflation, and closed chest cardiac massage (Kouwenhoven) are invoked in emergent states. Sodium bicarbonate is given intravenously. Isuprel has a prominent indication where chronotropic and not inotropic action is sought. Intracardiac epinephrine is deemed a ritualistic procedure by some; but, aside from its pharmacological action, mechanical stimulation by puncture of the myocardium may initiate independent contractions. Lidocaine should be given routinely in such emergencies. Again, teamwork and close coordination of the several efforts with a premium on time will assure the highest recovery rate.

Of the contributions of engineering to the medical effort, none is more impressive than the electronic pacemaker. This element, activated by a transistor implanted in the abdominal muscles, is connected to the heart by electrodes that are in turn imbedded in the myocardium. The impulses from the pacemaker take over the initiation of the cardiac contraction from the intrinsic neuromuscular apparatus of the heart and control the symptoms and signs arising from heart block (including the Adams-Stokes syndrome). One of the earliest and most efficient of these pacemakers was devised by Chardack and his associates (Veterans Administration Hospital, Buffalo, New York). To Central Office, Washington, there came an earnest appeal for help from the Czechoslovakian Embassy. Their Scientific Attaché told of a physician in Prague who suffered from heart block with severe cardiac decompensation. This physician had learned of the development of the Chardack pacemaker and sought its support. By chance, one of the surgeons from the Oteen Veterans Administration Hospital was in Russia on another professional mission. Mechanically minded, he had taken a Chardack pacemaker with him. We related the fortuitous circumstance of its ready availability to the Czech representative. After due deliberation with his superiors, he asked that we initiate the request with the Soviet authorities for the movement of our surgeon to Prague. When we indicated the impropriety of such a procedure, the Czechs apparently went into another huddle. Eventually, after several weeks, the Czechs arranged for the movement of the American surgeon to Prague. Significantly, several Russian physicians accompanied him on his mission of mercy. Fortunately, for all concerned, the procedure was expeditiously performed and the results were highly successful.

Surgery has not lagged in capitalizing on the physiological and diagnostic advances in cardiology. The heart and great vessels were actually the last structures of the human body denied surgical intervention. Certain desultory approaches to intracardiac lesions had earlier been attempted (Cutler); but ligation of the patent ductus arteriosus was the first modern major surgical success (Gross and Hubbard, 1939).

I was busy with problems of military medicine in my office in Paris when Professor Crafoord was announced. He merely wished to pay his respects. My wandering thoughts were brought sharply to attention, however, when he said: "I have just completed my fourth successful correction of coarctation of the aorta." When I asked him to explain, he repeated his statement, giving the technical details of his procedure. Realizing Elliott Cutler's sustained interest in the field, I called him into my office to hear the wonderful message at first hand— a second major breakthrough in cardiovascular surgery. With remarkable technical support, open heart surgery replaced the blind closed technique. Sound approaches to complex problems can be planned on the basis of remarkably accurate diagnostic procedures. Acquired cardiac lesions joined congenital lesions as objects of surgical attack. Prostheses were early used in the replacement of damaged heart valves and diseased vessels. Natural tissue has had a priority; but synthetic materials have perforce had a wider utilization than might have been the choice. More recently homographs of the heart valves have been increasingly used. Endarterectomy, vascular grafting directly or bypassing, and various efforts to replenish the myocardial nutrition have largely been planned by the cineangiography of the compromised coronary circulation. At the present time, implantation of the internal mammary artery is widely employed for the last named indication (Vineberg). By affording extracorporeal circulation, mechanical pumps have played an important role in these great advances. At this time, transplantation of the human heart, while revolutionary and spectacular in the extreme, is still in the experimental stage. Further control measures and wider experience will establish its ultimate place in medicine.

At an earlier period the stethoscope was subjected to ridicule by such outstanding American litterateurs as Oliver Wendell Holmes and S. Weir Mitchell. An eminent radiologist, Merrill Sosman of the Peter Bent Brigham Hospital, Boston, made easy mirth of "this contraption," a stethoscope prominently exhibited in the x-ray department (Pl. 8).

The stethoscope was most disrespectfully treated on a later occasion. I had repeatedly stated that I could not walk, let alone think, without it. One morning a few years ago, *the* stethoscope was missing from my white coat pocket. Was some curious-minded student putting me to the test? Or was there a conspiracy to put an end to the diabolic little tool with built-in murmurs, friction rubs, and the like? After several weeks, employees were cleaning the elevator well, and there in the pit they found *the* priceless stethoscope.

The moral of the story is to keep your trusted ally close at hand. It is an instrument that will not wear out with use. Using it faithfully, you will develop a confidence that it will never betray. There are nuances and shadings that come only to the initiated. Rather distressing than flattering is the too common reaction of the patient, who says: "Doctor, this is the first complete examination I have ever had." In a period when the glamour of new objective methods, reinforced by gleaming, complicated apparatus, captures the imagination, do not forsake your God-given senses, and the proven methods of our glorious past. Whatever the allure of the green pastures of the laboratory, remember—the most interesting object in the world is people. Preserve the vital patient-physician relationship at whatever cost. *The* stethoscope measures twenty inches (Pl. 9) and I permit nothing to extend this distance between me and my patient.

MEDICINE IN THE UNITED STATES: THE ROAD FROM YESTERDAY TO TODAY

This anniversary symposium affords the opportunity for reflection on the road medicine has traveled and the prospect of the way ahead.

Within a short distance of my boyhood home in Pennsylvania was a group of abandoned county fair buildings. One of these wooden structures served as an isolation hospital for smallpox from time to time. With bated breath, as youngsters, we scurried by the "pest house" on the opposite side of the road. The roping off of an area of a metropolitan city and the posting of guards armed with shotguns at the front and rear doors of a house quarantined for smallpox would now be deemed incredible. Yet I witnessed this scene in Philadelphia. The terms "black" measles and "black" smallpox convey a measure of their virulence and horror at that time. Diphtheria took a heavy toll of playmates, and the pervasive odor of asafetida in the classrooms and on the playgrounds bespoke the faith of the laity in unusual prophylactic measures. "Summer complaint" was still the designation for dangerous enteric infections in infancy. Typhoid fever was a persistent reminder of the unwholesome sanitary conditions of that period, when many rivers were literally open sewers. Tuberculosis was the feared white plague, with its awesome death rate and even greater drain on the health and the economy of the nation. Osler remarked: "I hope to live

Presented at 75th Anniversary Symposium—University of Minnesota, Mayo Memorial Auditorium, November 4–6, 1965. Reprinted from *The Journal-Lancet* (Minneapolis) 86 (November 1966): 523–29.

to see the true treatment of pneumonia." This prospect was not realized, and lobar pneumonia continued as a "captain of the men of death" for some years. In a cloud of Victorian prudery, venereal diseases were met with inadequate therapy, and their complications and sequelae opened a Pandora's box of pathology.

By modern standards, the hospitals of that period were quite primitive. This circumstance, coupled with their high incidence of puerperal sepsis, contributed in some measure to the survival of the midwife and deliveries in the home. Asepsis has replaced antisepsis. But as late as my medical school days, certain foolhardy surgeons eschewed the use of rubber gloves as an impediment to accurate tactile sense. Abdominal and pelvic organs were essentially the limits of visceral surgical approach. Cranial and thoracic surgery, by and large, awaited developments protective of the patient and techniques within the capabilities of the surgeon. Anesthesiology as a specialty was unborn, and the administration of these agents was almost exclusively at the hands of nurses. The examination of the patient had not been materially modified since the remarkable renaissance of the French school of Bichat, Corvisart, Laennec, and Louis. The x-ray had been discovered by Roentgen in 1895, but roentgenology was in swaddling clothes in the early twentieth century. Indeed, two pioneers in roentgenology from Philadelphia—Leonard and Kassabian—had the fatal marks of their exposure when we were medical students. Our laboratory support was defined by the routine urinalysis, hemogram, and examinations of the secretions and excretions. Cytology and bacteriology played their appropriate roles, but the laboratory still served in a purely supportive role. Although surgical pathology had made material advances by the 1890s, the diagnostic biopsy was still the exception.

EARLY TRAINING

The standards of medical practice commonly reflect the level of education of a given time. For perspective, the origins and the course of medical training in the New World must be explored. In colonial days, medical care for the settlers scattered on the Eastern seaboard was desultory and precarious. Preceptorial training under the trying conditions of the apprentice or house pupil status afforded the only door to the practice of medicine for aspiring young men until 1765. At the commencement of the College of Philadelphia that year, John Morgan, a native of the city and a graduate of Edinburgh, gave his classical "Discourse upon the Institution of Medical Schools in America." Its lofty principles and ambitious prospects were not to be realized for many generations, but he was named professor of medicine. Shortly thereafter William Shippen, Jr., also a graduate of Edinburgh, was elected professor of anatomy and surgery. One of the new medical school's Scottish hallmarks was the institution of clinical instruction at Pennsylvania Hospital under Thomas Bond, who said: "[The student] must join Examples with Study, before he can be sufficiently qualified to prescribe for the sick, for Language and Books alone can never give him Adequate Ideas of Diseases and the best methods of Treating them. . . . There the Clinical professor comes in to the Aid of Speculation and demonstrates the Truth of the Theory by Facts . . . he meets his pupils at stated times in the Hospital, and when a case presents adapted to his purpose, he asks all those Questions which lead to a certain knowledge of the Disease and Parts Affected; and if the Disease baffles the power of the Art and the Patient falls a Sacrifice to it, he then brings his Knowledge to the Test, and fixes Honour or discredit on his Reputation by exposing all the Morbid parts to view and Demonstrates by what means it produced Death, and if perchance he finds something unexpected, which betrays an Error in judgment, he like a great and good man immediately acknowledges the mistake, and, for the benefit of survivors, points out other methods by which it might have been more happily treated."

The initiative of Philadelphia was promptly followed by New York. In 1768, King's College established a medical school that, faring the fortunes of war and certain local dissensions, ultimately became the College of Physicians and Surgeons of Columbia University. Medicine was offered at Harvard in 1783, but its real fruition awaited the movement to Boston in 1810. In 1796, medical courses were first conducted at Dartmouth. The nineteenth century was marked by an astonishing wave of new medical schools—their numbers were prodigious and their locations unpredictable. From 1810 to 1840 there were twenty-six new medical schools in this country, forty-seven were added from 1840 to 1876, and 114 originated between 1876 and 1890. In Missouri alone there were listed at one time or other forty-two chartered medical schools! In the westward course of the tidal wave that was in many instances marked by brazen cupidity and flouted morality, several institutions stand apart. At Lexington, Ky., Transylvania University made an auspicious beginning in medical education (1817), but contentious personalities and local dissension closed its doors. Cincinnati (1820 to 1908) and Louisville (1837) had areas of great strength at various periods, but the early exploitation of their educational advantage was sacrificed to petty bickering and insignificant personal differences. In the Middle West, Daniel Brainard led the way to the formation of Rush Medical College in 1837. Aside from the flagrant diploma mills conducted without thought of the standards of education, other institutions were ostensibly set up for the purpose of legalizing human dissection, such as those at Evansville, Ind.; Freeport and Rockford, Ill.; and La Crosse and Madison, Wis.

It is estimated that, by the end of the eighteenth century, the medical schools of the country had graduated only 250 physicians. Several times this number had attended some courses in the medical schools. At this time, there were approximately 4000 practitioners in the United States and, although an appreciable number had had the advantage of foreign education, the majority were the product of the preceptor system. In this relation it should be remembered that William Beaumont followed this informal pattern of training for two years and never attended the sessions of a medical school.

With due attention to the limitations of transportation, forty-five years later Davis justified the earlier relative weights of the preceptorship and the instruction in the medical schools as an expedient of time and substance. He concluded: "The idea of the founders of medical schools, both in Great Britain and in this country, was to make them supplement, but not supersede the work of the preceptor and the medical apprentice." However, by this time too frequently the preceptorship had fallen to the low estate of a mere registry.

MEDICAL SCHOOL IMPROVEMENTS

Whatever may have been the contributing factors, overcrowded with the cheap product of woefully incompetent instruction, American medicine became a national problem. The American Medical Association was the natural outgrowth of this concern. Convening under Nathaniel Chapman in 1847, this constituted body urged increased entrance requirements and standard two-year curricula for the medical schools. Pennsylvania and Columbia extended their annual sessions from sixteen to twenty weeks. Although supplemental private courses were offered between the regular sessions, the subject matter of that period was so limited that, in many instances, the lectures of the second year duplicated those of the first. The first departure from this conventional plan came from the Middle West under the guiding hand of Nathan S. Davis, who broke with Brainard of Rush on this issue. With the establishment of the Chicago Medical College (later to become Northwestern) in 1859, a carefully graded three-year course was offered. Its junior, middle, and senior courses represented a logical adaptation of progressive academic instruction. Twelve years later,

Harvard accepted this principle and Syracuse followed suit. Beginning with the opening of the John Hopkins University Medical School in 1893 and Harvard's announcement in 1901, the requirements for admission to medical schools included certain levels of collegiate credits.

Into this sea of medical unrest the University of Minnesota College of Medical Sciences (under other names) was plunged. Of the state-supported medical schools of the Middle West, Ohio State (1847), Michigan (1850), and Iowa (1870) anticipated Minnesota. President William Watts Folwell, famous author of the Minnesota Plan (1870), successfully thwarted efforts to stampede the regents of the university into ill-conceived plans for a medical school. However, a licensing board for physicians, divorced from teachers of medicine, was authorized. By the selection of its members from a panel nominated by the university, the state was placed in an enviable position for the control of medical practice. A member of this Board, Dr. Perry Millard of Stillwater, played a leading role in the resolution of the problems of the establishment of medical education in the university. Not only did he initiate negotiations, but by personal financial support he was responsible for the ultimate amalgamation of four inadequate medical schools —the Minnesota Hospital College of Medicine, Saint Paul Medical College, Minneapolis College of Homeopathy, and Minneapolis College of Physicians and Surgeons—as the University of Minnesota College of Medicine (1888). Because of inadequate facilities, the movement to the University campus was deferred several years.

The birth date of the University of Minnesota College of Medicine found medical education in the United States at its lowest ebb. By general agreement, a careful study of the situation was long overdue. To this herculean task, Abraham Flexner, with the support of the Carnegie Foundation for the Advancement of Teaching, was called. Flexner encouraged the physical or geographic association of the preclinical and clinical departments of the medical school. His arbitrary listing of the elements of the preclinical and clinical curricula was to have an immediate impact on medical education and its repercussions are felt to the present time. The weakness of the large clinics and amphitheaters, as well as many administrative details, fell under his critical notice. The prospect of full-time appointments to major clinical posts, while remote, still offered much promise for the future. In this respect Frank Billings had anticipated Flexner. In the president's address to the American Medical Association in 1903, he advocated the full-time system with the reservation that there should be two types of representation in the clinical areas, namely, the full-time academic and the "clinical teachers who are in private practice."

Minnesota fared well at Flexner's hands. In his objective survey of May 1909, he described the laboratories as excellent, exceedingly attractive, and well organized in all scientific branches. The objective of full-time chiefs of the major services was applauded. Further, the prospect of a teaching hospital under university control had been strengthened by the provision of financial support that would assure appropriate staffing. Possibly another detail that attracted Flexner's attention was the annual budget of $71,336 for the College of Medicine at a time when fifty-six other medical schools operated on annual allotments of less than $10,000!

Obviously the season was ripe for the reform of medical education and practice in the United States. The fate of the less adequate medical schools was foreordained. Although the Flexner report had neither legal nor legislative sanction, public sentiment and professional conscience welcomed its revelation of glaring abuses and rank deficiencies. Its stark candor afforded no refuge for the most callous offenders. Forthwith the number of medical schools was reduced from 155 to eighty-five. Among the survivors, a wholesome spirit of self-searching scrutiny vastly improved the content and the quality of medical curricula.

DEVELOPMENTS IN PHYSIOLOGY

Morbid anatomy and its relation to the disease expressions dominated clinical medicine until Virchow's principles carried medical thought to the cellular level. With the advent of microbiology, the etiologic diagnosis took precedence, and medicine experienced one of its most exciting phases as one after another causal factor of the infectious diseases was disclosed. Not infrequently, such discoveries were tantamount to the evolution of a protective or therapeutic biological agent to combat the disease. The spirochaeta pallida was discovered by Schaudinn in 1905. The serologic test for syphilis followed the next year.

From the nineteenth-century emphasis on pathology and, latterly, bacteriology in clinical thought and practice, we passed almost imperceptibly into an appreciation of the important place of physiology and physiological chemistry in health and disease. Without loss of interest in the etiologic factors and their effects, increasing attention is paid to the changes in function and chemical reactions incident to disease. With the scientific advances in concept and methodology, such determinations have been transferred from the laboratory to the bedside at a breathless pace. To the elucidation of physiologic and chemical principles have come technological advances undreamed of a generation past. To cite an isolated example, serum proteins are characterized in many manners. In addition to the common biochemical tests, chromatography, electrophoresis, serology, immunochemistry, and ultracentrifugation may be invoked. Several radioisotopes have lent themselves admirably to the physiological and metabolic studies as tracers to establish the localization and the concentration of certain elements. Transferred to the clinical field, with the limitations imposed by their respective half-lives, these tagged elements have assumed an important role in diagnosis and therapy. Electron microscopy has opened an entirely new vista of normal and abnormal histology. With its wonders of magnification, chromosomes, microsomes, foot and brush processes, and a host of other details assume a reality that is lost to the familiar objects of light microscopy. Image amplification and cineroentgenography have greatly extended the range of diagnostic roentgenology. At an earlier stage, urography had revolutionized the study of the genitourinary tract. Cardiac catheterization with pressure and gas determinations, indicator dilution studies, and cineangiocardiography have brought a remarkable degree of objectivity to the field of cardiovascular disorders. Certainly the more exact definition of hemodynamic forces contributes inestimably to the assurance of successful cardiovascular surgery. This field of exciting proportions has been rendered accessible not alone by such physiological advances but by technological achievements such as extracorporeal circulation.

Cytogenetics is playing an ever increasing role in the understanding of human disorders. Familial and hereditary diseases have been the natural targets of such studies. Inborn errors of metabolism have been so related. Phenylketonuria, with the attendant mental deficiency, has followed this pattern. Aberrations of the Philadelphia chromosome (XXI) are associated with chronic myelocytic leukemia, and the absence of this fault has proved a sound basis for the conclusion of the leukemoid reaction. Most fruitful have been the explanations of certain hemoglobinopathies on genetic backgrounds. The breaking of the code of the double helix of deoxyribonucleic acid (DNA) and the appreciation of the messenger function of ribonucleic acid (RNA) have afforded a logical approach to the explanation of the origin of life. Transplantation of tissue and organ has been a coveted objective of surgery for generations. The prospect of its more regular achievement has been greatly enhanced by the elucidation of the basic mechanism of rejection reactions and the development of methods for their control. Immunochemistry offers the logical approach. With overlapping into the field of microbiology, the thymus gland and the lymphocyte have assumed renewed importance as the sources of clones of immunologically competent cells. The introduction of a simple test, such as fluorescein staining, has added a new parameter to the studies of immune reactions. The diagnostic biopsy had won its place in the clinic by the early days of the twentieth century. Histochemistry in the broader sense is a relative newcomer. Enzyme chemistry has played a prominent role in the advancement of medical knowledge. Its manifest operations in the digestive processes and elsewhere are apparent. The vital functions of enzymes in oxidation, phosphorylation, decarboxylation, and countless other directions are well understood. Less appreciated may be their essentiality in the transport of electrolytes or other solutes across biologic membranes.

AUTOMATION

The application of automation to medicine is already extensive and there is much more in sight. After fighting a long rearguard action against random probing by expansive laboratory studies to derive a diagnosis, evidence is accumulating that batteries of twelve to eighteen chemical determinations can be made rapidly and accurately by automatic analyzers on small specimens at a saving over conventional studies on highly selective materials. There is thus promise of a "chemical fingerprint" (Godber). The economy, comprehensiveness, and occasional serendipitous finding by this approach may eventually prevail over the psychological reservations. The Coulter counter has largely replaced the hemocytometer. The mechanical offices of the clinic offer an open invitation to electronics. Monitoring of vital signs by electronic means is an accepted procedure in modern surgeries and recovery rooms. The transmission of vital signs, blood pressure determinations, electrocardiograms, and electroencephalograms over great distances by telemetry is a marvelous demonstration of the advanced stage of this development. The cardiac pacemaker is a natural application of the transistor for the rhythmic stimulation of the myocardium in atrioventricular heart block with Adams-Stokes manifestations.

Automatic data processing has invaded many fields of human endeavor. Its inroads into medicine were first in the laboratory and then in administrative fields, where repetitive "hard" data invited the speed and accuracy of the computer. The ability of the machine to receive, store, and deliver information on command much more effectively than the unaided human mind is indisputable. Perceptive programming and accurate input will assure satisfactory retrieval. Already by appropriate techniques of transfer of the electrocardiographic signals to the computer, an accuracy of approximately 95 percent in reading has been attained. Automatic data processing will eventually revolutionize history-taking, hospital records, patient control, and the dispensing of drugs. At some future time, the automation of these procedures will pass from the individual institution to the community, then to the region, and to the nation so that the experience of the entire medical profession will supplement that of the individual practitioner. Already its principles are being applied in record linkage on a regional basis in Great Britain (Acheson).

PHARMACOLOGY

Therapeutic nihilism was abroad seventy-five years ago. Quinine, opium, and digitalis were the trusted sheet anchors of therapy. Mercury and the iodides held a limited but respected place. In general, galenical drugs prevailed. Vaccination against smallpox was the only widely accepted biological prophylactic measure in 1890. Diphtheria antitoxin was discovered that year (von Behring). Polytherapy on an empiric basis was the rule. With man's eternal interest in drugs, the advances in pharmacology and therapeutics on sound scientific grounds have attracted widespread notice. Assuredly, they have radically altered the practice of medicine. But in an evaluation of the total picture, the contribution of hygienic and preventive measures must be given due weight. Under their influence, diphtheria and the exanthems have shrunken in importance. Typhoid fever is now deemed a reflection on the good name of a community. Pneumococcus lobar pneumonia, a commonplace in my student days, is now rarely seen in its classical form in our major hospitals. Tuberculosis has lost its awesome significance. Most striking among the contributions of preventive medicine has been the virtual disappearance of tuberculous cervical lymphadenitis. tabes mesenterica, and tuberculosis of the bones and joints upon the eradication of bovine tuberculosis in this country.

Turning to the therapeutic advances of the past seventy-five years, one must exercise Procrustean prerogatives. One great breakthrough was discovery of salvarsan (Ehrlich and Hata, 1910). For the first time, the principle of therapia sterilisans magna was vindicated in the affected patient. Syphilis was rendered vulnerable to therapeutic control, but human frailty has denied its eradication. There followed the frenetic and frustrating quest for analogous agents to combat bacterial infections. The efficacy of sulfonamides (Domagk, Prontosil, 1935) brought a new concept and renewed hope to a fallow field. Sulfapyridine (Whitby, 1938) proved especially effective in pneumococcus infections.

Scarcely had these agents gained a foothold when new and unanticipated developments opened the virgin field of antimicrobial therapy. With a sustained interest in lysozymes, Fleming isolated penicillin in 1928, but its application to human ills awaited the catalytic force of World War II and the diligence of the Oxford group (Florey et al.) for its ultimate exploitation. Of the host of antimicrobial agents that has since been discovered, streptomycin (Waksman, 1944) deserves a special notice. To its virtues we owe the first aggressive attack against tuberculosis. Special tribute is due John R. Barnwell and Arthur M. Walker for their design of the cooperative chemotherapy study of the Armed Forces and the Veterans Administration that firmly established the efficacy of streptomycin. Their approach will serve as a model for all future mass therapeutic trials. Inviting as is the widening field of antimicrobial therapy, it must be dismissed with several broad generalizations. In certain respects, these potent agents have proven to be two-edged swords. Resistant strains of microorganisms have emerged. Sensitivity to these potent remedies has given not only serious and even fatal reactions but has denied their availability to patients sorely in need of their support. In their indiscriminate use, the profession must assume its share of the responsibility for this situation. In a more subtle fashion, the advent of the antimicrobial agents has altered the mode of infectious diseases. By the destruction of common bacterial forms, these marvelous elements have created a striking biologic imbalance. This dislocation is evinced by the ascendency and pathogenicity of unusual bacteria, fungi, and viruses. Most recently, idoxuridine (IDU), an analogue of thymidine, offers promise in combating certain viruses.

Substitution therapy for hypothyroidism was initiated by Murray in 1891. Thyroxin was isolated by Kendall in 1914. Osler commented on the miraculous relief of the asthmatic seizure by epinephrine (Abel, 1898). Parallel experiences attended the first injections of insulin (Banting, Best, and Macleod, 1922). The impact of this discovery of the basic understanding and management of diabetes mellitus cannot be exaggerated. Interesting, however, was the early revelation of the unanticipated complexity of the problem. Houssay's experiments from 1921 to 1930 demonstrated the interdependence of the hypophysis and the islands of Langerhans. Continuing to the present time, advances in the knowledge of this involved subject emphasize this circumstance. By immunoassay, Berson and Yalow (1959–60) have determined normal or increased levels of serum insulin in patients who developed diabetes mellitus at maturity. And so the exciting developments in endocrinology could be vastly expanded.

Hematinic agents were limited seventy-five years ago. Various forms of iron occupied a prominent place. With the experiences of World War I, renewed interest came to blood transfusions and their substitutes in the control of traumatic shock. Blood grouping gave security to the procedure and in the interwar period, transfusions took their proper place in modern practice. However, these measures afforded no sustained support for patients with pernicious anemia. With the fundamental work of Whipple and Robscheit-Robbins in 1925 came the evidence of the unusual virtue of liver in the regeneration of hemoglobin in standard anemic dogs. With characteristic alacrity and direction, Minot and Murphy (1926) successfully applied the principle to patients suffering from pernicious anemia. To Castle belongs the credit for elucidation of the interaction of the intrinsic and extrinsic factors by his classical experiments in 1928. The impetus of these contributions revitalized this aspect of medicine to culminate in the definition of the role of vitamin B_{12} (cyanocobalamine). Its force continues with unabated productivity. In spite of the promise of virology in explanation of some forms of leukemia in animals (Gross et al.), practically all therapeutic approaches are directed toward destructive or antimetabolic agents against the neoplastic process. Without minimizing the importance of this direction of attack, further progress may be anticipated through new and basic principles that hopefully might help solve the secrets of neoplasia in general.

The discovery of the adrenal steroids and the definition of the pituitary-adrenal axis have had a profound effect on medical thought and practice. Limiting the discussion to the adrenal cortical extract (Reichstein, 1936; Kendall and Hench, 1937), unquestionably the availability of cortisone gave medicine the most potent agent it has ever possessed. Its powers have operated both to the benefit and to the detriment of the subject, but the balance is strongly on the credit side of the ledger. In many instances, its actions have served to solve physiologic questions.

The tranquilizing agents have enjoyed wide and uncontrolled usage. Their beneficial action is unquestioned, but classical modern methods of control study are difficult. Certainly, they have rendered patients with mental illness more accessible to recognized forms of therapy, and the tide of bed occupancy for such patients is at last ebbing.

IMPACT OF SPECIALIZATION

Isolated as these cited instances of scientific advances are, with a vast number of other aspects, both basic and clinical, their burgeoning force toward specialization is inescapable. Not only is it impossible for the superior mind to grasp all medical progress but its possessor is fortunate to keep abreast of even a limited segment of medicine. Nevertheless, in this period of specialization, medicine must perforce take a long look at its proper place in society of the future. Studies have indicated the need for more physicians. Medical educators are frantically attempting to close the gap by increasing the students in existing schools and the number of schools. Physical limitations are encountered in both directions, but promises of substantial relief have been made. An even more serious obstacle to the successful assault on this problem is the difficulty in the recruitment of the medical staff. A recent survey disclosed over 900 funded vacancies in our medical faculties. Salaries are scarcely competitive with opportunities elsewhere, but a more telling argument is not difficult to find. In the presence of abundant money for research, often from federal sources, the young man of promise is hard pressed for reasons to accept a teaching assignment where academic advancement is less rapid and less assured. We must breed a generation of well-motivated young physicians for whom teaching is not a second-rate academic prospect—and make it stick.

In self-protection, medicine must seriously contemplate its proper place in society. No longer can we maintain our proud isolationism. The stepping stones on which the revered physician of the past precariously made his individual way are being swept from under his feet. More and more he has come to realize that he is a member of society— a servant, not a master. This statement is made without a feeling of denigration, but with a realization that health is the natural birthright of every human being. Medicine is the keystone, but not the entire arch, of the health team and every physician must be a member. No longer may he feel himself the sole custodian of this precious commodity, to which so many contribute in modern society. Indeed, to this protective circle nursing was first admitted. Dietetics was a natural partner. With rehabilitation, the early attention was directed to physiotherapy and occupational therapy. With due thought to the mental aspects of health and disease, clinical psychology joined the ranks. Social service had earned its place when due thought was given to the environmental and other social forces that operated on the person under study.

From a period when medicine was practiced in the home and office, we have witnessed a gravitation to the hospital. Urbanization and transportation have been active factors in this movement. Under voluntary insurance plans and federal support, this tendency will grow. Specialization requires the highly refined instrumentation and equipment that only a hospital can afford. These circumstances combine to encourage associate and group practice, but they do not deny the advantage of independent practice—with appropriate support.

Indeed, the need for the family counselor was never greater. With proper training he can give satisfactory care for 75 percent of the common ills and will relieve the highly specialized psychiatrist of 50 percent of his misdirected clientele. Obviously such a practitioner may function in the group or associate capacity as well as individually. This well-motivated practitioner may siphon an appreciable number of patients from our overloaded hospitals for appropriate attention in the office and home. Certainly, in the future as in the past, the family counselor will more distinctly reflect the image of medicine to the public than any of his more sequestered professional brothers in the larger medical centers.

SUMMARY

As one would anticipate, radical changes have occurred in the transition from the horse and buggy medicine to the space era. The empiricism that still marked the 1890s has given way to the scientific approach in the laboratory, clinic, and sickroom. The modern physician is capable of infinitely more exact practice than his grandfather. Therapeutic advances have vastly improved his care of patients. The surgical approaches to intracranial lesions, diseases of the lung, and disorders of the heart and vessels are essentially all developments of this period. Truly there are no secret hiding places that escape the modern surgeon. Specialization is basically a product of this period through the vast growth of medical knowledge. The manner of practice shows a steady movement toward the hospital. Although abundantly evident at this time, automation and mechanization will be increasingly utilized in medicine in the future. Let us consider: seventy-five years from now, some essayist will reflect on the backward state of the science and the art of medicine in 1966. Certainly, ever broader, brighter vistas are still ahead.

MEDICAL EDUCATION

SOME REFLECTIONS
ON MEDICAL EDUCATION

Medical education had its origin in the priesthood of antiquity. For many generations the shaman, or priest, and the practitioner of the healing art were one and the same individual. Under the Hippocratic oath, the knowledge of the medical skills was imparted only to physicians and to the sons of physicians. Chomel termed this the traditional method of medical instruction. In the evolution of Greek culture, medicine was eventually separated from the priesthood. The first medical school at Alexandria was founded by Alexander of Macedonia. Notable medical figures, as Herophilus, Erasistratus, and Galen, trained in this school. With the Roman conquest of Egypt, the school at Alexandria was disbanded. Interestingly, the church bridged the gap until the establishment of the next formal medical school at Salerno in the ninth century A.D. The monks at Monte Cassino assiduously copied ancient medical work, while at St. Gall the first medical botanical garden was maintained.[1]

The torch of medical education at Salerno was kept bright for at least four centuries, but its decline dates from the thirteenth century, when the medical leadership passed in turn from Bologna to Naples to Montpellier to Paris. The doors of the University of Salerno were eventually closed by Napoleon in 1811. True academic tradition in pageantry and

Address presented at regional meetings in Trenton, New Jersey, and Chapel Hill, North Carolina. Reprinted from *Annals of Internal Medicine* 34 (June 1951): 1457–62.

1. D. Riesman, *Medicine in Modern Society* (Princeton: Princeton University Press, 1938).

form dates from the University of Paris. The influence of the church in medicine waned very perceptibly when first surgery and then all forms of medical practice were denied the priesthood. In France, surgery was separated from medicine and taught at the Collége du St. Côme.[2] In turn, Leyden, Edinburgh, and London gained ascendancy in medical education in the late seventeenth and eighteenth centuries. The first medical school in North America was established as the Medical Department of the College of Philadelphia in 1765. Its founders, John Morgan and William Shippen, Jr., were both graduates of Edinburgh.

Before the establishment of the medical school in Philadelphia, the apprentice system of medical education prevailed. Among the most notable of the Philadelphia preceptors were John Kearsley, Sr., and John Redman. While formal medical education showed a mushroom growth in the nineteenth century, the pattern of medical apprenticeship persisted in varying degrees throughout this period. The opportunity to read in an established physician's office was a coveted method of introduction to the study of medicine almost to the end of the nineteenth century in this country. True, the house pupils were frequently required to perform menial duties, but the intimate contact with practicing physicians in the office and sickroom earned incalculable dividends in the attainment of the art of medicine.

The formula for the first organized courses of medicine in America differed in no wise from the European or the British pattern. Classroom lectures and demonstrations were the rule. Personal dissection by the medical student was exceptional, and prosectors were commonly employed by the professors of anatomy to demonstrate either the actual dissection or prepared anatomic specimens. Private courses were conducted not only by independent teachers but also by occupants of the respective chairs in the medical schools. So limited was the scope of medical knowledge that the short course of winter lectures was repeated in the second year, and only two such courses were required for graduation. Not until 1859 was the course lengthened to three terms of five months each, over the protest of many members of the profession. The four-year course in medicine dates from 1894–95.

The requirements for admission to medical schools had undergone an almost imperceptible improvement before the Flexner report (1910). Since that time, there has been a distinct trend toward vocational preparation. Indeed, in recent years the more vociferous sciences have seriously crowded the humanities from the scene. A majority of medical schools require three years of premedical preparation. Of ninety essential credits over this period, some seventy odd are actually required for

2. Ibid.

admittance by most institutions. With the science subjects in the ascendancy, chemistry is finding ever increasing weight.

The medical curriculum, like Topsy, "has just growed." Neither its length nor its content has been subjected to serious functional change in the past forty years. In its organization, too frequently compartmentalization prevails by reason of the overweening ambitions of special departments and skills. The movement toward overspecialization in medicine has made its impact felt even upon the undergraduate training of medical students. In many instances, highly refined specialties are taught to the medical student by teachers whose perspective is seriously distorted by their limited field of interests and vision. Mechanization has supplanted clinical acumen and judgment in many quarters. A medical wag has said: "Here lies the body of Hiram Smythe, born a man, died a gastroenterologist." Undoubtedly, this system has certain elements of strength in offering to the medical student in his formative period the latest knowledge within specific areas of medical endeavor. By the same token, such a student, pursuing this development to his ultimate practice of the profession, could never be expected to see the patient as a whole, the host of a disease, from such a detached approach.

The remedies for the present situation in medical education should begin with the college program. It is eminently unfair from a psychological as well as a practical standpoint to term this period of preparation "premedical." Rather, it should be "pre-professional," or general collegiate training with special weight, but without vocational implication. Medical administrators appreciate the mental hazard to even our superior aspirants for medical training when the tag of "premedical" is placed upon them from their matriculation in college. If, in the course of the next few semesters, other aptitudes present themselves, or a lack of proficiency in special sciences emerges, a serious dilemma confronts the unfortunate student. In all probability the designation of a "pre-professional" course will be the early answer to this problem. In the interest of sound educational tenets, the entire college curriculum should be reviewed with a thought to broadening its base. In general, medical educators are agreed that foreign languages should be eliminated as required subjects. A minority of students, those with either a proper background or the prospect of a future in medical research or academic fields, should be encouraged to acquire a good working knowledge of one or more foreign languages. For the vast majority, the current requirement of two years of college French or German is a sheer waste of time. The classical languages, Latin and Greek, offer much sounder educational disciplines, if this be the objective. Currently, the natural sciences have unsurped a lion's share of the college curriculum in the preparation for medicine. In the interest of broadening the product of such training, the humanities, social sciences, and psychology should be materially increased at the expense of the natural sciences. Futhermore, the natural sciences may properly be subjected to careful study. They should be taught as living sources, not as unsavory memory disciplines. The mere accumulation of isolated facts for regurgitation in more or less digested form at examination is not a measure of true education.

The next consideration, namely, that of the selection of students for admission to the medical school, is a very sensitive one. Particularly is this true when one represents a state-supported medical school in which preference must be given to residents of the state in the order of their academic accomplishment. Nevertheless, it is possible that such an experience may more properly qualify one for fair judgment in this matter. After forty years in academic life, I find it increasingly apparent that qualities of character and judgment are more important than mere intellectual attainment in the practice of medicine. Conversely, it should be equally evident that there is no logical basis for the assumption that, because an individual has unusual intellectual endowment, he need be lacking in these most significant attributes of the practicing physician. Since the function of the medical school is primarily the production of physicians, in the ideal situation one would leave only a small secondary space, constituting not more than 10 percent of the elected, for the potential research prospects. Undoubtedly this would be the more difficult group to select, and a 50 percent error would leave the very high figure of 5 percent of prospectively productive graduates in the field of medical research.

A careful evaluation of the medical curriculum, with the possibility of its rational revision, has long been overdue. Lest this circumstance be deemed a measure of complacency, it should be indicated that the medical courses have been continuously subjected to minor changes over the past generation. Indeed, among the professional disciplines, medical education is deemed the most progressive. Yet we cannot accept this position as satisfactory. Let us first look to our objective. The late Professor William H. Welch, of the Johns Hopkins University, related the following experience to me:

> Armed with letters from Doctors Janeway and Osler, I presented myself to Dr. James Mackenzie on an early visit to England. He read the notes and then turned to me and said, "I am well acquainted with some of your work in bacteriology and pathology, but are you the Welch

who has had something to do with medical education at Baltimore?"
When I admitted that I might be he, Dr. Mackenzie continued, "Well,
you are making the biggest mistake in the world." When I protested
mildly and asked whether he had a basis for such a statement, he said,
"Yes, when I was a medical student, we had a professor who took the
men out of the clinics and classrooms and put them in the laboratories,
and even sometimes took them out of the wards and put them in the
laboratories." I ventured to ask what was the result of this practice. Dr.
Mackenzie retorted, "I came out of the medical school knowing no
medicine." I interjected, "And knew that you knew none and wished
to learn more?" "Yes," he said, "and I wished to learn more." "Then," I
said, "Dr. Mackenzie, you have had the finest medical education I have
ever heard of."

From many quarters you will encounter proposals for the integration
and correlation of medical instruction. The movement for the vertical
coordination between the preclinical and the clinical subjects is growing throughout the medical world; but there has been little effort to
carry this principle into a horizontal integration at the preclinical levels.
For a generation, the basic sciences were taught as abstract sciences,
and any suggestion of practical application was offered apologetically.
The leaders in anatomy, histology, physiology, and physiologic chemistry, particularly, felt that they were losing caste among their kind if
their respective subjects had a popular appeal to the students. Without prostituting their ideals, and without seeking vocational levels,
such teachers should give increasing thought to the potentialities of
correlating information among the related subjects, so that the student
is confronted with a living unit. The opportunity for effective integration is even greater in the area of medical microbiology and pathology.
The elimination of detailed technic, as of dissection, staining reactions,
and cultural characteristics, except in the interest of a cohesive design,
should be seriously considered in all subjects. The routine lecture is a
relic of bygone generations. Occasionally there are special fields in
which the instructor may have unusual grasp or facility which will
offer insight and direction to the medical student. On the other hand,
the mechanical transfer of the pearls of wisdom from the instructor's
lips to the notebook of the student is one of the most wasteful of pedagogic procedures.

Unfortunately, about 85 percent of students at all levels must be
spoonfed, and only 15 percent (a liberal estimate) will think for themselves. Certain subjects, as pathology, are replete with theories. If this
preferred 15 percent might alone be stimulated by the theoretic considerations, the time and effort of the majority as well as of the instructor would be spared. To this minority group should also be afforded

the stimulating experience of the opportunity for the observation and experimental study of phenomena uncovered by their mental curiosity. Revitalization of the basic sciences by the appropriate introduction of clinical subjects is an expedient that is now widely and commendably employed. Even the most uninspired student might well be stimulated by this method, and would grow apace as source references are cited and explored. The introduction of psychobiology and medical psychology into the preclinical period is a wholesome sign of the times, but the social sciences have been seriously neglected in this newer development. Adequate exposures to the existing philosophies and practical examples of their operations will better prepare the medical student for the realities of a modern world when he is introduced to the practice of medicine. Above all, time for contemplation should be afforded. Perhaps no better means to this end than the continuance of nonscience electives into the medical school can be recommended. Even in education, a change of pace is an effective device.

Ideally, there should be no sharp division between the preclinical and the clinical disciplines of the medical student. Certainly he is in a much better position for thinking in terms of basic sciences when confronted with the clinical problem, and the converse is patent. Cross fertilization by an interchange of instruction among representatives of the preclinical and clinical fields insures a mutual advantage to both the students and the staff. In this day of overspecialization, it is most important to avoid a segmentation of medicine by the exposure of the student to the technic of specialists. The medical curriculum, particularly in the clinical fields, has grown by accretion. Much of the current crowding of the so-called clinical years depends upon this circumstance, which has obtruded itself without thought to its pedagogic unsoundness. For example, radiologic considerations may be attached to a series of clinical subjects if the student be given only a very slight insight into the principles involved in this highly specialized field. Certainly, undergraduate medical students should not be expected to acquire a profound mastery of these technical subjects. To insure the best clinical approach in the ultimate product, the physician, the patient should be presented as a unit. The patient, as the host of the disease, will be subjected to many forces. The student who is introduced to the consideration of medicine with due emphasis upon the effects of heredity, environment, nutrition, sociologic, and economic conditions, will be much broader beamed than one who approaches his ultimate clinical problems from a series of tangential specialties. From the inception of the clinical years at the University of Wisconsin Medical School (1925), a coordinate course of medicine and surgery has been afforded. Wherever possible, all hours and facilities are pooled. Every skill that impinges upon the ultimate management of a given disease is utilized in continuity. For example, if foreign bodies in the tracheobronchial tree be under consideration, in sequence the pediatrician, roentgenologist, and otolaryngologist will discuss the subject with the class. Effective as is such a simple device, periodically the members of the faculty must be briefed as to their respective responsibilities toward the total effort.

Singularly, medical educators have assumed that teachers are born. Until relatively recent years, there has been no studied effort to establish the validity of this position. Yet the technics of education have grown apace. It is high time that we invite specialists in the field of pedagogy to advise us in this matter. Growth in clinical medicine depends upon painstaking attention to details. Osler wrote: "To study the phenomena of disease without books is to sail an uncharted sea. While to study books without patients is not to go to sea at all." At the bedside, then, with careful supervision and increasing responsibilities, the student lays the foundation for his ultimate development to clinical maturity. The instructor has the added opportunity of inculcating in the student at this malleable period an appreciation of his reciprocal responsibility to society. In 1926, the late Dean Charles R. Bardeen introduced the Wisconsin Preceptorial Plan, which attempts to recapture the advantages of the old house pupil-preceptor relationship. By the expedient of extending the normal academic year of thirty-six weeks to forty-eight weeks in the senior year, an added quarter is gained to the student. During this period he is assigned to a recognized clinician in one of fifteen centers in the state. A single physician is made the responsible preceptor, although he may have any number of associates. Dr. Bardeen's design was to permit the student at this stage in his development to look over the shoulder of a tried clinician, and to observe his manner of handling the medical situation at its source. For the first time, these medical students realize the impact of environment upon disease expressions. At this very early stage in their development, their responsibility to society and many other sociologic, ethical, and economic implications are brought into relief. In our judgment, the extramural preceptorship is one of the most effective elements in the educational discipline of the medical student.

With this background, Professor Welch's philosophy of medical education must obtain. No student will leave the medical school with a sense of the fulfillment of his training. Brown has written: "Education is not something that is wrapped up and handed to the graduate rolled up in his diploma. Education is not a thing at all, but a process." May you enjoy this process to the end of your days; for then will your years be full and your life contented.

MEDICAL EDUCATION
– A PROJECTION

At a period when cellular concepts have given way to molecular biology, when the emission microscope has disclosed the separate atoms within the molecule, and the whole educational world is agog with the new vistas ahead, medical curricula will come under increasingly careful scrutiny and withering fire.

Miller (1962) wrote: "Despite the phenomenal advances in medical care that have come about in the last half century, changes largely attributed to the quality of medical education, the whole process of training physicians has since the time of Flexner taken on a strangely magical and basically immutable quality." In truth, the subject divisions and schedules recommended by Flexner (1910) did become a shibboleth to educators and legislators alike.

However, after a period of stabilization, medicine has been an envied discipline in university circles by reason of its relentless efforts to improve education. In the main, such progress as has been made depends on its insistence on higher entrance standards and curricular modifications. This ferment has been especially active in the post-World-War-II period.

The designation "premedical" by Flexner was unfortunate and its rigid coverage of the natural sciences afforded little latitude for the humanities, social and behaviorial sciences. Broad scholarship was not encouraged by the strictness of the collegiate curriculum designed for

Delivered to alumni attending the Association meeting in Chicago during the AMA convention. Reprinted from the *Wisconsin Medical Alumni Quarterly* 6 (Fall 1966): 20

progression to the medical course. In a highly competitive area the cultural aspects of the coveted profession were nipped in the bud. Psychologically the very designations, "premedical" or "preprofessional," fixed an objective at a stage of academic evolution when the student had neither the experience nor the maturity of judgment to determine his fitness or aptitude for medicine. Meanwhile, the tide of scientific advancement has been making increasing demands for the inclusion of further subjects at the college level. The stage of academic education at which such important topics as embryology, general physiology, physiological chemistry, histology, and anatomy should be taught, has been subject to discussion and decision in different colleges and universities. Among other disciplines, genetics, bionomics, biometrics, biostatics, mathematics, medical engineering, and psychopathology, to mention only a few, are clamant for recognition.

Assuredly the growing appreciation of the reciprocal role of sociology and medicine will require increasing attention among educators and physicians in the future. A Wisconsin man, Henry Baird Favill, like the prophet crying in the wilderness, eloquently charged this responsibility (1908):

> The time is already here where to be only a practicing physician is a discredit. Not only has the medical profession to furnish its full quota to the army of social service, but in many respects it must point out the way. The pathology of society is as much the function of the medical man as is the pathology of human disease. . . . Then it will come to pass that the physician will, as a measure of self-development and self-expression, become a sociologist, and while cooperating with his colleague in his medical labor, will cooperate with his community in its social needs.

The manifold experiments in medical curricula now current in this country are a brief for the gravity of the situation and the tangible evidence of educators' resolution to meet its exigencies. Material improvement has accrued to vertical as well as horizontal coordination of instruction at all stages of the medical course. Pooling of resources in the presentation of the patient as a unit has been rewarding in the teaching-learning process. The "core" program has found favor in some medical schools. The preceptorial plan in different forms has recaptured a measure of the art of medicine that eludes the most skilled instructor removed from the environment of the inception of the illness with all of its social and economic nuances. Family care and the early introduction of medical students to its ramifications have been pursued in other centers. The tutorial plan with highly individualized guidance has enhanced the depth of educational exposure in limited areas. And so the list might be extended. The breadth of some proposals patently negates the coveted depth of the undergraduate discipline. "Where there are many remedies, there is no cure," reads an ancient medical truism. In this era of unprecedented scientific growth that so intimately affects medical precept and practice, thoughtful educators realize that instruction in the medical school must undergo a radical revision or revert to a purely vocational level. Confronted with a basic question in any field of education, the teacher must ask: "What objective do we seek?" The primary mission of the medical school is the education of physicians. The hospitals of the medical schools are the largest and most complicated laboratories on a given campus. Except for the training of physicians and coprofessional personnel they would not be so located. Their superior human service is a most vital byproduct. Research is essential to the growth of education as well as knowledge; but balance rather than submergence of any element of this traditional triad should be sought.

Furthermore, the direction and depth of scientific advance in areas related to medicine are inevitably drawing the keen minds of our younger associates of the medical faculty further and further from their original position of support to the clinical branches of the curriculum. Where this traditional position is enforced, such instructors lack the infectious enthusiasm that marks the true teacher—and the student is the first to appreciate the disaffection. Since this gap promises to widen, the corrective measures must consider both sides of the coin. Viewed in a broad light, many of the lines of demarcation in the basic sciences have been blurred or erased. This circumstance becomes increasingly apparent as we move from cellular to molecular biology. Biochemical alterations dominate thought in many directions in health and disease.

In the inevitable transition with biologic concepts prevailing, a gradual phasing of the basic sciences into broader units will consolidate the educational front. As their scientific principles prove tenable, they may be expected to infiltrate clinical thinking and instruction. Incidentally, the physician product of such a firm discipline will approach his clinical problems with a deeper insight into the natural processes and their alterations in disease (Wagner).

In some quarters medical students are required to engage in research. The appreciation of such methodology and the critical analysis of evidence are invaluable assets in the practice of medicine; but they must not be permitted to dwarf the primary objective, i.e., training of physicians. Rather they should be designed to complement the essential teaching-learning formulae. A generous estimate would assign to 10 percent of the graduates of American medical schools possible future careers in medical research and education. Carefully selected at the end of the first semester (or year) in the medical school, these key men might thereafter be required to complete only the minimal essential laboratory or classroom work for the remainder of their medical course.

Their major effort would be directed toward an area of special interest of their own choice under the sponsorship of an inspiring faculty member. They would, however, stand the stated examinations with their classmates. Such a system would obviate the present pattern of multiple doctoral degrees and would assure a pool of competent candidates for the medical faculties. Their strength would be welcomed especially in the basic sciences, where the prospect of great advances is so bright for the early future. For a majority of students, a basic understanding of the research approach would suffice without serious encroachment on the primary objective.

If the signs are read aright, the medical schools will perforce assume an increasing role in graduate and postgraduate education. Indubitably the limitations of staff and finances have not encouraged the measure of such participation that might be anticipated in these important areas. By common consent the internship, as now constituted, is an essential transition in the preparation of the graduate for the practice of medicine. Certain of the current experiments in medical curricula incorporate this discipline in their program. The revival of the plan of the required internship with adequate material and moral support has some merit.

Organized graduate and postgraduate education has been quite limited in this country. The unprecedented growth of specialization has vastly extended the demand for graduate training through residencies and fellowships. Following the leadership of the American Board for Ophthalmic Examination (1916), eighteen other specialties have organized boards whose primary mission is to establish standards of acceptance for certification. They possess no legal authority of licensure. The Advisory Board for Medical Specialties fixes the basic principles for the organization of such boards; but, in turn, this body exercises only an advisory supervision of the operations of its constituent members. Viewing the current loosely organized status of the internship and residency (fellowship), the substitution of a broad phase of graduate medicine is offered. Such a design would place these elements squarely in the hands of the medical school for sounder organization and evolution on a graded educational basis for varying periods and objectives (McClaughry).

The physician in the field is constantly reminded of the rapid turn-over and obsolescence of medical knowledge. Painfully conscious of his personal shortcomings in this direction, the conscientious practitioner seeks every source of information. For example, the most accessible medium for the promulgation of the knowledge of therapeutic advances is frequently the detail man. Without disparaging the latter's effort, he is scarcely in a position to give professional guidance. And so the entire gamut of medicine may be reviewed with the obvious conclusion that the medical school inevitably must assume leadership in this area. Minnesota has had a head start through its Continuation Center. Kansas has done a splendid job and was the first to use the closed-circuit television. Albany has made a notable contribution with the radio-telephone conferences. Under the leadership of Assistant Dean Thomas C. Meyer, Wisconsin bids fair to close the gap in post-graduate medical education. Among other devices, great efforts are being made to reach even wider circles of physicians through radio-telephone conferences. The success of this plan depends on your participation. Do not be satisfied (but silent) listeners; use the faculty members as your sounding board through thoughtful questions. And this is just the beginning!

PRECEPTORSHIPS – A REVIEW

The unceasing scrutiny of the educational disciplines in medicine is a wholesome sign of the times. Medicine is a living and a live profession. Its alert practice reflects the vitality of its roots. In the feverishly, and frequently detached, search for methods to improve the educational formula, an isolated facet is occasionally seized upon as the cure for all of our pedagogical ills. No such "cure-all" exists. Regardless of methodology, three ingredients are essential for best educational results—intelligent, receptive students; inspired, well-motivated teachers; and ready, open channels of communication. The processes of teaching and learning may be facilitated by recognized pedagogical procedures; but we must realize that such devices are the means and not the ends of education. If such measures do improve the current curriculum, a progressive profession will anticipate their modification and replacement with newer developments from time to time. In this everchanging ebb and flow of medical education, it is inevitable that certain established techniques should lose favor and be replaced by other methods of instruction.

In this category of discarded plans for medical education falls the medical preceptorship. From the days of Hippocrates, the preceptorial plan played a dominant part in the training of a physician. The early history of medical training in this country is built upon the contribution of unofficial preceptors to the professional growth of housepupils. Indeed, before the foundation of the Medical School of the College of Philadelphia (University of Pennsylvania) in 1765, no formal medical

Reprinted from *Journal Student American Medical Association* 3 (October 1954): 24, 32, 49.

education was available in North America. With the rash of medical schools being formed in this country in the nineteenth century, the house-pupilship steadily lost favor. In the latter half of this period, this form of training had undergone a complete eclipse. Yet, assistantships in the offices and clinics of prominent physicians remained a coveted opportunity for graduate training until the ascendancy of the specialty boards that usually frowned upon such outlets.

With the establishment of the clinical years of medical training at the University of Wisconsin Medical School in 1925, the Preceptorial Plan was adopted upon the recommendation of Dean Charles R. Bardeen. The first class embarked upon this Plan in 1926; so that an experience of twenty-eight years in this educational area has been had at Wisconsin. I feel singularly qualified to survey this effort, since I opposed Dean Bardeen in his well-conceived plan at the outset. From 1912, he had repeatedly discussed the matter with me and I had raised all manner of objections that today seem so trite and theoretical. Fortunately, Dean Bardeen's position prevailed. Under the immediate supervision of Dr. Joseph S. Evans, the Preceptorial Plan received the support of a group of inspired leaders practicing medicine in Wisconsin. From its inception its success was assured. Most of my objections were refuted and as a convert I review the Wisconsin experience of the past twenty-eight years in this area of medical education.

From the beginning, the Preceptorial Plan was designed to take the senior medical student out of the academic environment and into the atmosphere of an active medical practice. Here he would see the practice of medicine over the shoulder of a trained physician. With the evolution of modern medicine, the great teaching centers and hospitals have become more impersonal. The patient removed from his home and native environment is psychologically a different individual. Try as we may we cannot reconstruct the local scene and its influence upon disease expression in our metropolitan hospitals. In the native community one must perforce see, or sense, the impact of the family, associates, and occupation without conscious readjustment. The economic, sociological, and environmental factors become primary considerations too frequently lost in the removed large hospital. The more highly organized the hospital, the more remote are its relationships with the patients apt to become. Certainly the unnatural position of the patient creates a serious psychological barrier to complete rapport.

The key to the early success of the Wisconsin Plan was the selection of the original group of preceptors. Largely through the efforts of Dr. Joseph S. Evans, a group of nine leaders of medicine in Wisconsin was selected to initiate the movement. They were men of vision who gave themselves unstintingly to the objectives of the Plan. Professional attainment, position in the community and the profession, and capacity to implement the Plan were some of the criteria for selection. Interestingly, three of the present preceptors in the Wisconsin Plan are sons of the original preceptors. In the intervening years, there has been one replacement and one withdrawal from the Plan. The latter defection arose from a difference of opinion relative to policy that did not involve the educational program. The nomination of the preceptors is a function of the dean and is free from political of corporate influence. The first preceptors were usually members or clinic groups. In turn, they nominated to the dean such practitioners as they might wish to serve as associate preceptors. In honoring such nominations there was no abrogation of the responsibility or authority of the chief preceptor.

To accommodate the added requirement of the Preceptorial Plan, the senior year of medicine was extended to forty-eight weeks. Twelve weeks, or a quarter, were assigned to the preceptorship. In the original scheme, two students were allotted to a given preceptor for the three-month period. So enthusiastic was the reception of the Plan both from the students and the preceptors that Dean Bardeen, in 1929, extended the period to twenty-four weeks, twelve weeks in each of two separate preceptorships. The experiment was uniformly unhappy and resulted in a prompt return to the original formula which still exists at present.

Dean Bardeen, in 1927, afforded general directions to the preceptors as follows:

> 1. A clinical apprentice is expected to be engaged along specified lines of work for five hours each week day, in ward work, clinical work, laboratory work, or in other work which puts him into immediate contact with patients or with procedures taken for the direct welfare of patients. This work should so far as possible be designed to give the apprentice an opportunity to be useful to others as well as to obtain a training personally beneficial.
>
> 2. At least half, and preferably more, of the practical work of the clinical apprentice as outlined should be devoted to general medicine or to general surgery from the medical standpoint. The balance of the time may be devoted to obstetrics if such service is available, and to one or more of the specialties with special reference to the problems of general medicine and surgery.
>
> 3. The time of the clinical apprentice should not be dissipated by permitting him to undertake work in more than two fields at a given period. Thus, if a student under the preceptorship of a general surgeon has major work in general surgery, he may work for a certain number of hours each day or every other day under the direction of a second or associate preceptor in urology, but so long as he does this he should not be assigned any further specified work in any of the specialties.

Thus, if he desires to devote more time to obstetrics, he should give up the specified hours with the urologist while on the obstetric service.

4. While on a given service, the clinical apprentice is expected to aid in history taking, in making physical examinations, in the laboratory work, and in such other ways as may be for the welfare of the service and beneficial to his own education.

5. When not on specified duty, the clinical apprentice is expected to do a large amount of reading and study, in part in direct connection with the cases seen while on service, in part along general lines designed to broaden his view of the field of medicine to which his work is related.

6. While on a given service the clinical apprentice should write up a case or group of cases with special care, at least once a month. Copies of these reports should be filed at the office of the Medical School in Madison [University of Wisconsin].

7. At the end of the three months' apprenticeship, the clinical apprentice is expected to submit to general examinations in the fields of work to which his services have been devoted and also to write a general report of the work which he has done and the benefits received.

An extended experience has led to a liberalization of the above program. At the request of the preceptors, a revision of the Plan has more recently been prepared from which the following is abstracted:

The senior student has had a period of premedical, pre-clinical, and clinical exposures that will appropriately prepare him for the practice of medicine. At this stage of his training the student will be found remarkably receptive to your reaction to your social responsibility. He will render such services as you may see fit to place upon him; but in the ideal pattern the following outlets are sought:

1. Contact with the patient in the home and office. Obviously there is no teaching outlet in any medical school in the country that can take the place of the family physician in these relations. Hence, we seek for our students at Wisconsin a superior training in the exposures that will come from supervised contact in the home and office.

2. Hospital contacts. In our judgment the student will have a greater spirit of usefulness, and will by the same token obtain much more from his hospital contacts if he is kept in a position subordinate to a house officer. It may be that there are special procedures such as the withdrawal of blood, of spinal fluid, gastric contents, and even of pleural fluid that will improve his facility and at the same time not encroach upon the prerogatives of the attending physician. Least of all do we desire assistantships in surgery. It is our measured judgment that the senior student is not far enough advanced to profit by such outlets.

3. Laboratory duties. In many instances the routine laboratory procedures upon the patient under his direct observation can be completed by the senior student. Such studies take on an increasing significance by reason of their application to the problem at hand.

Recapitulating, the Medical School requests no special privileges for senior students except the opportunity to observe the patient under natural conditions in the hands of a trained recognized clinician who is willing to lend his effort to this unusual educational outlet.

The implementation of the general design of the Preceptorial Plan varies widely with the local situation and conditions of practice. Six of the present fifteen preceptors are located in towns of less than 15,000 populations, and an added five in cities with less than 30,000. A single preceptorship is maintained in Milwaukee to utilize the talents and facilities of a member of the staff of the hospital for communicable diseases. The earlier plan of the integration of the preceptorship in a clinic group still exists in eight of the fifteen; but, there is a studied design to center this activity in the small community under a sound family counsellor. Interestingly, five of the clinic-connected preceptors have included general practitioners in outlying smaller communities in their associate group with a distinct broadening of the educational outlook for our students.

Dean Bardeen's early vision stressed the externship aspect of the preceptorial opportunity. The clinical faculty indicated the inherent danger of the premature internship. The Wisconsin experience has supported the validity of this objection. Without making invidious comparisons, the educational opportunities of preceptorship without fixed hospital responsibilities have been adjudged superior to the conventional externship arrangement. Certainly, the Medical School would not condone the prostitution of its students in the sole interest of maintaining hospital records without an educational objective. Indeed, a conscious effort has been made to keep this restricted use of the preceptee constantly before the preceptors. The readjustments in their educational interest have been most gratifying. In many communities of the Middle West the hospital is the natural refuge of the emergent sick and injured. In such instances, the best interests of the preceptee have been served by residence in the hospital, but his duties and responsibilities are subsidiary to the house staff and the visiting physicians. In recent years, a concerted effort has been made to limit the surgical exposures of the preceptees, who are not prepared for major responsibilities at this stage of development.

The greatest advantage accrues to the impressionable senior who is taken under the wing of the seasoned preceptor. This apprentice may take the original history and do the physical examination of a new patient in the office, hospital, or home. The preceptor in turn checks these findings and discusses their adequacy and accuracy. The supporting laboratory examinations may in part be performed by the student. The diagnosis may be derived in such intimate conferences and the subsequent conduct of care discussed. The home calls are an enlightening experience, and such intimacies afford an excellent opportunity for the preceptor, as an elder brother, to indoctrinate the novitiate in the philosophy and ethics of medical practice. Assuredly, precept and example are much more effective than formal presentations, spoken or written. As is clearly understood among all contracting parties, the preceptor may assign any duty to the preceptee during his period of training. The preceptor is answerable only to the administration of the medical school.

The opportunities of the Preceptorial Plan are not measurable solely in the clinical outlets. However ideally situated and staffed the mother University Hospital may be, the patient-physician relationship must perforce be somewhat artificial. Attempts to bridge this widening gap are encountered in the various social service agencies. In a small community the family counsellor is the sole repository of such confidences that may spell the difference between understanding and health on the one hand, and detachment and illness on the other. Certainly, here to the greatest degree exists the wedding of the art and the science of medicine. An intimate knowledge of the family life, ambitions, and frustrations gives the physician, working under these conditions, a perspective denied his fellow practitioner in the large metropolitan clinic or hospital. The conflicts of the home, office, and shop are an open book to him. The social and economic factors in a simple or complex situation are readily invoked by a preceptor to the edification of the student. For a period of three months the preceptee becomes a part of the community. The continuity of his duties is established by the preceptor who, as a rule, spells himself and his associates by a rotation of the assignments.

Inherent in the Preceptorial Plan are certain weaknesses. Obviously, there will be a wide variation in the type and even the quality of instruction. The interest of the preceptors has been remarkably sustained. Admitting certain discrepancies in the educational pattern of the several preceptorships, the students themselves effect an equalization through their frank criticism. Upon reflection, every physician is a teacher. He questions his patient for the dual purpose of informing himself and of purging his patient. His instructions to the sick individual and the attending persons must be carefully geared to their intellectual level for the faithful execution of directions. In no other field is a sound knowledge of human nature and psychology more essential for effective practice. The preceptee-preceptor relationship affords an unexcelled opportunity for the unobstrusive demonstration of this vital interchange of knowledge.

At an early period the Preceptorial Plan encountered a serious hazard in the assumption of a control of the student's activities by certain hospitals. Naturally, this prerogative gained added force when a given preceptor had arranged for the board and room of a preceptee in a hospital. This pattern carries with it the obvious implication of the performance of certain functions in return for the benefits received; but the administration has looked askance upon such arrangements and has held the preceptor completely responsible for their educational value. At no time has the University of Wisconsin entered into a contractual relationship with any hospital of the State for the accommodation of its students.

Upon his visit to the University of Wisconsin in 1949, Prime Minister Nehru of India became greatly interested in the Preceptorial Plan. Aside from its educational content, its support was especially surprising to him. The preceptors are volunteers whose services to medical education are rendered without fee—nor does the student pay a special fee. Rather, his total University fees are lowered $90 in the senior year to compensate in some measure for the dislocation. Actually, this sum does not bridge the financial gap of the married student who must maintain a separate establishment in Madison, but it does adequately meet such minor readjustments as the geographic change of scene may impose upon the unmarried man. In neither instance has a paid externship without due thought to its educational promise and performance provided a satisfactory solution to this problem.

Each preceptee prepares a daily log of his activities. In general, these reports are most effective instruments in evaluating the educational opportunities of a given preceptorship. Bearing in mind the relatively uninhibited reaction of a medical student at this stage of development, his constructive criticisms are given full weight. To avoid personal differences between the preceptor and the recent guest in his home, the preceptee, such issues are never immediately raised. If they recur, the opportunity to confer with the affected preceptor has inevitably led to a reconciliation of the differences.

From the inception of the Preceptorial Plan at Wisconsin, periodic tours of all of the preceptor centers have been made. A party, composed of the Superintendent of the State of Wisconsin General Hospital, the Associate Dean, and the Dean of the Medical School, visited all preceptors once a year. These calls became rather perfunctory by reason of the extended distances and the available time. Three years ago a plan, utilizing a group of senior members of the Medical Faculty for independent surveys of the several preceptorships, was initiated. At the mutual convenience of the preceptor and the assigned staff member, an appropriate date is arranged. The staff member goes as the guest of the preceptor, not as an inspector. The primary function is the observation and the evaluation of the teaching opportunities of the preceptorship. A full day or longer may be spent in this survey, and he will have close contact with the student in this capacity. To broaden and cement our relations with this extramural Associate Teaching Staff of the Medical School, these representatives of the intramural staff hold themselves ready for conferences and consultations. In a majority of instances they have given stated lectures or clinics for the local profession on these occasions.

In the autumn, the preceptors are invited to Madison for a scientific meeting prepared especially for their needs. The subject matter, wherever possible, is arranged at their request. Newer developments in medicine receive due consideration. Dinner is served in the evening and the next morning is devoted to clinics of their own election. The preceptors are again invited to the University at Commencement time in June. On this occasion, matters of policy and procedure are discussed and the preceptors meet their prospective preceptees of the succeeding year. These students have previously been briefed in the significance and the opportunities of the preceptorship. The preceptors then give them specific instructions. The further design of this meeting is to afford the preceptors the opportunity of acting as escorts to the medical graduates. A growing number of the seniors elect preceptors for this distinction. Honoraria are afforded to two representatives of each preceptorship to attend both of these important sessions.

From the preceptorial experience our students return to Madison with a new viewpoint of the practice of medicine. They have worked shoulder to shoulder with physicians in the home, the office, and the hospital. The impact of environment upon disease expression is a living experience, not a philosophical thesis. The intricacies of insurance and industrial relations stand revealed by actual observations.

The patient-physician relationships are cherished memories of awakening responsibilities. The place of the physician in the body politic and social is amazingly clear to a majority of them for the first time. Significantly, an appreciable percentage of the ranking men of each graduating class elect general practice in small communities as a result of this experience. In a word, maturation in a professional and a social sense is a natural result of the preceptorial training. The byproducts of the Wisconsin plan in improved professional relationships and patient care through this coordinate effort are imponderable, but widely recognized, in the State. In the judgment of a convert, the Preceptorial Plan in one form or another is here to stay!

CONTINUING EDUCATION IN MEDICAL RAMBLING

The discipline of medicine has a very dignified and revered background. If we were to start from the beginning, perhaps we would go beyond the 2400 years that are represented in the Oath of Hippocrates. Hippocrates said that "by precept, lecture, and every other mode of instruction, I will impart a knowledge of my art to my own sons, to those of my teachers, and to disciples, bound by a stipulation and an oath according to the law of Medicine, and to none others." This is a very weighty oath that is taken by everyone who enters into the practice of medicine. It imposes upon each of us an appreciation that, as Chomel, the great French clinician, indicated, there is a "traditional" formula of medical education. This pledge becomes exceedingly important as one visualizes what has happened over the ages past and has come down to us in these past 2400 years. In every medical school, there is a faculty dedicated to the principles enunciated by Hippocrates. These teachers, to whom you and your past have been exposed, to whom we in the future will be exposed, are men who adhere to the precepts of Hippocrates. I have no doubt that the "traditional" method will prevail through time. In its basic tenets, there will be a sense of responsibility on the part of every faculty member, and it does not stop with the Medical School. In the hospitals of all civilized countries, at the operating table there is a transportation across that table of all the details of accumulated skills and experience from the master surgeon to

Presented as the Alpha Omega Alpha Initiation Address in September 1963. Reprinted from *The Pharos of Alpha Omega Alpha* 28 (January 1965): 16 ff.

the apprentice. The physician at the bedside attempts to carry the same transportation of experience to the undergraduate, the recent graduate, and the young physician. The roentgenologist, the pathologist, and the clinical laboratory worker will have the same motivation in his contact with the young undergraduate and physician. In truth the "traditional" method of medical education goes forward; each and every one of us has participated in it, either as the recipient or the donor. Currently we are preoccupied with the charge and the fear that under the existing formula of medical education there may be a fixed mold, into which we are attempting to pour every student who comes before us. If I were to pass among this group, I am quite certain that the medical professional fathers would admit that they have some difficulty in recognizing their offspring. In other words, there is so much variation in the personality of the staff and of the student, and there is such latitude in this process that we call teaching and learning, that the recipient is as frequently molding the donor, as is the donor molding the recipient. This circumstance is ever stimulating and challenging to the teacher.

As has been indicated, teaching does not stop in the halls of the Medical School; but it is found in every walk of professional life, if a physician is truly fulfilling his highest ideals and ambitions for his profession. Clearly this tenet is the basis of our continuing education. While we are all concerned with the advancement of our profession, the dividend from personal participation encourages a continuation of medical education from our first exposure as undergraduates until the last chapter in our careers is written. So when, in my rambling comments, I have occasion to refer to certain personal contacts with men of great stature and to men less conspicuous in the profession, and when I cite incidents that are apparently light and others that have a weighty impact, you will not count this an autobiographical recital but rather one medical man's experience in continuing education.

For example, a medical student who went to the University of Pennsylvania in the year 1907 and for four years was exposed to its faculty will perforce select certain individuals who had a distinct influence on his own point of view and an impact on his philosophy of life. Among these I would cite, first of all, Dr. Allen J. Smith, Professor of Pathology, a man with an encyclopedic grasp of medical knowledge. His flair for parasitology excited his students to explore this field for themselves. So when I reconstructed the *Opisthorchis sinensis*, there was no doubt in my mind that I was destined to become a parasitologist. Certainly when, between my second and third, and third and fourth years of the medical course, I worked in the laboratory of pathology at the State

Hospital for Insane in Norristown, Pennsylvania (that is the last time I shall use the word *insane;* they are emotionally or mentally ill in the present parlance), there was a continuity of interest which was to persist through the remainder of Dr. Smith's life. Beyond his noteworthy propensity for stimulating his associates there was a tremendous capacity for friendship with medical students. His interest and apparent absorption in one's problems, petty though they must have appeared to him in the composite, left a lasting impression. It is one of the great opportunities of the teacher to share with the youth of the land their ambitions, their trials, their problems, and to attempt to lighten the burden and to point the way.

The contact with certain of the surgeons at Pennsylvania was illuminating. In 1910, Dr. J. William White, Professor of Surgery, was a dynamic but stereotyped lecturer. After he had completed his general discourse of the conventional treatment of syphilis with potassium iodide, mercury, and bismuth, he said that there had come to his attention the discovery of a new arsenical called salvarsan. From his dependable sources, this discovery of Ehrlich and Hata was the six hundred and sixth arsenical compound and it was reported to have been highly effective in the treatment of syphilis. "But mark you, gentlemen," he added, "I wager you that twenty-five years from now you will still be treating syphilis with potassium iodide and mercury." I cite this episode as a measure of the strictures of arteriosclerosis in limiting the vision of an aging teacher.

Professor White's successor was Dr. Edward Martin, a very ebullient surgeon, who had once visited England with a letter of introduction from Dr. William Osler. The latter had warned his British friends that Martin was a most gregarious individual who would find welcome in all homes and clubs; but he added that his friend had "bird legs." The British friends did not understand the inference until Osler later explained that this meant that his femora were hollow, and therefore in taking up alcohol he would probably outdrink any of them. One day, on the steps of Houston Club across Spruce Street from the Hospital of the University of Pennsylvania Dr. Perry Pepper, heir-apparent to the chair of medicine, greeted John Gilmore, a contemporary intern at Philadelphia General Hospital, and me. Shortly Doctor Martin joined us and said: "Hello, Perry; hello, Gilmore." When I was introduced as a medical man, he said: "You're practicing medicine, and Gilmore surgery." He proceeded: "Perry, of course, you and Middleton are of entirely a separate clan. Gilmore and I are craftsmen. We work with our hands. We can see the results of our handicraft. But you internists, you are metaphysicians; you deal with logic and all sorts of esoteric subjects. The good or harm you do, God only knows!" Such was the attitude of that generation of surgeons toward internists.

The man who influenced me most, my father in medicine, was Doctor David Riesman. In my plans I was a confirmed surgeon until my third year in medicine when I attended Doctor Riesman's ward classes and saw the light. From that time on, I availed myself of every possible exposure to his instruction. To this day he is still the most erudite, the most compassionate, the most learned of all physicians of my acquaintance. He was not only learned in medicine, but in the classics and in medical history. Astrophysics was his hobby. As I looked behind the scene for the explanation of his broad interests I found that his wife, a brilliant woman, was the one who led the conversation at the dinner table into fields entirely foreign to Doctor Riesman's professional calling. Her special areas of interest and study would be explored by Doctor Riesman to afford a high level of intellectual interchange.

Leaving Philadelphia, the influence of my father in medicine was to follow me to Madison in 1912. I still have the memory of my first meeting with the Dean of the Medical School of Wisconsin. At Pennsylvania, the dean was held in some awe. Meeting Dean Charles R. Bardeen, coming out of the University Club, after the Eastern custom I tipped my hat. His ill-concealed amusement disconcerted me on the moment; but I came to have a high respect for him. By his alphabetical listing in its first class, Dr. Bardeen was the first graduate from the Johns Hopkins Medical School. He always maintained that he was given his degree on the condition that he would not practice medicine. A student of Mall, he became one of the outstanding anatomists in this country. In 1926 he revived the preceptorship plan over the protest of many of us in the clinical fields who did not deem it practicable. Dean Bardeen prevailed and today the system of undergraduate preceptorships is applied in some twenty-four medical schools across the country. Dr. Bardeen once told me that he felt that the basis for the early success of the Medical School at Wisconsin was in the selection of its first faculty. He felt that the strength of a faculty should be primarily in the basic sciences. There is no strong medical school without a strong basic science faculty. Regarding the clinical faculty he said: "Middleton, do not buy names." This admonition repeatedly comes home to me, as I contemplate the present trend in certain quarters. Men-on-the-make have much greater potential in medical education than men already-made. All too frequently when you recruit them after their name is made, they are over the hump and on the way down. Dean Bardeen was a very wise man and I gained a great deal from my association with him. I could spend much time in Madison; but the recital would be so colloquial in interest that the University of Wisconsin is relegated to a subordinate place in my thinking for purposes of this discussion.

The Chicago group of the period when I went to Wisconsin (1912) was an extremely strong one. One of my close friends of later years was Dr. James B. Herrick, a small man physically but large of intellectual and professional stature. As you will recall, he was the first to describe sickle cell anemia (1910). In 1912 he described the syndrome we now know as coronary thrombosis with myocardial infarction. He had two fine feathers in his clinical cap. He was a cultured individual and wrote a classical essay on "Why I read Chaucer at 70." He continued to read Chaucer and repeatedly gave this speech, as "Why I read Chaucer at 72, 75, 80 and 82." It was always very warmly received and worthy of re-hearing. For a time he served as physician pro tem at the Peter Bent Brigham Hospital. On his return he said: "Middleton, I had a most unusual experience in Boston." I asked: "What might that have been, Doctor Herrick?" He said: "I was walking along a corridor, you know just contemplatively, when I was greeted by one of the bright-eyed, eager young men who grasped me by the hand and said, 'Doctor Herrick, I'm so glad to meet you. I'm so glad to shake your hand. You're one of the passing generation, one of the type of bedside clinicians that we no longer see.'" He added: "You know, Middleton, for the moment I felt as though he had put me in a specimen jar on one of those shelves in the Pathology Museum."

Almost in diametrical contrast, physically, psychologically, and in many other respects, was his friend, Dr. Frank Billings. In my judgment, Dr. Billings was the strongest man of his period in American medicine; a man, physically and mentally large, whose heart was just as large as his body. He was known as a builder largely through his efforts at the University of Chicago. One of his errors in judgment was his strong espousal of the theory of focal infections. Focal infections now have a very limited place in clinical thought and practice; but in the past largely through the efforts of Rosenow, Dr. Billings was a conspicuous proponent of this cause of many ills. In the educational field, because of his interest in Chicago and his devotion to President Harper, he strongly supported the latter's suggestion that the University of Chicago develop a Graduate School of Medicine. A major benefactor of Chicago, John D. Rockefeller, had been indirectly approached. Finally Dr. Billings decided to see him in person. On appointment he went to Cleveland. When he arrived, Mr. Rockefeller was having his bath and asked whether Billings would go and see his wife who was suffering from rheumatoid arthritis. In an hour and a half Dr. Billings returned to report. He sat down at the breakfast table with Mr. Rockefeller and outlined his findings on the wife. After this detailed report, he said: "Mr. Rockefeller, my mission is entirely different. I have come from Chicago with a mandate from President Harper to approach you relative to the establishment of a Graduate School of Medicine at the University of Chicago. Dr. Harper is in his declining years and this would be a crowning glory to his very illustrious career." The old gentleman listened for a moment, then shook his head and said, "I will not support this project, not one bit." Dr. Billings, relating this encounter to me, said: "Middleton, if John D. Rockefeller was in hell and my little finger extended would pull him out, he would stay in hell." A rugged individual, Frank Billings.

The third of this Chicago group of that period to whom I would direct your attention was Dr. Henry Baird Favill. Dr. Favill was to the manner born. Physician-father in Madison of a socially prominent family, he had every educational advantage. With great pride in his Indian lineage, he was a very fine figure of a man, handsome, swarthy, tall, straight as an arrow. He never wore a topcoat. Dr. Herrick told me that on one occasion late in Dr. Favill's life he saw him with an overcoat and he said: "Harry, you must be feeling badly." And he said, "How can you tell that?" Dr. Herrick answered, "For the first time in your life, I've seen you with an overcoat." I would call your attention to a single quotation of Dr. Favill that deals with a subject important to all future generations of medicine as well as the present. Although he was the society favorite and wealthy in his own right, Dr. Favill was extremely social-minded. I refer to his sense of social consciousness and equity. In 1909, in addressing a meeting of the Alumni of Rush Medical College, his topic was the "Place of the Physician in Conservation." There is one sentence from this speech that I wish engraved on each of your minds. "The pathology of society is as much the responsibility of the medical man as is the pathology of human disease." This charge is extremely important to all of us. Medicine has too regularly sat at the common table of society, while its other members looked askance at us, because of our aloofness in assuming social responsibility. We have been perfectly satisfied to see patients more ill, surgery more difficult, and have not looked to the source. We have not gone behind the scene to the family and to society at large to determine just what might have been their contribution to these diseases. I think that this is one of the most serious charges against modern medicine.

The scene changes quite rapidly, and there is an epidemic of violence. World War I and some of the experiences of that period undoubtedly, consciously or subconsciously, had their influence on me.

One of the first contacts dealt with a passage in the Ypres Salient, when as an American medical officer I was detached from the Fourth Division, British Expeditionary Force, to a Casualty Clearing Station where Dr. Harvey Cushing was stationed. He was doing a great deal of surgery for wounds of the head. His technique was superb. The medical man who could appreciate the artistry of a master, of course, held full sway at his hands. However, there was a circumstance that I shall never forget. Dr. Cushing was the most selfish man with whom I had ever dealt. As a young man I was astonished that this great surgeon could be so unmindful of the mere comforts of his associates. He would talk to me over afternoon tea until 4:00 or 5:00 o'clock. Then he would go into surgery and keep the team that had been standing by scrubbed up and ready for two hours working into the small hours of the night. A small detail but in my judgment it was a measure of his shortcomings.

The opportunity of association with Dr. Walter B. Cannon and Dr. Hans Zinsser evolved in a rather unusual but intimate manner. I had been recalled from the British Expeditionary Forces by Dr. John Lawrence Yates, who was heading a chest surgical team, to serve as his medical man. Dr. Robert Drane of North Carolina was chosen as the roentgenologist. These associates desired to foregather in a breakfast mess. They chose one room that Robert Drane and I had in our billet for this purpose. In the intimacy of this mess I came to know these men very well. Dr. Cannon was the most gentle soul, compassionate, warm, and genuinely interested in anything that you might be doing. One day we were walking along a street in Dijon where our laboratory for experimental chest surgery adjoined Dr. Cannon's shock laboratory when Dr. Cannon asked: "Bill, what is the most serious problem that you have in clinical medicine back in Madison?" I answered: "The most difficult differential diagnosis that I know is between effort syndrome or neurocirculatory asthenia and hyperthyroidism." He said: "When you get home, Bill, the work of DuBois is going to make available to you basal metabolism and you will have an answer." I relate this interchange simply to give you a temporal relation and to cite a physiologist who thought in clinical terms.

Dr. Cannon would announce an experiment in shock to the class of medical officers. To induce shock he filled the pericardial sac of the cat with normal saline. Upon increasing the intrapericardial pressure and limiting the inflow of blood to the auricles and the outflow from the ventricles, the peripheral arterial pressure fell and a shocklike state of the circulation could be demonstrated in the capillary bed of the omentum and the mesocolon. Thus, he announced his experiment:

"This, gentlemen, is a sterile (he did not say, aseptic) operation." If a former Harvard student came into the laboratory, he would shake hands with him, wipe his hands on his gown, and go on with his "sterile" operation, as he termed it. In his naivete Dr. Cannon was a prime target for Dr. Zinsser.

Of all scientists Dr. Zinsser was the most poetic, most volatile, most voluble, and, I think, the most brilliant of my knowledge. He would carry the weight of the entire military operation on his shoulders. If things went well with the Allied Forces, he would come in the gate at the bottom of the garden singing at the top of his voice; but, if the reverse were true and things were going against the Allies, he would have entirely a different attitude. Depressed, his shoulders drooping, he was unnaturally silent and withdrawn. One morning he came in singing "It was Christmas Eve in the Harem." Things were going very well with us on that occasion. Dr. Cannon said, "Won't you sing that again, Hans? I never heard that song before."

There were many other incidents of like order, so that when I read "The Way of an Investigator," by Dr. Cannon, and the autobiography of Dr. Zinsser, *As I Remember Him,* those rare days are recalled. There was one characteristic detail in Dr. Zinsser's evolution of a practical joke that should be recorded. He billeted with Jack Yates, who had been in the field with his team on the Aisne-Marne offensive of the French and Americans. When we returned to Dijon their demure little French landlady kissed Dr. Yates on both cheeks and then said in bland tone: "Go to hell, you . . . !" Jack Yates' jaw dropped and he said: "I know. That pink-eyed Dutchman, Hans Zinsser, has been teaching you." Indeed, Hans Zinsser had spent hours on end teaching this benignant French lady how she should properly greet an American officer returning from the battlefield, in the low vernacular of the doughboy.

The picture changed and the Armistice signed, we were pulling loose ends together, and one of our memorable meetings was a luncheon for Dr. Anton J. Carlson, who will appear in other relations later. Dr. Carlson had been in Great Britain to evaluate the food situation. Dr. Cannon, Dr. Zinsser, Dr. Yates, Dr. Drane, and I were at this lunch. Dr. Cannon asked: "Well, A. J., just what is the food situation in England?" "Well," he said, "they are low in protein." When this situation was the rule in British reports, he pursued the matter further. Dr. Carlson proceeded: "What do you mean?" "We don't have enough meats or eggs to go around." "Well, what about fish?," Dr. Carlson asked. "We have fish, but we get tired of it," the Britisher replied. "How do you cook it?," Doctor Carlson asked. The Britisher said: "We boil it."

"Well, what do you do when you get tired of boiled fish?" "There is no other way but to boil it." Dr. Carlson exploded: "They should starve to death!"

The evacuation of the chest wounded, for whom our team was responsible, imposed a problem in the evaluation of the later results of surgery. Finally Dr. Yates decided that the best plan would be for us to go to each evacuation port to examine the patients with chest wounds in the hospitals that were collecting the casualties for clearance to the United States. With Dr. Drane, I was charged to go to Headquarters at Neufchateau to discuss this proposal with Dr. Finney, the Chief Consultant in Surgery, American Expeditionary Forces. Since Dr. Finney was his brother-in-law, Dr. Yates did not wish to compromise him. We talked the matter over with Dr. Finney. Twice offered the presidency of Princeton University, one of the outstanding laymen in the Episcopal Church and in my judgment by every quality of mind and character, he was one of the truly great Americans of all times. After our recital General Finney said, "It sounds good; but, let's put the question before the mess.' 'It was about dinner time and we went into the mess. Present about the table were Drs. Finney, Fischer, Thayer, Cushing, Boggs, and Salmon, Consultants to the American Expeditionary Forces. When we were through dinner Dr. Finney said: "Now, Bill, what is your proposition?" Thereupon I outlined Dr. Yates' plan. When I was through, Dr. Cushing, sitting directly across the table from me, said: "But, Bill, there is a much simpler way to get the answer." They all asked, "What is that?" "Well," he said, "Draw up a questionnaire and send it around to all of the hospitals and have them fill it out." Robert Drane and I had just come from the Roosevelt Base Hospital at Chaumont, where Dr. Eugene Pool was chief surgeon. Dr. Pool had had such a document. He said: "See here what Harvey Cushing is circulating." We asked: "What is this?" He answered: "He has two foolscap sheets with questions he wants answered on all of the patients, upon whom he has operated." He added: "I'll be damned if I'm going to write Harvey Cushing's next textbook for him." With this reaction the questionnaire went into the wastebasket. I couldn't tell Dr. Cushing this; but I did tell General Finney. He said: "Well, why didn't you tell it at the mess? Nothing would have pleased me more than to have Harvey taken down a peg."

The medical contacts of World War I were with men whom I should never have met in the ordinary course of events; and on terms that for a young man were certainly most unusual. Which recalls that shortly later at the Association of American Physicians meeting in Atlantic City, I had listened to all the papers that I could absorb and I walked out as quietly as I could, only to encounter Dr. William H. Welch at the exit. He said: "Middleton, you're saturated too, are you?" I said: "Yes, sir," a little shamefacedly. He said: "We all come to such a point; let's take a walk." We walked down the boardwalk and he said: "I'd rather walk out on the sand." The interchange of a man of his stature with a youngster, of course, meant a great deal. On another occasion he told several of us that as a young man he had gone to Britain for the first time with letters of introduction from Dr. Osler and Dr. Janeway to Dr. Mackenzie. James Mackenzie had not yet been knighted. Dr. Welch thus related the encounter:

> Upon reading the notes he turned to me and said, "I am well acquainted with some of your work in bacteriology and pathology, but are you the Welch who has had something to do with medical education at Baltimore?" When I admitted that I might be he, Dr. Mackenzie continued, "Well, you are making the biggest mistake in the world." When I protested mildly and asked whether he had a basis for such a statement, he said, "Yes, when I was a medical student, we had a professor who took men out of the clinics and classrooms and put them in the laboratories, even sometimes took them out of wards and put them in the laboratories." I ventured to ask what was the result of this practice. Dr. Mackenzie retorted, "I came out of the medical school knowing no medicine." I interjected, "And knew that you knew none and wished to learn more?" "Yes," he said, "and I wished to learn more." "Then," I said, "Dr. Mackenzie, you have had the finest medical education I have ever heard of."

This interchange measures a great deal of what we are attempting to do at the present time; cram and crowd youngsters with facts. In the last analysis this is not our primary mission. Our approach should be directed toward the basic principles of determining and evaluating evidence. You will recall that William Osler said: "Give him good methods and a proper point of view and all things will be added as his experience grows." In my judgment, it is very important for us to appreciate this basic premise from our vantage point. A special mandate to realize: Principles, principles, principles!

The time changes, the civilian picture becomes more vivid in the discovery of insulin. The opportunity to work with the first commercial product, Iletin, was exploited at Wisconsin. Into my personal care came a physician, Dr. MacLachlan, eighty-four years old, who had graduated when he was forty-two, and had practiced in a small community, McFarland, Wisconsin, for forty-two years. He had a complete heart block and had begun to show signs of cardiac decompensation. To encourage conversation with Dr. MacLachlan I said: "I'm so delighted to hear that your nephew, Dr. Frederick Banting, has won the

Nobel Prize for his discovery of insulin." He said: "Doctor, he is the dumbest of all the Bantings. Mark my word, he'll never discover another thing!" So that your own kin will bring you to your proper level.

The mention of the discovery of insulin takes me back to an interchange with Dr. A. J. Carlson in 1932. We had attended the annual sessions of the American College of Physicians in San Francisco. As we crossed San Francisco Bay on the ferry to Oakland he was in a reminiscent mood, and I asked: "Doctor Carlson, how did you miss insulin?" Here was the experiment: Dr. Carlson had found that if he pancreatectomized a bitch, she developed diabetes mellitus. If the bitch were pregnant when she was pancreatectomized, she would go through her pregnancy until the litter was delivered; and then only after a period of days would she become diabetic. Right in his hands he had the evidence that the litter of puppies in utero was producing something that was sustaining the function of the pancreas in the mother. And he said: "I missed it. Damn fool, blind damn fool." So you have the reaction of an objective scientist who missed an obvious target. Yet Dr. Cannon said, "I never present a paper before the American Physiological Society without waiting to hear Carlson's comments. If he does not discuss it, or if he comments and does not tear the paper to shreds, it is a very successful meeting for me." In other words, he was held in respectful esteem. When he presided at a meeting of the American Physiological Society, a participant reported the results of an experiment on one dog. Then he continued to say that he proposed to carry these experiments further and projected such and such results. He went on to the completion of his fifteen minutes. When he sat down, Dr. Carlson arose and in his devastating manner said: "What we want is more dogs and less words."

On one occasion I was on a visiting faculty at the University of Washington with Dr. Carlson. Obviously he was most restive, moving around in his chair and quite distracted. Finally when he was given the floor, he rushed to the lectern and said: "Gentlemen, gentlemen, I have yust heard of a product of the thyroid gland that is nontoxic. A thyroid extract that is not toxic is yust so much hay, yust so much hay!" That was the honesty and the devastation of Ajax Carlson.

The development of liver therapy and its application to pernicious anemia is a story of great interest. Its evolution has opened new vistas in hematology. I will touch on a single issue. Here was a man, Dr. George R. Minot, who was a severe diabetic, who certainly would have died between the years 1921 and 1926, when with Murphy he discovered the liver treatment of pernicious anemia, had he not had insulin. Dr. Minot was academically bent, *The Inquisitive Physician*, as he was termed by his cousin Rackemann. Dr. Francis Rackemann's biography is interesting; but his cousin's inquisitiveness was even more interesting. Enroute to Atlantic City from Philadelphia for the Association meeting, I engaged him in conversation on an absorbing topic. Beams of Cleveland had suggested that insulin would lower the blood sugar if it were dropped into the eye. This idea attracted Dr. Minot because he was faced with the necessity of injecting himself or having Mrs. Minot give the injections of insulin. I suggested to him that he might try the expedient that the Borgias had used—dropping the poison into the ear of their victims. When at length we came to the salt flats west of Atlantic City, he exclaimed, "Oh, my God, I've got a wife in the other car," and rushed back to find her. He was an intellectual grasshopper to me. No matter when I talked to him, he was always three or four jumps ahead. The story of his application of liver to the treatment of pernicious anemias is noteworthy. Learning of the observations of Whipple and Robscheit-Robbins on the value of liver in the standard anemia dog, he had called in his patients with anemia and had recommended large feedings of liver. To me, he said: "You must have done the same." I replied: "We did the same; but, in any event, we did not come on the same results." Whereupon he said: "I'll show you the first example." He called in a nearby pharmacist, who was quite florid of face. Dr. Minot said to him: "Tell Dr. Middleton just what happened." He said: "Dr. Murphy and Dr. Minot called us in and told us that liver was good for anemia. I like liver and I ate from half to one pound of liver a day. When I came back at the end of a month my red count was up a million and a half. They called me back and asked me just what I had done differently." Herein lay the story. The basic laboratory work of Whipple and Robscheit-Robbins, the prepared mind in Minot and Murphy, a man who liked liver, and the establishment of the efficacy of the liver therapy of pernicious anemia.

The impact of World War II altered the face of medicine. By this time (1941) the medical officer had come to appropriate stature in the military program of the Armed Forces, particularly in the Army where I was privileged to serve. Then, too, there was the opportunity to work intimately with certain leaders in British medicine. I will not regale you with accounts of our fellow countrymen; but I should like to tell you of certain contacts with the British that mark the quality in this particular branch of the profession. In the early days of October 1942, I spelled Colonel Hawley, later General Hawley, in a reception at Christ Church, Oxford, for the American medical officers of the vicinity. Here I met Professor Howard Florey (not yet knighted) who invited me to visit the Dunn Laboratories to see his work on penicillin. I

was naturally anxious to accept his invitation. Colonel Hawley so delegated me. On October 24, 1942, I found Dr. Florey quite concerned and
a little preoccupied. The production of penicillin in the racks of earthen
flasks was obviously at a meager level. In 1941 with Heatley he had
visited the United States and was assured that there would be immediate mass production by our pharmaceutical houses. Instead, in over a
year he had only three samples and they were all of low potency. He
was naturally disillusioned. Yet before I left him he promised two-
thirds of his total production and the instruction of our staff by his wife
for the care of the American troops. The Americans then in combat
were the crews of Flying Fortresses, engaged in high level daylight
bombing. The casualties from these flights had the earliest advantage
of penicillin therapy. In my opinion this is the answer to the objections
to Lend Lease; it was Lend Lease in reverse and we were greatly the
benefactors of Dr. Florey's magnanimity.

Dr. Alexander Fleming was an acquaintance of later date; but we
had several interesting interchanges. I attended a meeting of the Medical Research Council in the School of Tropical Medicine in London
when the work of Raistrich on patulin and the work of Enoch and
Wallerstein on vivicillin were discussed. I never saw this little banty
of a fighting Scotsman so angry. He said: "And they did nae have the
decency to find a root for themselves." In other words they used -cillin
for the root and he felt he had a sort of copyright on that designation.

One of my good British friends was Sir Henry Tidy, who rendered
such splendid service as an organizer and presiding officer of the Inter-
Allied Conferences on War Medicine that did a great deal to dissemi-
nate medical information among the officers of the Allied Forces. On
one occasion I was his dinner guest at the Athenaeum in London. Perhaps the atmosphere was not particularly stimulating; but with a
thought of directing his attention to his favorite subject, glandular
fever, I said: "At Wisconsin we have found the maintenance of a normal platelet count in infectious mononucleosis a good point of differential diagnosis from acute lymphoblastic leukemia, where the platelets
are almost invariably decreased." Sir Henry was silent for a few moments and then said: "Strange, I never thought of it. Can't be too important." It is helpful to have such devaluation from time to time.

And so we might continue to relate the experiences with our medical
counterparts in foreign service. The rapport with the British, Canadi-
ans, Australians, and Norwegians was intimate. Complete confidence
and mutual respect led to professional interchange without reservation.
Gradually the understanding with the French attained a similar level
of cooperative effort. Always with the Russian representatives there

was a reserve that arises in a one-way street. Certain experiences in this area cast their shadows before, and subsequent international events have amply confirmed these first-hand forecasts.

I have attempted to indicate that there are continuous experiences, contacts, and interchanges in our professional lives that mold our careers. The words of Jim Waring, my beloved friend, are particularly cogent in this respect: "Once one has put his hand to the medical plow, he is not fit for the Kingdom of Heaven if he does not ever look forward." Medical education is a continuing process. It does not stop when one is given a diploma at graduation. It continues for the rest of one's life and hopefully with growth. This growth will come in greater measure if one cultivates sound and lasting friendships and if he budgets his time carefully, for this is a precious element. One cannot regain what he lost yesterday. It is most important that when one reads, he read carefully, with design and with direction; that he digests and takes time to assimilate; that he give himself the opportunity for contemplation. The hour out of the twenty-four of the day that is given to contemplation is time well spent. It may be called daydreaming or mere looking into space; they may say you are attempting to see what is beyond the stars. But significantly you are assimilating what you have attempted to digest from the day. It is important that you have sound bodies with your sound minds, which means you will as carefully attend your recreation as you do your study.

"Make no small plans, they have no magic to stir men's souls."

MEDICAL PRACTICE

THE NATURAL HISTORY
OF DISEASE

Appropriately, we are met today to honor the memory of a great clinician and medical statesman, Frank Billings, in Chicago, where his fine professional stature and eminence were attained. In 1878 a sturdy farm lad from Iowa County, Wisconsin, matriculated in the Chicago Medical College (now Northwestern University Medical School). Of splendid Anglo-Saxon stock, he was superbly endowed physically and intellectually. Upon completion of a common public school education, young Billings had attended the Platteville (Wisconsin) State Normal School for two years. Thereafter, he taught a country school in the town of Eden. His prompt advancement to the principalship of the Platteville High School was, in retrospect, a true forecast of his driving ambition and capacity.

Upon graduation from the Chicago Medical College, Dr. Billings served an internship in Cook County Hospital, a coveted post for the young physicians of that period. The investment of postgraduate studies in London, Paris, and Vienna gave his career an impetus that brought him shortly to the forefront of medicine in Chicago. Aside from Dr. Billings's personal attributes, his activities in the introduction of laboratory methods into clinical practice were probably the "open sesame" to his initial success that eventually carried him to a position of preeminence in American medicine.

Dr. Billings was a born leader. He literally dominated every gather-

Presented before the Section on Internal Medicine at the 105th Annual Meeting of the American Medical Association, Chicago, June 12, 1956. Reprinted from the A.M.A. *Archives of Internal Medicine* 98 (October 1956): 401–8.

ing he attended by the force of his presence and personality. Both at Northwestern University Medical School and at Rush Medical College, his efforts brought fruit in the improvement and the expansion of the physical plants. He was particularly effective in enlisting the financial support of wealthy Chicagoans in medical philanthropy. From his vantage point, Dr. Billings led the attack on nostrums and subnormal medical schools. The Council on Pharmacy and Chemistry and the Council on Medical Education and Hospitals of the American Medical Association were natural products of his energetic representations. His thoughts on medical education were especially advanced in the advocacy of the utilization of full- and part-time clinical teachers in an integrated program. His recommendations for the coordination of public and private hospitals in a teaching plan are still valid and might be reviewed with profit in the light of a changing picture. With characteristic prescience, Dr. Billings urged the establishment of a national examining board.

Lest the erroneous impression of an impersonal austerity be gathered from this recital of achievements, it should be recorded that Dr. Frank Billings was fundamentally a warm, kindly man. Physically massive, he was just as large of heart. Out of the abundance of his life and substance he gave unstintingly to every worthy cause. The connotation of the term "builder" that is so regularly applied to Dr. Billings in this community may deprive posterity of a measure of the deep humanity of the man. Rarely are the dominant qualities of accepted leadership so blended with the depth of human sympathy that characterized him. His students, nurses, interns, and associates adored him. Dr. Billings died in his seventy-ninth year (Sept. 20, 1932). His memory is held in reverence by a host of friends, both lay and professional, who were privileged to associate with him in his manifold activities.

DEVELOPMENT OF THE STUDY OF DISEASE

Health is no longer viewed in the negative sense as the mere absence of disease. Health connotes a harmony of mind and body with self and environment. This balance will obtain with the normal activity of every vital and supporting function. The nice adjustments of the body to its surroundings have been grouped under the term homeostasis by Cannon. Selye has extended this concept in his theory of adaptation. The internal milieu of the mammalian body is a complex, ever-changing medium of physical, physiological, and chemical factors so integrated in health as to maintain a sense and a presence of well-being. The present viewpoint, for example, emphasizes the continuous alterations in chemical constituents upon momentary changes in bodily or tissue requirements. Such changes may involve simple chemical reactions, or they may invoke complex physical, enzymatic, and steroid mechanisms. As long as the reserve of the involved elements is adequate, physiological equilibrium may be maintained. To this harmonious balance, the term eucrasia (eucrasy) has been applied.[1] An unnatural imbalance through an exhaustion of the reserves or an inability to meet demands from normal or abnormal sources results in a disturbance of functions. Such disruptions find expression in symptoms and eventually in signs arising from pathological changes in tissues or organs.

From the beginning of recorded time, man has endeavored to interpret the manifestations of disordered function. The concepts reflect the state of human knowledge of a given period. From time to time, medical advance has been impeded by attempts to apply rigid criteria in the grouping of diseases. Nosology has, on occasions, been viewed as an end rather than an instrument in our hands. Indeed, systems of practice have been built on such insecure foundations. With the ascendancy of morbid anatomy and the splendid dividends from clinical-pathological correlations in the early nineteenth century, "dead-house" medicine dominated the scene for a period. In fact, in certain quarters no diagnosis was complete without the autopsy findings! Microbiology came into high estate in the late nineteenth and early twentieth centuries. With its rise came the clinical fixation upon etiology. The last three decades have witnessed an upward surge in the physiological and the physiological-chemical knowledge of bodily reactions in health and disease. The impact of physical, physiological, steroid, enzyme, and nuclear physical-chemical observations on medical thought and practice has been stupendous in recent years and will increase.

In this advance, medicine must never lose sight of fundamental facts. Sydenham wrote: "A disease, however much its cause may be adverse to the human body, is nothing more than an effort of Nature, who strives with might and main to restore the health of the patient by the elimination of morbific matter."[2] In this light, disease must not be considered as an isolated phenomenon nor a series of more or less related phenomena. Man is rarely the passive host of "morbific matter" but reacts more or less violently, dependent upon the nature of the alteration induced locally or generally. Regardless of whether the inciting factor be mi-

1. T. Laycock 1862, "Physiognomical Diagnosis of Disease," *M. Times & Gaz.*, *1*:101.
2. T. Sydenham, *Works*, trans. R. G. Latham, 2 vols. (London: Sydenham Society, 1848–50), 1:29.

crobial, nutritional, metabolic, degenerative, or neoplastic, there are always contributing circumstances in the evolution of the state of inequilibrium termed disease that must be given due consideration in the true comprehension of its natural history.

Within the memory of many physicians still active in the practice of medicine, there have been many radical changes in the mode of infectious diseases and in the clinical expression of specific infections. The exanthems are waning in incidence and severity. Black measles, black scarlet fever, and black smallpox are now only terrifying memories. Diphtheria, with its toll of morbidity and mortality, is largely controlled. Typhoid no longer recurs each summer and autumn to reflect the limitations of sanitation and the contamination of the water (and milk) supply. Lobar pneumonia is a rarity in our teaching hospitals. Suppurative mastoiditis and empyema are relics of a past that medicine would forget. Tuberculosis is losing some of its terror, but it is by no means a vanquished threat to health and life. Syphilis and gonorrhea are more adequately treated than ever before, but the failure to eradicate these diseases reflects the limitations of purely curative medicine. Moreover, man is paying a penalty for the disruption of the biological balance of nature through the introduction of antimicrobial agents. Resistant strains of pathogenic bacteria are appearing. Rickettsial and viral infections have increased with the abatement of bacterial diseases. With the change in the flora of the body under antimicrobial therapy, fungal infections have emerged in increasing frequence.

OBSERVATION AND EXPERIMENTATION

The time for reflection is now at hand. Before the countenance of certain of these diseases has vanished from the earth, we must attempt to commit to the printed record every detail of their course. At best, our observations are fragmentary. The published accounts of diseases too frequently represent the subjective reports of the patient, supplemented by the periodic examinations of the physician. From these bits and pieces, a composite picture is reconstructed. This reproduction is frequently at variance with the autobiographic accounts of physicians suffering from the same disorder. Sydenham's (*Works,* 2:124) account of his own gouty attacks is a classic example of this truth. A physician should be a "minister [or servant] and interpreter of nature" (Hippocrates). By observation and experimentation, medicine must strive to fill the gaps in a comprehensive understanding of the natural history of disease.

Sir Thomas Lewis, while deploring the cleavage, bespoke the separate training of physicians for clinical medicine and for clinical science: "This science seeks, by observation and otherwise, to define diseases as these occur in man; it attempts to understand these diseases and their many manifestations and, here especially, makes frequent use of the experimental method."[3] In his evolution of the thesis, Lewis indicated that two different types of psychological attributes were involved: "Self-confidence is, by general consent, one of the essentials to the practice of medicine, for it breeds confidence, faith and hope. Diffidence, by equally general consent, is an essential quality in investigation, for it breeds inquiry." Obviously, an acceptance of this position would spell a sharp limitation to the observational approach of which Lewis stated: "Eventually, however, the fertility of this method greatly declines by a process of exhaustion and, for those who can read the signs, this time has come in medicine." Trotter voiced a similar reservation thus: "This limitation is the circumstance that the observer must wait upon the natural occurrence of the phenomena he wishes to study. The phenomena may be too infrequent for their significant recurrence to come within the span of human life, they may be too complex and too closely mixed with irrelevant events for the invariable sequence they possess to be detected."[4]

Actually, the contention that observational and experimental skills are incompatible is untenable. The ramifications of the scientific approaches to the study of man in health and disease exceed the capacity of any physician to encompass, much less to apply them to the multitudinous clinical problems with which he is confronted. Wherever possible, these scientific methods must be invoked in the elucidation of covert situations, but a proper sense of proportions must be preserved. Mackenzie said: "When I see the modern cardiologist getting his assistant to take an x-ray photograph of the heart and an electrocardiogram, and even a blood-pressure reading, and then behold him sitting down to study these reports, I am truly amazed. I never could have realized that the practice of medicine could have become so futile and ineffective."[5] Certain of the random chemical probings in the guise of medical practice are even more astounding. Without depreciating these studies one iota, let it be clearly understood that the only individual competent to direct the care of the patient is the physician. If he be

3. T. Lewis 1930, "Observations on research in medicine: its position and its needs," *Brit. M. J.*, 1:479–83.

4. W. Trotter 1930, "Observation and experiment and their use in medical schools," ibid., 2:129–34.

5. J. Mackenzie, quoted in R. M. Wilson, *The Beloved Physician: Sir James Mackenzie* (London: J. Murray, 1926), p. 80.

wise, he will welcome the support of his associates in the basic sciences for coordinate clinical study. From their joint efforts will come a more complete understanding of the patient's problems and more intelligent treatment.

Indeed, out of such cooperative efforts have come material advances in the clinical appreciation of certain disorders in very recent years. Pheochromocytoma was a poorly understood neoplasm until physiologists and pharmacologists clarified the background. Aldosteronism emerged as a distinct clinical entity upon the definition of its steroid responsibility. Agammaglobulinemia awaited electrophoretic fractionation of the serum protein for elucidation of the attendant recurring infections. The unusual symptoms and signs attendant upon carcinoid of the intestinal tract with hepatic metastasis represent an extraordinary example of the interdependence of observation and experimentation in the explanation of disordered function. With Charcot we may say: "Disease is from of old and nothing about it has changed. It is we who change, as we learn to recognize what was formerly imperceptible."

Hence, it behooves the physician to preserve his clinical acumen, as he accepts and extends the application of newer laboratory methods to the study of his patients. Indeed, his position must be fortified from a psychological standpoint to avoid the impersonality of the laboratory. If the physician is to capitalize on this advantage, however, the time is ripe for a new approach to the natural history of disease. With due attention to the experimental and laboratory contribution to this vital subject, there remains a vast area for reexploration and inquiry. John Brown wrote: "Symptoms are universally available; they are the voices of nature."[6] Mackenzie[7] said: "When we search for the recondite and the obscure, we fail to recognize the simple and the obvious." The English school has produced a number of great clinicians in the Hippocratic pattern. Thomas Sydenham said:

> In writing the history of a disease, every philosophical hypothesis whatsoever, that has previously occupied the mind of the author, should lie in abeyance. This being done, the clear and natural phenomena of the disease should be noted—these, and these only. They should be noted accurately, and in all their minuteness, in imitation of the exquisite industry of those painters who represent in their portraits the smallest moles and the faintest spots. No man can state the errors that have been occasioned by these physiological hypotheses (Works, 1:14).

6. J. Brown, *Horae Subsecivae* (Edinburgh: T. Constable & Co., 1858).
7. Quoted in Wilson, *The Beloved Physician.*

Thomas Willis was a true seeker for knowledge, as witnessed in the following statement:

> After I had not found in Books what might satisfy a mind desirous of truth, I resolved with myself to reach into living and breathing examples: and therefore sitting oftentimes by the Sick, I was wont carefully to search out their cases, to weigh all the symptoms and to put them, with exact Diaries of the Diseases into writing; then diligently to meditate on these; and then begin to adapt general notions from particular events.[8]

In a similar spirit, William Heberden afforded the following plan:

> The notes, from which the following observations were collected, were taken in the chambers of the sick from themselves, or from their attendants, where several things might occasion the omission of some material circumstances. These notes were read over every month and such facts as tended to throw any light upon the history of a distemper or the effects of a remedy, were entered under the title of the distemper in another book, from which were extracted all the particulars here given relating to the nature and cure of diseases.[9]

Heberden's account of diabetes serves as an example of the application of his method:

> An unusual thirst is first taken notice of, with a tongue rough and furred, and a bad taste in the mouth; the appetite fails; the pulse is too quick; the strength and flesh waste; the skin is in a burning heat, without the least tendency to sweat; the thirst makes these patients drink immoderately, and of course they make water much more frequently than is common to them, and in much larger quantities, like hysterical persons. . . . The urine in a diabetic is said to have a honey-like sweetness; but, in my judgment, formed upon the most perfect cases of this distemper, it ought in most persons rather to be called insipid; in one joined with a fever, I found it sweetish.[10]

Even more illustrative of Heberden's clinical portraiture is the account of angina pectoris first published in 1768. Indeed, this account may be taken as a proper model for the natural history of disease. Abstracted in essential detail, it reads:

> The seat of it, and sense of strangling and anxiety with which it is attended, may make it not improperly be called angina pectoris.
> They who are afflicted with it, are seized while they are walking (more especially if it be up hill, and soon after eating) with a painful and

8. T. Willis, quoted in C. Symonds 1955, "Circle of Willis (Harveian Oration)," *Brit. M. J.*, 1:119–24.
9. W. Heberden, *Commentaries on History and Cure of Diseases* (London: T. Payne, 1802), pp. vii–viii.
10. Ibid., pp. 141–42.

most disagreeable sensation in the breast, which seems as if it would extinguish life, if it were to increase or continue; but the moment they stand still, all this uneasiness vanishes.

In all other respects, the patients are, at the beginning of this disorder, perfectly well, and in particular have no shortness of breath, from which it is totally different. The pain is sometimes situated in the upper part, sometimes in the middle, sometimes at the bottom of the os sterni, and often more inclined to the left than to the right side. It likewise very frequently extends from the breast to the middle of the left arm. The pulse is . . . not disturbed by this pain. . . . Males are most liable to that disease, especially such as have passed their fiftieth year.

After it has continued a year or more, it will not cease so instantaneously upon standing still; and it will come on not only when the persons are walking but when they are lying down, especially if they lie on their left side, and oblige them to rise up out of their beds. In some inveterate cases it has been brought on by the motion of a horse, or a carriage, and even by swallowing, coughing, going to stool, or speaking, or any disturbance of mind. . . .

Some have been seized while they were standing still or sitting; also upon first waking out of sleep; and the pain sometimes reaches to the right arm, as well as the left, and even down to the hands, but this is uncommon: in a very few instances the arm has at the same time been numbed and swelled. . . .

The termination of the angina pectoris is remarkable. For, if no accidents intervene, but the disease go on to its height, the patients all suddenly fall down, and perish almost immediately. Of which indeed their frequent faintnesses, and sensations as if all the powers of life were failing, afford no obscure intimation.[11]

INFECTIOUS DISEASES

Unfortunately such accuracy of clinical observation is the rare exception in modern medical writings. This deficiency becomes increasingly apparent in the welter of laboratory data, relevant and irrelevant, that so frequently clutters papers in the medical journals. The natural history of the infectious diseases has been reasonably well recorded. Particularly is this true where the etiological agent has been isolated. Contributing to the adequacy of the natural history of the acute infections has been their clear-cut definition and their self-limiting course in many instances. The knowledge of exposure and the routes and portals of entry of the etiological agents has been quite comprehensive. The ability to establish incubation periods, prodromes, symptoms and signs of the fastigium, and the manner of defervescence to convalescence for the acute infectious diseases has lent great impetus to this effort. In most instances, the laboratory has afforded material

11. Ibid., p. 292.

support to the completion of the individual picture. Great hiatuses still exist in the knowledge of susceptibility and immunity. Actually, the advent of the antimicrobial agents, while a great beneficence to humanity, has delayed the attack on some unsolved problems in this area. In the first place, the opportunity to study the natural history of a given bacterial infection is limited by the almost universal administration of antimicrobal agents at the earliest moment. Not infrequently, the broad-spectrum antimicrobial agents have been given on suspicion before the etiology has been established. The vis medicatrix naturae is overlooked in the medical thought of many contemporary physicians. Certainly, Gairdner's admonition is completely outmoded in modern medicine: "There is one stipulation that I must make with those who desire to follow out this inquiry with the view of testing the normal mode of the crisis in typhus fever. It is, that *as many cases as possible should be left to their normal course, unaffected by either drugs or stimulants.*"[12] Assuredly, the effectiveness of the antimicrobial agents in the treatment of lobar pneumonia, typhoid, and a host of other bacterial diseases seriously delimits any prospect of extending the knowledge of their natural history. A further deterrent to advances in this area has been the shifting emphasis in interest and study. This circumstance is doubly unfortunate in the unexplored fringes of this broad field.

CONSTITUTIONAL DISORDERS

The case of the constitutional disorders is much more involved. Many of the factors formerly attributed to heredity are now viewed as environmental and even infectious in origin. The area is wide open for a frontal attack. The degenerative and neoplastic diseases afford a fallow field for this approach. Mackenzie forsook a lucrative practice and an assured future in Harley Street to pursue this angle in St. Andrews, Scotland. He had two objects: "(1) understanding of the mechanism of symptoms, and (2) understanding of their prognostic significance."[13] In his biographer's phrase he urged his contemporaries "to forsake the study of death for that of life."[14] The way is not easy, but the future growth of clinical medicine is inextricably bound with a refinement and a discriminating use of the proved methods of clinical observation. The pathogenesis of atherosclerosis, for ex-

12. T. W. Gairdner, *Physician as Naturalist: Addresses and Memoirs Bearing on History and Progress of Medicine Chiefly During Last Hundred Years* (Glasgow: J. Maclehose & Sons, 1889), p. 165.
13. Mackenzie, quoted in Wilson, *The Beloved Physician*, p. 52.
14. Ibid.

ample, will be more clearly understood when all contributing factors in its initiation are brought into focus and their relative importance fixed. The familial occurrence of vascular degeneration is a commonplace observation, yet heredity has been discredited in some studies and dietary factors have been given increasing responsibility. The exact part of faulty cholesterol metabolism in the ultimate atherosclerotic process is still uncertain. The pendulum is apparently swinging toward a secondary relationship. In developing the natural history of this degenerative disorder, increasing attention must be devoted to the detailed history, with especial reference to the occurrence and the complications of past illnesses, social history, including habits and exposures, family history, and the evolution of the referable complaints. Since physicians have a conspicuous predisposition to atherosclerosis, they might render a conspicuous service by affording clinical autobiographies in this direction. Added to this approach would be the invaluable laboratory studies that anticipate and measure gross changes in pathological physiology. Billings wrote: "Medicine today is applied science. If we utilize the knowledge of today in an attempt to cure and prevent disease, it must also be an experimental science. . . . Experimental medicine must be the means of removing the ignorance which still embraces so many of the maladies which afflict manhood."[15]

Neoplasia arises from so many causes as to render a generic factor difficult of definition. Yet there may prove to be a single basic etiology with a number of variants responsible for the development of specific new growths. Painstaking studies of patients with neoplasms may add materially to our knowledge of their inception and course. Furthermore, especial attention to departures from the rule in apparent susceptibility and resistance to given tumors in certain strains may afford leading clues to the fundamental origin of neoplasia. While great progress has been made in this direction, the clinician is woefully deficient in the tools for the early recognition of a majority of visceral tumors. Surface or accessible neoplasms will receive early and appropriate attention in most instances, but carcinoma of the pancreas, for example, has usually reached an inoperable stage when surgery is proposed. Deep-seated upper abdominal pain radiating to the back, painless progressive jaundice, sudden diabetes mellitus in individuals past forty-five years of age, and unexplained phlebothrombosis are late manifestations of carcinoma of the pancreas. Yet they may be the first symptoms or signs that bring the patient to the physician. Frequently,

---

15. F. Billings 1903, "Medical education in the United States," *J.A.M.A.,* 40: 1271–76.

cachexia has already become manifest. In a few patients, vague upper abdominal discomfort, coupled with marked introspection and nervousness, has anticipated frank symptoms and signs of carcinoma of the pancreas by months in our experience. In carcinomatous involvement of the head of the pancreas, melena, occult or overt, may be a guidepost. In such instances, roentgenologic confirmation may be anticipated. The chemical studies directed toward the quantitation of the digestive ferments of the external secretion of the pancreas afford little support to the early diagnosis of carcinoma. Here, then, lies one of the unsolved mysteries of medicine whose solution may be expedited by an "exact Diary of the Disease." Its parallels are innumerable.

If Hippocrates be forgiven his sententious vein, the following quotation affords an excellent argument for a profound knowledge of the natural history of disease:

> And he will manage the cure best who has foreseen what is to happen from the present state of matters. For it is impossible to make all the sick well; and this, indeed, would have been better than to be able to foretell what is going to happen; but since men die, some even before calling the physician, from the violence of the disease, and some die immediately after calling him, having lived, perhaps, only a day or a little longer, and before the physician could bring his art to counteract the disease; it therefore becomes necessary to know the nature of such affections, how far they are above the power of the constitution; and, moreover, if there be anything divine in the diseases, and to learn a foreknowledge of this also. Thus a man will be the more esteemed to be a good physician, for he will be better able to treat those aright who can be saved, from having long anticipated everything; and by seeing and announcing beforehand those who will live and those who will die, he will thus escape censure.[16]

Obviously, prognosis is a vital element in the practice of medicine. Its cultivation and acquisition are avidly pursued by all clinicians worthy of the name. Recently, Bloomfield wrote a cogent editorial on the subject, in which he evaluated the factors in deriving such conclusions. With experience, he stated: "the analytical process may become lightning fast and indeed may be largely carried on subconsciously. The young doctor, however, may well profit by deliberately taking into account the various factors in prognosis . . . and by making a conscious analysis of the situation in case of his patients. Such a running of mental scales will help develop later virtuosity."[17] With incisive in-

16. *Genuine Works*, trans. Francis Adams, 2 vols. (New York: W. Wood & Co., 1886), 1:194–95.

17. A. L. Bloomfield 1956, "Prognosis, editorial," *A.M.A. Arch. Int. Med.*, 97: 267–68.

sight, Ryle remarked: "Prognostic ability is born largely of pathology and patiently gathered clinical experience. It evolves even more slowly than diagnostic ability. Minute and careful clinical observation, a good visual memory, and that necessary inquisitiveness about the subsequent course of cases which is nowadays systematized in the follow-up inquiry may all be numbered among the handmaidens of prognosis."[18]

CONCLUSIONS

In a word, there is no royal road to success in the prognosis of human disease. Feeble though the reed may appear when tested by strict scientific standards, the patient or the family may properly expect general information as to the probable course of a given illness from the physician. Fortified by extended experience and careful study of the problems presented by the patient, the true natural historian, supported by discriminating laboratory studies, will become increasingly proficient and accurate in assembling the evidence for the diagnosis and prognosis. Futhermore, with a sound basic knowledge of the natural history of disease, he will not fall into the uncritical habit of therapeutic sophistry, but, with a broad perspective, his therapy will have direction and his conclusions of its effectiveness will reflect measured judgment.

"Sit down before fact as a little child, be prepared to give up every preconceived notion, follow humbly wherever and to whatsoever abysses nature leads, or you shall learn nothing" (Huxley).

18. J. Ryle, *Natural History of Disease* (2nd ed., London: Oxford University Press, 1948), p. 422.

MEDICAL PRACTICE:
A CASE REPORT

The literary allusions to medicine and its practitioners have been a part of your educational heritage. You will not have been misled by the fulsome praise that elevates the practitioner beyond his human limitations. Conversely, as you have read the works of Voltaire, George Bernard Shaw, and others, you have come to realize that barbs have been directed toward our profession for centuries past. They will undoubtedly continue. However, it is an unusual circumstance that the present time finds medicine and medical science of a stature never before conceived, yet confronted by an attitude of the laity that holds the profession at large in questioned status and the individual practitioner in deep respect. Phrased mildly, medicine does not have a kindly press. Moreover, in the United States the military draft affects the physician at an age period beyond that of the ordinary citizen. By reason of the medical demands of the services, a further discrimination is observed in the call-up of physicians. Nor has medicine fared well in the political arena. Assuming that voluntary health insurance is not an adequate means to meet the medical requirements of the aging population, compulsory insurance has now become a political chess match and the aging ill or disabled citizen the pawn. Certain of the most pressing problems of the present congress center about this issue. One element of government advocates compulsory health insurance under

Presented to members of the third-year class at the University of Oklahoma School of Medicine during an Interdepartmental Conference in 1964. Reprinted from *Oklahoma State Medical Association Journal* 62 (June 1969): 236–39.

the Social Security Program closely patterned after the systems of Great Britain and countries of Europe.

Medicine has been placed in a compromised position in its Fabian policy toward social reform. The American Medical Association early opposed prepayment health insurance. Hospitalization insurance was also resisted by this body. In the early 1930s during the depression, I encountered an amusing change of attitude midstream. With the general counsel of the Wisconsin State Medical Society, I was scheduled to speak before the Portage County Medical Society in Stevens Point, Wisconsin. As we traveled north my friend offered many arguments against the acceptance of the delivery fee of $35.00 by physicians from federal sources. The program had been developed in the interest of maternal welfare. He stated that he had been instructed by the American Medical Association to denounce this governmental subsidy of medical practice. After he had presented his case before the Portage County Medical Society, the secretary of that group arose and said: "Gentlemen, I would like to read you a letter that I have just received from the American Medical Association, which says that physicians of the country at large should get behind this movement and accept fees from the federal government for the delivery of mothers at the rate of $35.00." I cite this as concrete evidence of a short-sighted attitude of organized medicine under specific conditions in the past.

My remarks are directed to you, because you are the medical leaders of the future and must be acquainted with some of the factors that have contributed to the deterioration of our public and personal relations. You have had much information regarding the shortage of physicians. At one time in Wisconsin, had I been given the authority to move fifty physicians from overcrowded urban areas on Lake Michigan to points of inadequate professional coverage, we could have had a physician within twenty miles of any habitation in the state. Obviously under these circumstances, the problem was one of distribution and not numbers. In a constructive sense, efforts should be made to afford adequate distribution as well as total numbers of physicians. When you are ultimately considering your permanent scene of practice, you will take into account many factors besides the actual professional advantage of a given location. In this respect I would earnestly advise you to make your wife a complete partner in the selection of your permanent home and the site for your medical career. Then, too, the availability of physicians must be a primary consideration, both from an altruistic and an ulterior standpoint. The conventional habit of an afternoon or a weekend off will depend upon the practice of the community; but, whatever may be the custom, under no circumstance should it impose a hardship upon any member of the community requiring medical service. By the same token, in the interest of personal health and hygiene, the physician is ill-advised who does not arrange for a periodic surcease from his practice. Mutual interest has led to arrangements for available coverance when the physician himself is not on call. In one neighboring state, however, over 60 percent of the private practice outside of hospitals is in the hands of osteopaths. To my dismay, as I have traveled through a prosperous farming area of Wisconsin, upon death or retirement regular physicians have been replaced by chiropractors or osteopaths. Furthermore, in certain communities, chiropractors advertise: "I Make Night Calls."

Some years ago, Dr. Sheldon, a revered practitioner over eighty years old, came into the Madison General Hospital weary and bedraggled one morning. Upon meeting several of the young physicians in the doctors' dressing room, there was the general query: "Well, what's up, Grandpa?" He answered: "This morning a little mother called me at three o'clock and said her baby was sick with the colic. She did not know what to do about it and had called four or five physicians who were not available." Red faces went about the circle. Doctor Sheldon continued: "When I got there, the baby really needed attention; but the mother was generous. She said the other physicians doubtless had other calls to make." The lesson to be drawn from this episode is that, were the patients or their families able completely to interpret the symptoms of illness, there would frequently be little occasion for professional advice. You must not neglect your duty in the care of the individual patient who will be your responsibility of the future.

Much of the deterioration of personal relationships has been laid to the rapid spread of specialization and to group practice. In neither instance is there a valid basis for these charges. Specialization does not eliminate personal professional responsibility. Group practice must not become impersonal, lest it destroy the foundations of clinical practice. A given individual within the group should assume continued responsibility for the immediate care of the given patient, whatever may be the requirements for consultation.

With the tremendous scientific resurgence of our day, there is an increasing tendency to lean upon the laboratory in deriving answers to our clinical problems. In fact, the laboratories have made cowards of us all. When we deal profoundly in milliequivalents and millimols, let us not lose sight of the true object of our study . . . the party of the first part, the patient. Confronted by difficult clinical problems we would do well to keep our patient advised of the direction and significance of proposed studies. Let us never be deluded by random probing. This practice has atrophy of discernment as its first byproduct. My appeal is for thoughtful, directional laboratory studies to supplement and extend clinical observations. In this frame of reference, not only is the vital function of the laboratory protected, but the attending physician grows in professional stature.

With the growing lay interest in medical advances, there has been a radical change in the dissemination of medical knowledge. Newspapers, magazines, and periodicals of every order respond to the demands for such information by articles of varying weights and measures. While much of the contained technical data is beyond the ken of the average layman, his appetite will not be satisfied by bland commonplaces or overt evasion. A considerable body of science writers has arisen in our midst, and many of the articles in the lay press are well written and factually accurate. As physicians we will do well to adjust ourselves to the changing pattern. The day is past when the physician may set himself aside, write a prescription in illegible Latin, and alienate himself from the patient by assuming that the patient and his family are incapable of appreciating properly tempered medical information.

An important lesson in reverse may be drawn from a consultation on a famous patient whose two physicians related the following contrasting reactions to me. Sir John Parkinson, the eminent cardiologist of London, beamed with satisfaction as he told me of his recent consultation on Sir Winston Churchill with Lord Moran. A few days later, my surprise was great when Lord Moran said: "Middleton, I had John Parkinson see Winston Churchill the other day and he took an hour and a half, or two hours, for the job. As you would expect, it was a thorough going examination; but when he got through he did not say a word to Winston regarding his condition. When I returned to see Winston, he said, 'What goes here? Parkinson spent an hour and a half examining me; and, when he was finished, he did not tell me a blasted thing!'" Clearly silence may limit or destroy your usefulness. In contact with the patient, remember that he is the party of the first part and should have as much information as he can assimilate usefully in cooperative therapy. In this partnership there should be only a reservation as to the elimination of information that may harm or seriously discourage the patient. We must not alienate the patient by the use of high sounding technical phrases without imparting a clear picture of the underlying basis of his symptoms or disabilities.

Perhaps one of the most serious factors in disaffection between the patient and the physician is financial. Traditionally physicians are poor businessmen. While I would not perpetuate this unfortunate circumstance, by the same token I would be disappointed were the monetary objective the primary motivation of your generation in medicine. The servant is worthy of his hire and I bespeak for all of you a secure and comfortable income during your careers in medicine. This hope for your future does not include the biggest house or the biggest car in town. Do not attempt to live up to the Joneses. In the opinion of some, the apparent disproportional income of certain physicians has set our profession apart from the mass. This situation, that renders us more vulnerable to criticism, should lead us to condemn all irregularities in practice. The image of medicine has been seriously impaired by fee-splitting and phantom surgery.

After we have diagnosed certain of the ills of medical practice, as physicians we naturally look to their prognosis and treatment. The recognition of ill health by the patient is the first step toward its treatment. Since our profession is held sub judice by a questioning public, we must take steps to remedy the situation. It has been a source of deep satisfaction to find that many of the circumstances that I have outlined have been recognized and treated in your community. The coming generation in medicine must take its place in society as servants, not masters. The time is long past when physicians can assume that they have the exclusive vested interest in health. This commodity affects the entire population and problems of health must be met by all of the social agencies that can assure its maintenance. In 1909 Dr. Henry Baird Favill said: "The pathology of society is as much the responsibility of the medical man, as is the pathology of disease." In a word, you cannot divorce disease from the patient, the family, the community. Its total impact on the social fabric may be all pervasive and overwhelming. Instead of maintaining our archaic attitude of responsibility for the sick person alone, we must perforce accept the partnership of all who are affected in the family and community. In a word, this is a two-way process and the ecology of disease involves intimately its sociologic origins and impacts. While at the bedside there is a single person in whom you are interested; before the total picture can be clarified you must know the influence of the personal contacts, family life, industrial and social exposures on the patient who is the present subject of your study.

Granting these circumstances, as you enter the practice of medicine, you will have reconstructed your approach and prospect with the broader concept of the place of medicine in the social fabric. You will maintain the intimacy of the patient-physician relationship by encouraging intelligent interchange relative to the patient's status, progress and prognosis. A few extra minutes of conversation at the bedside or in the office may be as revealing to you as it is comforting to the patient. One of the conspicuous psychological byproducts of illness is the increased need for support. Without maudlin sentimentality, rapport with the sick may be a determining factor in the restoration of health. A number of years ago, the Colorado Medical Society initiated a movement that has spread to cover the entire country. At the county or community level, a grievance committee receives and resolves complaints of varying orders; but, psychologically their influence is much broader in affording the public a forum for resolving differences with our profession. The solutions to personal and financial difficulties can be derived by the application of a common ethical code. In many of the issues that we have raised, the direct answer lies in a considerable measure in the compassionate heart. At times it is the difference between health and disease, life and death. Francis Peabody once said: "The secret of the care of the patient is in caring for the patient." In the clear conception of your opportunity and responsibility of the future, you will maintain the credo that "Medicine exists for the benefit of the afflicted, not the afflicted for the benefit of medicine."

THE PATIENT–PHYSICIAN
RELATIONSHIP

"The art consists in three things—the disease, the patient and the physician. The physician is the servant of the art, and the patient must combat the disease along with the physician." This relationship is as vital to good medical practice today as it was when Hippocrates expounded it in 400 B.C. Since the accepted thesis implies a bilateral responsibility, its logical analysis must begin with an objective survey of the respective places of the contracting parties. If we begin with the patient we may assume that disquieting or disabling symptoms have led him to seek the professional service of a physician. From this moment a chain reaction is initiated which may result in the closest rapport or, conversely, in misunderstanding and recrimination.

Let us view the patient from a detached standpoint. Beset by unfamiliar evidences of disordered function, he seeks the advice of a physician. We trust that this medical counselor may establish easy rapport since the patient is constitutionally a selfish individual. Essentially introspective, the patient becomes very egocentric in the presence of pain or less obvious symptoms, to which he naturally ascribes the most serious explanation. Of course, there are notable exceptions to this major tenet. In fairness to the thousands of sufferers who bear adversity, pain, and disability bravely, may I say I wish their fortitude and forbearance might have a wider audience than the devoted families and physicians who gain inspiration and strength from their glowing examples. Whatever may be the factors involved, Parkinson strikes

Reprinted from *The Wisconsin Medical Journal* 54 (June 1955): 288–92.

the proper note when he says: "Confidence is the hallmark of the good patient." The very existence of this sense of dependence constitutes a sacred trust to the medical profession. As Parkinson states: "Truly the best [patients] will keep faith when things go wrong, and what a stimulus that firm trust can be." Indeed, to the conscientious physician, its implied ramifications may be almost overwhelming.

The physician, as a party of the second part, has been born to a life of human service. His adjustments to the individual psychology are the reflection of a natural acceptance of his role as an adviser. Appreciating the profound concern of the patient, he will avoid any attitude or expression that may augment or fix fears. Whatever may be his natural reaction to a grave situation, he will steel his nerve and discipline his vasomotor and facial controls to dissemble his concern. Remembering that the patient is basically a human being, he will maintain those contacts that reflect his immediate personal interest. However profound may be his scientific background, the physician will do well to remember that patience, sincere kindliness, and forbearance will weigh much more heavily in the balance of reciprocal understanding than the most comprehensive knowledge of isolated scientific data. Parkinson expressed this thought: " 'And whosoever shall compel thee to go a mile, go with him twain.' The good physician will accompany his patient on the second mile and to the end of the road." As John Brown wrote: "that gentleness and compassion for his suffering fellowmen without which no man need hope to be a great physician."

Obviously, the traditional patient-physician relationship has undergone a serious deterioration within recent years; but the movement is not new. Superficial observers have found medicine an easy prey through the ages. Voltaire wrote: "A physician is one who pours drugs of which he knows little into a body of which he knows less." In a more constructive vein, Plato said: "For this is the great error of our day in the treatment of the human body, that physicians separate the soul from the body." This theme is repeated in the quotation from the contemporary Eduard Rist: "How many errors have been committed because the physician has not been able to discern, behind the masque of the invalid, a man." Although the feckless rantings of self-appointed judges, without and within the profession, have shaken the temple of medicine from time to time, certain events suggest an augmentation of discord and a perceptible weakening of the public support of medicine within recent years. Significantly, many serious students of the subject trace the acceleration of the decline of the patient-physician relationship to the ascent of the curve of specialization after World War I. Simultaneous increases in group practice are given a share of the blame by some observers. The inevitable outcome of these movements in the interest of improved professional service has been a decrease in general practitioners.

Before ascribing a causal relationship of this modern trend to the deterioration of professional relationships and the consequent sacrifice of public support, let us carry the inquiry a bit deeper. Medicine is clearly on the defensive. We have openly been charged with reducing the output of our medical schools in the interest of a monopoly of services. The decision of a high court of the land has found medicine to be a trade. Hospitalization insurance was belatedly accepted by organized medicine as a sound economic policy after a delaying action of several years. Voluntary health insurance followed on its heels. Discriminatory action in the registration of physicians up to fifty years old is enforced by Selective Service. The draft beyond the legal age limit applies only to medicine. Federalization of medicine has become a national issue.

Perhaps we would do well to look to some of the sources of individual disaffection and frank opposition to medicine. A lack of geographic coverage is perhaps a more cogent basis of serious criticism of the medical situation in this country than the numerical inadequacy of physicians. Admitting the wider sphere of activity of the modern physician by reason of improved facilities, roads, and transportation, there remain certain areas, usually marginal in economic, social, and educational outlets, in all states without adequate medical coverage. The local community and the responsible representatives of medicine have not realistically resolved their mutual problem (and responsibility) about a common board. Indeed, as in many other areas of public welfare, the physician has too frequently been the led rather than the leader.

An ominous answer to the withdrawal of regular practitioners of medicine from the rural areas is appearing widely over the country. Through the years my duties have taken me into a prosperous agricultural district of Wisconsin. From time to time an older physician has retired or died in one of the small towns along this highway. In each instance his place has been taken by an irregular practitioner, i.e., osteopath or chiropractor. In one of our neighboring states over half the country practice is in the hands of osteopaths. Heed well the signs at the crossroads. The affection of the people lies close to the hearthstones of their homes.

In urban communities, in the interest of preserving a semblance of hygienic life, physicians have placed a limit upon their office hours and have attempted to free an afternoon or a day for rest or recreation.

Such a protective device is universally applied in all trades and professions; yet a hue and cry goes up when the physician seeks surcease from his daily tasks. What would occur were a forty-hour week decreed for or by medicine? Seriously, until very recently no assurance of medical coverage was given. With characteristic rugged individualism, each physician went his way—and the devil (or the chiropractor and osteopath) took the patient!

With the stupendous growth of medical knowledge, a premium has been placed upon technical details. In the approach of the physician, the etiology of disease apparently replaced the personal interest in the human host of the disorder. At the same time the public was afforded a certain measure of information on medical matters through the press and radio that prepared him for closer rather than more removed professional confidences. Naturally he resented being treated as a human test tube or the innocent vehicle of interesting scientific findings. The physician in honest absorption in the clinical problem overlooked that essential to sound medical practice; namely, an understanding heart. Unfortunately, finances raised their ugly head to mar the idealistic tradition of medical disregard for material reward. While altruism in medicine has always been a cherished and natural inclination, the exploitation of the physician's weakness in monetary matters has not redounded to the credit of the profession. The reaction of recent years has been even more distressing. Two children, eight and nine, respectively, were riding in the rear seat of an automobile through a small Wisconsin town, when one said flatly: "That's the doctor's house." "How do you know that?" queried the other. "Why, it's the biggest one in town," she answered. Try the test in your own community and then ask why medicine has become the singular target of criticism. Not only is this factor a dominant argument, but it has become a boomerang in our efforts to obtain adequate support for medical education.

To this important question must be attached the very devastating practices of fee-splitting and "ghost" surgery, since they have their roots in the mire of unethical financial arrangements between physicians who have wandered far from the basic precept of our profession: "Medicine exists for the benefit of the afflicted, not the afflicted for the benefit of medicine." To traffic in human suffering is as immoral as it is unethical. To these financial excesses and irregularities medicine owes much of its current difficulties. However, let it be clearly understood—the whole profession suffers from the sins of a few who should be unmercifully exposed in their infamous pursuits.

Although many patients have a fragmentary knowledge of their medical conditions, they are almost devoid of knowledge of the devices that medicine has through the centuries developed for their protection. Psychologically, complete frankness on the part of the physician may render him a serious liability to the sensitive patient. Rarely is absolute candor helpful to the desperately ill patient. Contrary to the recently expressed thesis, few patients can really take it when the cards are down. We must "temper the wind to the shorn lamb." I hasten to add that a responsible member of the family must always be apprised of the true situation. "He is the best physician who is the best inspirer of hope." Careful explanations of the probable course of events will often prepare the patient and the family for unanticipated reverses or delays in convalescence. Appropriate consultations are a measure of strength, not weakness. Moreover, pains in explaining the place of records and x-ray films may spare both contracting parties discomfiture at a later date. Legally, such records are not owned by the patient; the physician is the trustee or custodian of a constructive trust in which the patient is the real beneficiary, but the latter has no proprietary rights.

Having in some measure outlined the problem, let us turn to the prognosis. Frankly, without a reconciliation of the differences, individual and collective, between the public and the medical profession, the prospect of reclaiming lost ground is remote. Serious consideration must be given to the primary advantage of the reestablishment of such rapport; namely, an assured improvement of medical care. Selfish and ulterior motives are unworthy and predicate the ultimate defeat of our aims. Medical economics translated into terms of personal advantage has carried our profession far from its objective. With prompt and adequate treatment, medicine may reclaim its lost ground and rise to new heights in the public esteem.

If you have accepted these tenets, American medicine in its most vaunted position of scientific advancement is socially ill. Its neighbors at the common board look askance at our manners and behavior. Before a patient can be treated effectively, he must admit that he is not well. The first step in treatment thereafter is a rededication of medicine to the service of humanity. Short of this fervid declaration of faith, no disciple of medicine is worthy of his calling. Since general practice constitutes over 80 percent of medical service, it must be given the dignity in the medical family that it merits. These worthy practitioners have manned the ramparts and outposts of medicine from the beginning of historical time. The fawning attention paid to their essential functions by "Johnnies-come-lately" in frock coats and dinner jackets on appropriate occasions must be revolting to the thoughtful physicians in general practice, who until recently were supposed to find full sustenance in the crumbs from the tables of the mighty. If these newly found friends in the profession be really serious, may I suggest that they find sections in their state medical societies and staff positions in their hospitals for these worthy fellow physicians. As family counselors, they will grow in numbers and usefulness with just a modicum of sympathetic support from the profession at large. Since specialization has been responsible in a considerable measure for the shrinkage of medical coverage in smaller communities, the expedient of requiring an apprenticeship of one to two years of general practice before admittance to a residency or fellowship might well fill this hiatus. From such an exposure would come the natural byproduct of improved patient-physician relationship among specialists. To those who elect general practice as a career, facilities should be made available to practice medicine on a modern plane. A health center or a cottage hospital with a minimal auxiliary staff would enable a young physician to maintain standards of medical service commensurate with his training. Associate practice, involving the pooling of resources, material and professional, of two or more young men has operated satisfactorily in certain removed areas of Wisconsin.

The necessity for twenty-four-hour coverage would seem too obvious to require comment. Yet the failure to afford medical service upon enforced absence has constituted a major breach with the public. Tradition has given to the young members of the profession the prerogative of night calls. In many communities this formula is no longer considered a natural entrée to practice. Indeed, in some of our Wisconsin towns the older practitioners are more responsive than their juniors to these importunities. Regardless of the unreasonable nature of many of these interruptions of one's rest, we must remember that the layman is not equipped to give sound judgment in such situations, else there would be no need for physicians. In some towns of my acquaintance, osteopaths and chiropractors advertise that *they* answer night calls. A word to the wise!

The medical profession must take a positive stand on the financial activities of its fellows. The Principles of Ethics of the American Medical Association read: "The prime object of the medical profession is to render service to humanity; reward or financial gain is a subordinate consideration." The fees of family counselors have not risen proportionately to the general economic scale or the cost of living. On the other hand, fabulous incomes have been derived in certain of the specialties without justification upon grounds other than the ability of the patient to pay. The sliding scale has been defended upon the specious contention that the rich pay for the poor. These modern Robin Hoods have made state medicine seem a natural solution to many superficial students of the subject. As one writer states, the defense that the wealthy man's life is worth so much more constitutes "biologic blackmail." Fee-splitting is openly condemned and secretly condoned in certain quarters. If medicine does not clean house, a Kefauver will do it for us. As slimy as is this practice, "ghost surgery" offers even greater potential danger to the patient, who neither sees nor knows the surgeon who sells his mechanical skill and moral integrity for a price. Medicine cannot survive these subversive practices. Incubuses on our moral fibers, either they are sloughed off or we perish.

Fortunately, medicine has come to realize that the public has a place in the consideration of its own welfare. In 1947, Colorado instituted the grievance committee to which patients and the public in general were invited to bring their complaints. Notices to this effect were placed in physicians' offices and in the public press. At first the "crackpots" and psychoneurotics dominated the scene. Then sound criticisms were received and promptly considered at the community (county) level. Financial misunderstandings were not common. The plan has spread over the country, and the results have justified the effort. Not the least of the favorable effects of its operation has been an improvement in professional relations. Medicine has opened its doors to the direct criticism of its constituent members.

George Bernard Shaw exclaimed: "Independence? That's middle-class blasphemy. We are all dependent on one another, every soul of us on earth." Medicine has maintained a position aloof from the body politic. We have been conservative to the point of isolationism in our reactions to social responsibility. "The time is already here where to be only a practicing physician is a discredit. Not only has the medical profession to furnish its full quota to the army of social service but in many respects it must point out the way. The pathology of society is as much the function of the medical man as the pathology of human disease." This pronouncement did not come from Soviet Russia or socialistic Britain yesterday, but from Chicago in 1909. Henry Baird Favill, a distinguished physician with a large and wealthy clientele, was addressing the alumni of Rush Medical College. His challenge has passed unheeded in the main because medicine and medical men are still more interested in curative than preventive measures. Posterity will acclaim the prophet Favill years hence. But our objective is none the less clear. Before a truly effective job in preventive medicine can be done, medicine must align itself with the social forces now assembling to limit or eliminate the hereditary, nutritional, environmental, and occupational factors in the production of disease and disability.

Medicine has been backward in fostering so-called public relations. In recent years, press-radio conferences have been encouraged at state and county levels. Many of the fancied differences may be resolved about a round table, when the common objective of the public weal is met by the participating representatives. Furthermore, such gatherings afford the opportunity for the education of an important source of lay information on medical matters. In such details as privileged information from a medical standpoint, there is a woeful lack of understanding by the fifth estate. Time was when the physician was the center of civic activities. This position obtains only in smaller communities today and, significantly, in the person of the general practitioner. Physicians would render the profession, as well as the public, a superior service by active participation in voluntary health forums and other civic projects in the interest of the advancement of community health and happiness.

To reclaim the enviable patient-physician relationship of the past, we must maintain an interest in the patient as a human being. Let him never feel that his misfortune is your intellectual or financial gain. Share that portion of your knowledge of his condition as he should understand in the interest of cooperative therapeutics. The psychological lift may be a determining factor in the battle—and he *is* the party of the first part. In this day the design of detailed laboratory tests may be imparted; but it must never imply abysmal doubt to be resolved only by random probing. Prognosis is a most unfaithful ally. Yet cautiously used with a background of wide experience, an accurate forecast of a clinical disorder brings great dividends of confidence and cooperation. As previously indicated, in all serious conditions some dependable member of the family must share the burden of knowledge of the gravity of an illness. It is axiomatic that the survival of a loved one for whom an unfavorable prognosis has been given is a happy circumstance; but rarely is a fatal termination overlooked when a favorable prospect has been vouchsafed. The thoughtful physician will maintain contact after the discharge of a patient, especially if the illness has been serious or protracted. In larger institutions and communities, social service will maintain this continuity; but I submit that this important agency must be an instrument, not the end to our design. Preferably, by personal telephone call or note, the physician may manifest his interest in the patient's progress—without fee! In no other manner may patient-physician relationship be more solidly cemented.

Maimonides (1135–1204), the great Jewish physician, left one of the gems of medical literature in his prayer. Engraved on the heart of every physician should be his words: "Let me see in the sufferer the man alone. . . . Let me be intent upon one thing, O Father of Mercy,

to be always merciful to Thy suffering children." Rededicated to service
to humanity and stripped of mysticism and pomposity, medicine will
take its proper place in the social fabric. In mutual confidence and
respect, medicine will be restored to its lost estate as the most humane
and affective agent for the advancement of mankind.

THE HUMAN TOUCH
IN MEDICINE

To me this is a memorable and an arresting occasion. The
Wisconsin Society of Internal Medicine has flouted convention on several scores. In the first place, our Society has voted to initiate a lecture-
ship named for a fellow member. Furthermore, this member is still
living. Then, to complete the cycle of nonconformity, the named member has been invited to give the first lecture. If I appear to be speaking
to myself, I know you will understand and will be indulgent. I am
truly appreciative of the honor and distinction you, my friends, bestow
upon me and I will discharge my responsibility to the best of my ability.

René Sand wrote that "the place of medicine is in the stream of life—
not on its banks." In recent months many thoughtful people have been
preoccupied with the development and the fate of earth satellites. For
some time the Veterans Administration has been studying the application of electronic data processing to its operational and research activities. The analog and digital computers are being utilized to resolve some
of the problems in spatial vectorcardiography. Conditioned by this
background, the invitation of International Business Machines, Inc.
(IBM) to a private demonstration of a model of Vanguard by their
experts was eagerly accepted. Absorbing as was the project for the
exploration of space, my attention was diverted by a statement of one
of our scientific guides: "Do not think me completely mad, Doctor,
when I say that some day the electronic data processing machine will

The First William S. Middleton Lecture of the Wisconsin Society of Internal
Medicine, presented September 20, 1958, at Janesville. Reprinted from *The Wisconsin Medical Journal* 58 (September 1959): 553–56.

prove useful in answering questions in the diagnosis and the treatment of obscure clinical conditions."

The natural reaction of the clinician was, "fanciful, visionary, preposterous." I parried: "Abrams had the same idea. One fed a few superficial facts into an electrical machine which returned the diagnosis and treatment." The physicist admitted that the data afforded the highly developed electronic data processing machine must perforce be accurate and tailored to meet the assumptions of an adequate answer. In other words, the product is determined by that which human intelligence supplies at the intake. Even granting the psychologic and the physiologic variables in a biologic subject he maintained that the objectivity of the procedure would one day determine its availability and utilization in clinical medicine.

This expert is not alone in his contention. Indeed, the literature on this phase of electronic data processing and its projection is growing. "And coming events cast their shadows before" (Campbell). Electronic methods have, in fact, infiltrated widely in experimental and clinical medicine. They have, for example, replaced the silvered glass string in the electrocardiographic apparatus. It is no longer a string galvanometer. The phonocardiogram has reinforced auscultation of the heart. The cathode ray oscilloscope has broad applications in physiologic and clinical studies. The electron microscope extends the range of visibility 30,000 to 100,000 times. The expansion of the several branches of chemistry in their application to research and clinical medicine has been especially conspicuous. The spectrophotometer is indispensable in the routine laboratory. The flame photometer extends its range for the determination of sodium and potassium levels in the serum. The color strips in paper electrophoresis are resolved into an amazingly accurate curve by the analytrol. Colorimetric methods have been refined by electronic devices. Newer electronic developments now bid fair to replace the hemocytometer in blood counts. Extending the base, radioisotopes have come to occupy an assured place in medical research and practice. Labelled iodine, chromium, cobalt, and iron have proved especially useful in diagnosis. Radioisotopes of iodine, gold, and phosphorus have recognized therapeutic positions in the modern practice of medicine.

"Keeping an open mind is like keeping an open mouth. Sometimes you have to shut it in order to chew and survive" (Chesterton).

Out of the mechanization of certain phases of medical practice has grown the natural suggestion that its basic evaluation might be accomplished by appropriate mathematical means. Yet recent efforts to assess the quality of medical care solely on objective criteria have fallen far short of their mark. The clinical records have regularly been utilized as source materials. The adequacy of histories and physical examinations, intelligent utilization of laboratories, diagnostic accuracy, therapeutic and operative results, complications and mortality figures have afforded much food for thought and projection. By common consent among students of the subject, the medical audit remains an incomplete and inadequate instrument for the exact measurement of the actual care rendered the individual patient. With all the advantages of statistical methodology applied to modern medicine, this approach in the evaluation of the quality of medical care has proved incapable of general application. Its material contribution has been the stimulation of self-analysis. However wide may be the ultimate acceptance of its tenets, there is no prospect of the quantitation of the quality of medical care that can be universally applied to the individual patient.

The students of this important subject must look to the evolution of modern medicine for the explanation of this elusive circumstance. From the earliest accounts of medicine elemental fear of supernatural forces dominated the prevailing concepts of disease and its control. The propitiation of beneficent spirits was invited by votive offerings. Magic and amulets were invoked to fend the forces of evil. Medicine was subordinated to religion in India and Egypt. Greek culture separated these elements; but Hippocrates, the father of medicine, was an Asclepiad. The priests at the temple of Asclepius enjoined the incubation sleep before administering to the sick and disabled. The inception of modern medicine, as currently recognized, may properly be dated from the French school of the late eighteenth and nineteenth centuries. Bichat emphasized the bedside-deadhouse correlation of disease manifestations as a most rewarding medium for the advancement of clinical knowledge. Corvisart, physician to Napoleon, revived the neglected *inventum novum* (percussion) of Auenbrugger. In his train followed a galaxy of Parisian clinical teachers who were to make this city the Mecca for curious-minded physicians from every quarter of the civilized world. Among these Laennec and Louis should be especially noted. Laennec invented the monaural stethoscope. By this epochal correlation of physical signs with necropsy findings he placed the diagnosis of pulmonary diseases on a firm basis for the first time. Louis evolved the numerical method in clinical practice. A symptom or a sign was significant in direct proportion to the frequency of its occurrence in a given disease. This principle is still generally applied in medical practice.

The leavening of the French school was early disseminated to Dublin, Edinburgh, London, Berlin, Vienna, Philadelphia, Boston, and New York. The intervening years have witnessed revolutionary changes in medical practice. As implied, morbid anatomy dominated medical thought for the early half of the last century. Indeed, Skoda, leader of the new Vienna school, considered few diagnoses clinched without a necropsy! The work of Virchow brought cellular pathology to the forefront, whereupon the microscopic definition of disease displaced gross pathology in medical thinking. The pioneer efforts of Pasteur, Koch, and Lister gave substantial form to the science of bacteriology. Forthwith the etiologic diagnosis became the objective of clinical medicine. Time tempered this fixation; but the advent of the sulfonamides and the antimicrobial agents brought renewed attention to this significant aspect of human disease.

Meanwhile many other basic sciences, impinging on human life in health and disease, have grown apace. Particularly cogent in the present relation have been the developments in physiology and physiologic chemistry. Moreover medicine recognizes the increasing impact of psychology, genetics, anthropology, and sociology on the problems of health and disease. It may be truly claimed that the aim of modern medicine is holistic. As an unwholesome byproduct of the highly technical support to clinical medicine, a certain impersonality in the patient-physician relationship confronts us. Several aspects of this problem emerge from a growing dependence on purely objective methods. Without detracting an iota from the importance of newer laboratory measures, their very availability imposes a serious responsibility for intelligent, discriminating utilization. The so-called batteries of functional tests smack of shotgun rather than rifle fire on a diagnostic target. Random probing in the feckless calls upon the laboratories for the whole gamut of examinations and tests without fixed direction is as devastating to the medical growth of the physician as it is to the effectiveness of the laboratory. With the temptation to lean inordinately upon this support comes a distinct trend toward scientific abstraction. Enmeshed in his scientific absorption the physician may overlook the fact that the object of his study is not merely the unhappy host of chemical aberrations, physiologic deviations, and electronic eccentricities, but a human being seeking surcease from the psychologic as well as the physical traumata of disease and disability. In the patient's debilitated state of mind and body, an air of detachment on the part of the physician may perchance serve to erect an insuperable barrier to effective therapy.

"The secret of the care of the patient is in caring for the patient" (Peabody). The potency of the laying on of hands is attested in the Holy Bible. "Then touched He their eyes, saying, 'According to your faith be it unto you'" (St. Matthew 9:29), was the Master's statement to the blind. Their sight was restored. Other references to healing by faith are encountered in the Bible. A recent account of the outstanding work of the Sisters of Maryknoll in Pusan, Korea, depicts the simple faith of the natives. A moribund child was brought to the clinic merely to be touched by a Sister. At least spiritual comfort was afforded the distraught parents. Particular interest in *Her Name is Mercy* stems from the fact that Sister Mercy is the sister of Dean John Hirschboeck. A graduate in medicine from Marquette University, her good works in many areas have redounded to the everlasting credit of her Alma Mater and to the glory of God.

Without ascribing divine power to the physicians, personal contact with the patient is admittedly an important factor in psychologic rapport. Not only will a painstaking history afford invaluable information to the physician but the patient will ordinarily gain composure and ease. The complete physical examination remains the most essential ingredient in the comprehensive study of the patient. By the physician's "quietly efficient thoroughness he will convey the comforting assurance of his interest and competence" (Middleton). Yet, how often have you heard the patient say: "This is the first complete examination I have ever had"? So serious an indictment of medical practice must not be lightly treated nor condoned. It must be met by precept and example. Indeed, this thesis is one of the foundation stones of the American Society of Internal Medicine. By the same token, the very technique of the physical examination, conducted with precision and dignity, establishes a relationship between the patient and the physician unattainable by any other means. To digress for a moment, a careful inquiry leads to the conviction that the actual physical contact of the examination and the treatment (?) constitutes a major explanation for the defection of patients to osteopathy and chiropractic. Here the parallel ceases; but too little attention has been paid to this significant factor in medicine. Of course, beyond the psychologic significance of the physical examination comes the establishment of the presence or absence of morphologic and physiologic changes incident to disease.

The physician who denies to himself the information disclosed by the carefully elicited history and the meticulously conducted physical examination immediately sacrifices insight and perspective. Certainly the inevitable impersonality of the patient-physician relationship under such circumstances must prove most prejudicial to successful cooperative therapy. As we have indicated, presently there is no prospect of resolving in a mathematical formula the actual quality of medical care to the individual patient. The objective criteria, now under consideration by the several agencies engaged in its study, are incapable of measuring the imponderable values of human sympathy and compassion. The output of the understanding heart of the true physician and the good nurse cannot be measured or approximated by any available method. Nonetheless this intangible force may be a vital, yes, a determining, factor in life and death.

FROM THE PATIENT'S VIEWPOINT

To the Chapter of Alpha Omega Alpha at Howard University my greetings and felicitations. Especially do I address myself to the new initiates. You have been signally honored. In acknowledging your academic attainment your associates and their faculty advisers have paid you an unusual tribute. By the same token, you have assumed a new responsibility. Such academic honors will impel you to even higher achievement in the future. Complacency may never place its staying hand on the throttle of your efforts.

The privilege of an audience of my peers always invokes a sense of deep humility in me. Perhaps this reaction is accentuated by the span of years and by the overwhelming advances in science and medicine that I have witnessed. Upon reflection, I realize that I must be guarded, lest my conservatism reveal my age and the status of my cerebral circulation! Of one detail I can assure you—I shall not speak of the good old days when the kerosene lamp was the student's source of light, before the Ford and the Jaguar had displaced the horse and buggy. Nor do I feel that the quality of medical students has deteriorated over the years, as one hears in certain quarters. I am reminded of an incident in Dartmoor Prison. A riot in that forbidding institution had brought the Chairman of the Royal Commission posthaste from London. To get at the roots of the affair he had a long-term prisoner called before him. "What brought about this mutiny?" he asked. "Quite frankly, what?

Address at the Initiation Banquet, Gamma Chapter of the District of Columbia, Howard University College of Medicine, April 13, 1957. Reprinted from *The Pharos of Alpha Omega Alpha* 21 (April 1958): 3–6.

The food, the discipline, what?" The old lag replied, "Well sir, I have been a member of this prison, man and boy, for forty years. I think, sir, I may properly claim this place my 'ome. Now some says one thing, sir, and some says another; but," lowering his voice, "it's my belief, sir, we're not getting the stamp of man in 'ere we used to."

While I do not accept this contention applied to medical students, I do recognize certain manifest trends that may jeopardize the preferred position of medicine and physicians in the fabric of modern society for the future. Moreover, I admit to a certain strain of perversity—a whimsical turn, if you please. For example, I have spoken on behalf of the pathogenic microorganisms. I have borne witness to the dislocation of biological balances in nature by the antimicrobial agents. Now with your indulgence I should like to develop certain basic aspects of the medical situation from the patient's viewpoint.

In *Horae Subsecivae*, John Brown has carefully delineated certain advantages of illness that were denied his father by reason of his robust health:

> This was all the worse for him, for, odd as it may seem, many a man's life is lengthened by a short illness; and this in several ways. In the first place, he is laid up, out of reach of all external mischief and exertion; he is like a ship put in dock for repairs; time is gained. A brisk fever clarifies the entire man, if it is beaten and does not beat; it is like cleaning a chimney by setting it on fire; it is perilous but thorough. Then the effort to throw off the disease often quickens and purifies and corroborates the central powers of life; the flame burns more clearly; there is a cleanness, so to speak, about all the wheels of life. Moreover, it is a warning; and makes a man meditate on his bed, and resolve to pull up; and it warns his friends and, likewise, if he is a clergyman, his people, who, if their minister is always with them, never once think he can be anything but as able as he is.

However, when illness befalls, the patient must, perforce, experience certain strictures upon his normal activities. Especially if he be bedfast, he will undergo limitations or modifications of his normal movements that, under other circumstances, would be intolerable. His very clothing is replaced by hospital bed clothes. From the morning recording of the temperature, pulse, and respiration to the evening medication, every detail of his waking hours is subject to professional control. Not the least of his trials are bathing and toilet—in bed. Little wonder that the patient in a modern sense is a displaced human being! This situation is accentuated by the psychological reaction of a majority of patients. Singularly, the average person, regardless of his normal outlook, becomes introspective, egocentric, and selfish when ill. This reaction is sharply accentuated by the impersonality of modern medicine. The more intricate the technical and scientific advances in diagnosis and treatment become, the more serious the danger of detachment may be. The larger and the more perfect the hospital refinement, the less personal human interest is apt to emerge in the care of the patient. Since our period has witnessed such epochal developments in this area, we would do well to look to our own house in the interest of the affected patient.

Medical education has advanced apace in the past half century. The progress in the United States has been greatly accelerated since the Flexner Report (1910). Not only are the standards of admission to medical schools high but no other educational discipline has more avidly sought to improve the quality of instruction at the undergraduate level. Many new patterns of teaching are under study and trial in various medical schools at the present time. In our zeal for innovation and perfection let us not overlook the fundamental ingredients of sound education, namely, "intelligent, receptive students; inspired, well-motivated teachers; and ready, open channels of communication" (Middleton). Presently, we are paying the penalty for ignoring these simple basic principles in staffing our medical schools. The premium on other qualifications of the medical faculty at the expense of teaching ability has, in certain areas, lowered the standards of instruction. Having paid the piper, we are returning to sounder tenets in the planning of undergraduate medical curricula.

Admitting the superior intellectual qualifications of the modern medical graduate, we have merely opened the listing of his essential attributes. True, intelligence beyond the average is required for the adequate practice of medicine. I would be the last to lower this baseline; but mere mental superiority will qualify no one to practice the healing art on his fellowman. Indeed, abstraction in the minutiae of scientific investigation may definitely alienate the physician from the patient whose egocentric propensities are in the ascendancy at this time.

A bedside manner carries the connotation of a studied approach to the sick or disabled patient. Such attitudes may be basically affected and insincere. Unless the interest of the physician be heartfelt, his superficial attention will surely find him out. Maudlin sympathy is as much out of place in the sick room as is cold detachment. Close personal observation of the bedside approach of many physicians has led me to the conclusion that a deep compassion for suffering humanity motivates the most successful of our profession. Francis Peabody said: "One of the essential qualities of the clinician is interest in humanity, for the secret of the care of the patient is caring for the patient." For the period of the professional visit, the patient must be and must remain the object of the physician's attendance. His movements must be unhurried and his attention undivided. Regardless of the triviality or the inconsequence of the patient's or the family's recital of historical details of the illness, he must never permit his impatience to create barriers to facile communication. By indirection he will lead the discussion into relevant channels. Clearly the first professional visit may set the pattern for all subsequent relationships. If easy rapport is established, future cooperation and understanding are usually assured. Conversely, unnecessary friction even in minor details may delay or preclude a free interchange between the patient and the physician.

Since the matter of rapport has been emphasized, let it be remembered that the patient is always right (with mental reservations!). Attitudes that might properly be resented in the sound and healthy are ignored or tolerated in the sick. The physician must exercise extreme forbearance in the face of unbelievable affronts. His equanimity will bridge many situations in human relations that would ordinarily create insuperable chasms. With tact and composure the physician will meet crises in human affairs, undreamed of by laymen.

Regardless of the weight on his heart, the physician will bring cheer to the sick and the oppressed. His quiet dignity and serenity will soothe the troubled in body and spirit. Renewed confidence is afforded by the physician who adds a smile to his potion. Force must supplement these simple virtues. Hippocrates recognized the effectiveness of cooperative therapy in: "The art consists in three things—the disease, the patient and the physician. The physician is the servant of the art, and the patient must combat the disease along with the physician." So sacred is the trust imposed in the practitioner of medicine that a single word properly embraces his most essential attribute, i.e., character. There is no substitute for intellectual integrity.

Whitehead said: "Medicine is not a field in which sheep may safely graze." Certainly medicine is not looking for men and women of sheep-like qualities. The career you have chosen requires a stout heart and firm resolution as well as a keen, perceptive mind. Hippocrates wrote: "We must also bring to the task a love of labor and perserverance, so that the instruction taking root, may bring forth proper and abundant fruit." To Osler's four attributes for the physician, "The Art of Detachment, The Virtue of Method, The Quality of Thoroughness, and The Grace of Humility," I would add respect for the "dignity of man" and "reverence for life" (Schweitzer).

Nor would I consider your future in medicine a bed of roses. You will meet obstacles, real and fancied, fair and unfair, within and without our profession. "Opposition is the best mordant to fix the color of your thought in the general belief" (Holmes). My chief concern is that such experience may not embitter nor degrade you like John Bunyan's man with the muck rake who "rakes to himself the straws and sticks and dust of the floor and can look no way but downward regardless of the crown which is being held over his head." To each and every one of you is offered the crown of universal approbation through your unexcelled opportunity for human service. I salute you and bid you Godspeed in your lofty mission of mercy.

GOOD METHODS AND
A PROPER POINT OF VIEW

"Give him good methods and a proper point of view, and all other things will be added as his experience grows."

WILLIAM OSLER

Granting the wisdom of Osler's position, perspective must be afforded to project the future. Santayana said: "Those who cannot remember the past are condemned to repeat it." Within the memory of man, the very face of medicine has been so altered as to merit a review of some of its notable changes as a basis for probable developments in this sphere of human interest and activity.

Perhaps the decline of infectious diseases, both in incidence and gravity, has been one of the most remarkable changes in the past half-century. Preventive measures of sanitation and vaccination have rendered typhoid fever and smallpox relatively rare diseases. Asiatic cholera and bubonic plague now have a circumscribed endemicity, although the speed and range of modern transportation by air hold an ever-present threat of a sporadic spread of these exotic diseases. Singularly, the exanthems have lost their terror. Immunization may be credited with much of the ground gained in limiting the occurrence of diphtheria. The education of the laity and the profession, early recognition, hygienic measures, chemotherapy, and surgery all have contributed to the gratifying success in the control of tuberculosis. In this area, a note of caution must be sounded. With the advent of antimicrobial and treponemicidal agents, the death knell of gonorrhea and syphilis was presumed to have been sounded. Instead, recent surveys have indicated a serious recrudescence in this important field, so the battle must be renewed with intensified vigor to regain lost ground.

Reprinted from *The Journal-Lancet* 84 (August 1964): 261–65.

Basically the same principles apply to the control of tuberculosis. The fight is not won. We must press our advantage relentlessly.

Another aspect of this matter excites further attention. The antimicrobial agents have created a profound disruption of the biologic balance of Nature. Smith thus expressed the situation prior to their introduction: "The normal microbiologic flora of man is varied and complex but seems to have been stabilized by a long process of evolution in such a manner that the organisms have a happy home and man is not injured. The microorganisms, bacteria and fungi are properly designated commensals and not saphrophytes. They are antagonistic to and prevent pure saphrophytes from joining the normal ecologic flora." So it has come to pass that strains of pathogenic bacteria have emerged that are resistant to the action of antagonists to which they were once sensitive. With the imbalance induced by the antimicrobial agents certain bacteria, fungi, and viruses have assumed unaccustomed pathogenic prominence in human disease.

Added to this expanding field, a clearer understanding of the part played by lesser or greater changes in the chemistry of life has greatly widened the horizon of medicine. Claude Bernard wrote: "The physician is one who studies the sick man and uses physiology to enlighten and advance the science of disease." Pausing for a moment to reflect on the course of medical progress, one is impressed by the transitions of the domination among the several disciplines in medical thought and practice over the years. Through Bichat, Corvisart, Laennec, and Louis, among others, the bedside-necropsy correlation of disease manifestations marked the dawn of modern clinical medicine. Thereafter the cellular pathology of Virchow revolutionized medical thought by transferring the emphasis from gross morbid anatomy to minute histological changes. In turn, the ascendency of microbiology under Pasteur, Lister, and Koch for the time placed the etiology of disease above all other considerations in practice. The professional attitude was not unnatural or unreasonable. By appropriate studies in the satisfaction of Koch's postulates, the exciting causative agents for a series of infectious diseases were disclosed. The etiology of a given disease afforded a cogent point for attack, but shortly the limitations of this approach became apparent. Ehrlich's side-chain theory was a provocative link in contemporary thought and study, but his magic bullets (antibodies) did not prove to be the panacea that had been anticipated. However, his discovery, with Hata, of arsphenamine (Salvarsan) for the treatment of syphilis was the first breakthrough in the application of an agent that destroyed the invading pathogen without harming the host. There followed a period of frantic search for substances with an analogous action against bacterial invaders.

Meanwhile, the advances in physiology, physiological chemistry (including the more esoteric fields of chemistry such as physical, enzyme, and steroid), and pharmacology were leading the practice of medicine perceptibly to Claude Bernard's characterization. The spectacular entrance of the sulfonamides and antimicrobial agents on the scene reoriented the clinician in the etiologic requirements of practice. Radioisotopes vastly expanded his vista in physiological and clinical studies. The new tool of tagged elements afforded an unprecedented insight into such basic functions as calcium, iodine, protein, and iron metabolism. Upon closer scrutiny, many of these observations merely served to refine earlier principles. The discovery of adrenocortical steroids initiated an astounding expansion of the knowledge of the physiology of this gland and its relationship to organs and tissues, connected and removed. In few other areas have the basic studies had a closer or more prompt application to clinical medicine. Hereditary traits and the actual transmission of derangements of bodily structures have long been observed. Orderly studies in medical genetics are, however, a development of the present generation. Already inborn errors of metabolism, mental deficiency, and certain organic faults have been traced to faulty chromosomal patterns. Traditionally, the physician experiences some difficulty in assimilating a new area of scientific study and understanding. The unfamiliar language and vocabulary of the geneticist shortly will become a working tool of the practitioner as he gains confidence in his competence in this area.

The past generation has seen surpassing advances in anesthesiology. With scientific teamwork among physiologists, pharmacologists, and anesthesiologists, a technological approach to this important area now assumes its appropriate place among the clinical sciences. After this limitation had been removed, or at least minimized, there remained the threat of wound infection. True, notable contributions had been made from the antisepsis of Lister to the asepsis of modern surgery, but the danger persisted and technical growth was impeded by postoperative infections under predictable conditions. With the discovery of the efficacy of sulfanilamide against gram-positive cocci, new hope arose. The replacement of the sulfonamides by penicillin marked a further advance, to which significant steps have been added by the discovery of many other antimicrobial agents. A dramatic contrast was afforded by the limited supply of penicillin in World War II. Such penicillin as was available was given to the American sick and wounded of the armed forces. In southern England, a United States Army general hospital was set up immediately across the road from a prisoner-of-war hospital. With available penicillin, the wards of the American hospital were free of offensive odors, whereas the prisoner-of-war wards, lacking antimicrobial therapy, reeked with the heavy odor of suppuration, reminiscent of World War I when the olfactory sense was widely employed in directing the treatment of war wounds! The emergence of resistant staphylococci in the setting of the hospital has kept us humble and relatively clean. To this time there has been no suggestion of a congressional study such as the book *Silent Spring* incited in the use of insecticides.

With the support of advanced anesthesia and antimicrobial agents, not only has surgery consolidated its position in the abdominal and neurological fields but it has sought new worlds to conquer. The first of these areas to capitulate was the lung, where infection had been a limiting factor in World War I. The availability of streptomycin and other antituberculosis drugs, particularly, was to prove most important in a protective sense. The cardiovascular system was the last anatomic stronghold to resist surgical attack. The brilliant successes that have attended the surgical correction of congenital and acquired structural defects of the major and more peripheral arteries are some of the brightest pages in medical progress. Eventually all components of the heart, beginning with the pericardium, then the endocardium, and finally the myocardium, have come under surgical reparative attack. One of the major contributions to the success of intracardiac surgery has been the assurance of effective extracorporeal circulation that permits a direct approach to affected valvular or septal fault. A number of prosthetic devices have been developed for the correction or replacement of defective valves. It is merely a matter of time, experience, and ingenuity until the ideal substitute is found. Visceral transplantation has intrigued man for centuries. The rejection of homologous tissues and organs after an apparent "take" has baffled man's attempts in grafts and transplants for years. From an understanding of the basic principles involved has come a plan of procedure that minimizes the rejection reaction and permits the successful transplantation of lung, liver, and kidney. Indeed, so confident are the workers in this field that they maintain that eventually hemodialysis will be merely a preparation for renal transplantation. Philosophers are projecting the moral as well as the psychological impact of such human chimeras as may ultimately emerge from such procedures.

All of this indicates the increasing complexity of the modern practice of medicine. If this were not enough, the armamentarium of the modern physician includes the vital support of the laboratories and radiological department with the burgeoning force of their refined methods. The intelligent use of these important services, while indispensable to the proper practice of medicine, constitutes one of the serious paradoxes of the day. Unfortunately, impressed as clinicians are by the objectivity of many laboratory determinations, they seek refuge in blanket requests for laboratory examinations without discriminating thought of their applicability to the problem at hand or their cost. Truly the laboratory has made cowards of us all. The time is ripe for self-analysis in this matter. Basically the clinical pathologist and the roentgenologist are our personal consultants and should be so treated. Every consultation request should have our studied consideration with relation to the clinical problem at hand. Viewed in a detached judicial light, they fall naturally into three groups, that is, those essential, desirable, and excessive to the needs of the situation. If the individual request is put to this test, the results will prove much more useful. The staff of a hospital with a teaching program may seek refuge in rationalization on the specious score of the completeness of study, whereas in truth they should afford guidance to the rising generation by the intelligent economy of greatly abused resources. It is necessary to strive for a balance in the application of scientific methods to clinical practice.

Inexorably, medicine is being swept into the maelstrom of automation. In the interest of accuracy and time, many laboratory procedures naturally are coming under automation as a realistic solution to the growing load. The application of electronic measures has invaded the clinic in increasing degrees for cardiologic, central nervous system, auditory, and other routine studies. The monitoring of blood pressure, pulse, respiration, and electrocardiography by telemetry is commonplace in many clinics. The spectacular success of an implanted cardiac pacemaker has minimized the terror and danger of the Stokes-Adams syndrome in auriculoventricular heart block. Automation has been extended to the dispensing of drugs and to the control of certain operational elements of the modern hospital. Toynbee asked: "Can computing machines come to the rescue of human minds that are in danger of being drowned in an ocean of information?" For the hospital record, at least, an early answer may be anticipated. Several agencies, federal and private, are assiduously applying data processing techniques to this important aspect of the hospital operation. Revolutionary changes may be anticipated, and we must be prepared to implement them in the interest of improved service. Projected a step forward, similar methods are being pursued in the diagnosis and prognosis of disease. Promising as such prospects may be, their ultimate utility will rest upon human intelligence. The retrieval value is obviously dependent upon the accuracy of the input. Strictly quantitative information lends itself readily to arbitrary coding and programming, whereas many clinical data are subjective. Herein lies a zone of human judgment that renders the process less exact. Be that as it may, the next generation will witness a drastic modification of the clinical approach and procedure through automation.

Insidiously, yet inevitably, medical practice has been confronted by the changing social philosophy of the public. Admittedly, medicine has not kept pace with the trend. Yet as early as 1909, Henry Baird Favill, in a prophetic speech before the alumni of Rush Medical College, had sounded the advance: "The pathology of society is as much the responsibility of the medical man as the pathology of disease." Instead of taking the initiative in the frontal attack on the problems with the evaluation of appropriate remedial measures, organized medicine remained aloof. Now this situation has become a major political issue in which the smoke of the emotional emanations befogs the light of reason. Indeed the programs of hospitalization and of the care of the infirm and aging citizens have lost a measure of their humane motivation in the clouds of political expediency.

The rising generation must recognize its place in the body politic. The attitude of isolationism on the part of our profession has incurred the debt of public misunderstanding that we must discharge without delay. Its first concession is an appreciation of the interdependence of all forces interested in the health of our citizens. Health is not the exclusive vested interest of any segment of the population. Yet, in the past, medicine has grudgingly lent its support to community health enterprises. The more recent coordination of effort by all interested elements of society has paid great dividends in the improvement of public health and welfare. This bridgehead will be consolidated and extended by thoughtful, public-minded physicians of the future.

Within organized medicine there has arisen a new force in the past half-century. When life was simple and medical societies less formal, the officers of organized medicine, with committee support, sufficed to meet the requirements of more or less orderly procedure and operation. As our membership grew and legislative and other extraprofessional functions cast their shadows on us, the necessity for lay support in key positions became apparent. At first, legal advice was extended from the occasional opinion to meet a passing issue or to influence legislation. Soon such counselors were retained on a full-time basis by many state medical societies. The lay secretary has established his important function in a majority of the state medical societies. In this capacity, more and more duties have devolved upon him. The inevitable result is the development of a highly organized secretariat that soon becomes indispensable. Moe aptly expressed the situation: "In your own world, I fear your little administrators, and especially your would-be administrators, your coordinators, your integrators, your setters-up of plans and charts and tables of organization and mechanisms. You are letting the smart operators get into the drivers' seats."

So eager is the busy practitioner to avoid the tedium of medical organization that he has abrogated many of the former obligations and prerogatives of keeping our house in order and representing the position of medicine to the public and to legislative bodies. Admittedly the advice of staff members skilled in the law and in public relations is necessary to orient our representatives in a modern society, but the true image of medicine can never be conveyed to the public by anyone except the physician. In a singular aspect of the activities of state and county medical societies, the influence of the lay secretariats has been manifested. Traditionally these societies have afforded a forum for scientific and clinical discussions. Insidiously, so-called medical economic subjects came to monopolize these programs. The discussions that usually were led by laymen involved the monetary affairs of medicine, insurance, and hospitalization and rarely entered into the basic principles of the socioeconomics of medical care. Admitting the increasing demands of the required attendance of busy practitioners upon hospital meetings, we see a heartening sign of the times in the greater thought and attention being given to the scientific contents of county and state medical meetings. To paraphrase Zinsser, "The administrative camel [must not] crowd the intellectual pilgrim out of his tent."

The occasion does not admit of a comprehensive discussion of the manner of practice of the oncoming generation of physicians. The period following World War II has witnessed a tremendous upsurge of the hospitalization of the sick and afflicted. Prepayment health and hospital insurance has contributed materially to this movement. Patently there are advantages both to the patient and to the physician in the centralization of such medical services, but to our dismay certain deterring factors arise from this approach. No complete answer to problems of the very short- or the very long-term illness has been derived. By court action insurance carriers are relieved of the financial responsibility for their beneficiaries who obtain medical care in certain tax-supported hospitals. By this decision, the companies (and their insurees) are relieved of this obligation and are granted a bonus that all other taxpayers cover in their hospital care. Unnecessary hospitalization is an abuse of the covering insurance which will constitute a major problem of the future in this area. The mounting cost of hospital care not only threatens the security of the program but affords a vulnerable point of attack by proponents of compulsory governmental insurance. The Achilles heel in the medical crisis that led to the adoption of state medicine in Great Britain was not the medical profession but the voluntary hospital system.

In our connections with the hospitals of the community, we are regularly confronted by the interdependence of the several interested elements. Admittedly, these institutions are designed for the care of the sick and disabled. Rarely have they been erected independently by physicians. Their sustained support in a majority of instances depends upon public, private, and sectarian funds. Accepting the joint partnership of the participating members of modern society in health affairs, we should welcome their active interest and counsel in the administration of the hospitals. In certain quarters of our profession, physicians have been reluctant to accept this basic tenet when, in the last analysis, sources outside of our ranks are affording physicians the physical plants and facilities for their practice. Perhaps the adoption of the radical suggestion of a charge to the physician for each patient-day of hospitalization might bring this issue into proper perspective.

Since the prospect of the utilization of hospital care appears to be increasing for the early future, attention should be directed to certain problems, great and small, inherent in the situation. Middleton said: "Almost inevitably, in the mechanization and sophistication that we term the modern hospital, there has arisen a certain impersonality that threatens its greatest service to humanity." Indeed, the larger and more complex the hospital organization, the more abstract and removed from the intimacy of the environment in which the disease had its seeding is it apt to be. In recent years, many advances have been made to relieve the chill of the hospital setting. In a satirical mood, Ruark was constrained to write: "Hospitals are not run to heal the sick. They are run for the convenience of nurses, technicians, doctors, and dieticians, who are paid varying salaries to torture the patients into exerting will power to escape with a breath of life still in their labored bodies." Appreciating the excesses of this generalization, every physician should lend his efforts to correct manifest faults in our hospital routines in the primary interest of improving patient care.

From personal experience, hospital routines are traditionally so deeply rooted as to be difficult to change. Yet the very intimate detail of dispossession of personal belongings upon admission can be quite distasteful unless its protective design be explained. The schedule of hospital hours is quite peculiar to that setting. Few patients accept the early awakening and toilet with equanimity. Perhaps the most frequently expressed objections are to the diet. Since this element of the patient's care is therapeutic, periodic surveys of the rejected foods on the returning trays by the attending physician can be quite illuminating in the interest of economy as well as nutrition. If the scheduled hours of nursing care prove a trifle unconventional and disturbing to the average patient, the vote of objection to the lack of efficiency in programming appointments in x-ray and special laboratories would be unanimous. Perhaps the hour has not arrived, but it cannot be far removed when our hospitals will operate on a seven-day week rather than a five-and-a-half-day basis. "Illness and disability know no moratorium in time," said Middleton. In the interest of sustained patient care and the utilization of precious hospital beds, these facilities will ultimately be operated on a full-time basis with an avoidance of the weekend ineffectiveness. By staggering the hours and days of personnel service, this objective can be attained with a minimum of trauma. Meanwhile, a careful assessment of all routine procedures affecting patients should be initiated by every staff physician of all echelons to determine their design and the effect upon the patient. Where there has been a deleterious influence on the patient merely for a trival and inconsequential advantage to the member of the medical team, such measures should peremptorily be modified or abolished.

Westcott's David Harum said: "A certain amount of fleas is good for a dog. Makes him forget he is a dog." If the problems of medicine, existent and projected, dismay you, my purpose will have miscarried, for the challenge and opportunities for human service in the practice of medicine have never been greater. Certainly "good methods and a proper point of view" have been instilled into you by the faculty members and preceptors. These dedicated teachers are the catalysts. You are the springs of medical strength of the future. Recently, while waiting for the elevator in the Veterans Administration Hospital, I engaged a veteran patient in a wheelchair in conversation. Two medical students chanced by and stopped to inquire of the patient's health. When they left, he asked, "Are you a teacher?" When I answered affirmatively, he continued, "Those men will be good doctors. They have the touch. They are interested in people." My anonymous friend had the answer to success in medicine. Never lose the touch. Maintain your interest in people. Keeping the faith, the future of medicine is assured in your hands.

BALANCE IN MODERN MEDICINE

My sincere congratulations on your clearance of the second and third hurdles of your medical education, respectively, for the Interns and Residents. Such recognition is as well deserved as it is hard won. Particularly would I publicly express my gratitude for the year of grace given to me to work with you. It has been a most rewarding experience.

The late James Waring wrote: "Once one has put his hand to the medical plow, he is not fit for the Kingdom of Heaven if he does not ever look forward."

Medicine is a discipline of continuing education. Upon the background of primary and secondary education, you have undergone a stern preparation for your professional careers in the undergraduate college and the medical school curricula. Your graduate exposures have taken you through the internship and, in most instances, into areas of specialty training as residents. Particularly at the graduate level have you come to realize that the physiognomy of disease can be learned only at the bedside. Classroom exercises, lectures, laboratories, and libraries are merely tools to cement your observations of the sick and disabled patient. In such observations objectivity, pertinacity, and the intellectual curiosity of the inquiring mind will carry you a long way toward your ultimate goal. May I indicate that discernment comes to play a most important role in your growth as observations become more and more refined; for the capacity of fine discrimination marks

Remarks made at the Certificate Granting Exercises for the Interns and Residents, the Veterans Administration Hospital, Oklahoma City, June 12, 1964. Reprinted from the *Oklahoma State Medical Association Journal* 58 (March 1965): 84–86.

your potential for development. The support of laboratories exercises an increasingly important part in your continuing education. Intelligently and discriminately used, this element is essential to the modern practice of medicine. However, random probing without direction is the refuge of the mentally destitute that should be assiduously avoided. In no other human endeavor is directional reading so important. The immediate clinical situation will in most instances dictate the area of study. Particularly would I commend its careful relation to the problem of the day by references to the elucidation of disease phenomena, in the basic sciences. A short time past, great systems of medicine or other areas were popular. With the present pace of medical advance, when even the most modern texts are five years behind time, recourse must be had to current literature. Choose well the medical journals regularly studied and do not limit your reading to your special field. Budget your time so that at least one hour a day is given to the study of the medical literature. For ready reference, abstract cogent articles and maintain a cross-indexed file by disease and system. To change the pace, cultivate the habit of nonmedical reading.

The revolution in science has changed the face of medicine. With some temerity, therefore, one attempts to prophesy the image of medicine twenty years hence, when you will reach the peak of your professional competence and stature. With the advantage of more than fifty years in the vineyard, with some trepidation I will undertake this task in broad general principles. When I entered medical practice, over half a century ago, the clinical study of disease had undergone little change during the preceding century. History taking perhaps had been somewhat refined, but the principles of physical diagnosis laid down by the French school of Corvisart, Laennec, and Louis had undergone no significant change in this period. The simple laboratory procedures available to us could be listed on the fingers of one hand, and x-ray study was indeed primitive.

The last fifty years have witnessed revolutionary changes in medicine. In the main these have arisen through the increasing application of advances in biology, biochemistry, physical chemistry, enzyme chemistry, immunochemistry, genetics, physiology, pharmacology, microbiology, and pathology. If we stop to consider a single area, namely, that of pharmacology, this period has seen the introduction of insulin, liver, vitamin B_{12}, sulfonamides, antimicrobial agents, and steroids. (Salvarsan was discovered just before this period [1910].) These elements alone have revolutionized the practice of medicine. With the better understanding of the double helix or deoxyribonucleic acid (DNA) and the messenger, ribonucleic acid (RNA) the very secrets of life may be disclosed shortly. The demonstrations of disturbances and distortions in the arrangement and configuration of chromosomes have elucidated certain structural faults and inborn errors of metabolism for the first time. Truly we are moving steadily from cellular to molecular medicine and the pace is accelerating.

Extracorporeal circulation has rendered open heart surgery very effective in correcting intracardiac septal and valvular faults. Peripheral vascular surgery has attained a level of effectiveness undreamed of a generation past. The replacement of diseased or functionless organs by normal members has been the subject of intensive study for many years. While the recent successes have led to overenthusiasm in certain claims, the basic understanding of the mechanism of rejection has advanced apace and the prospect for avoiding such adverse results has become brighter and brighter with measures of suppression of the reaction.

The age of automation is upon us. As might be expected, the application of electronic devices to laboratory procedures led the way. A few years ago a heavy blizzard isolated Boston. Many of the essential laboratory technicians could not reach the Veterans Administration Hospital. In their absence, for two days, resident physicians of the staff through the available electronic devices such as the Coulter counter and the autoanalyzer conducted the essential laboratory examinations without interruption. Monitoring vital signs, electrocardiography, and electroencephalography by telemetry and other electronic devices are widely used today. Spectacular results have attended the control of heart block by the implanted electronic pacemaker. Dispensing drugs now can be accomplished with a minimum of error by automation. Several years ago the Veterans Administration engaged the services of the Systems Development Corporation in Santa Monica, California, to study the feasibility of the application of automation in several directions, i.e., hospital operation, research support center, and patient data processing. A simulated ward was set up and its operation in the admission, movement, and discharge of patients, together with pertinent information as to personal data, cardinal symptoms, diagnosis, laboratory returns, and treatment was controlled by a computer. The success of the experiment has led to its transfer to the actual operation of a ward at the Wadsworth Veterans Administration Hospital in Los Angeles. In the sophisticated area of modern medical research, it is obviously impossible to duplicate all skills at every one of the 140 hospitals in which research programs are currently being conducted. The centralization of special skills in geographically strategic points over the country affords advice and guidance, not control and supervision, to the host of workers in this system who are seeking the widest application of newer methods to their studies. The medical record is a point of natural attack for data processing. In my mind's eye the future in a given hospital, then an area, and finally nationally will so reconstruct the history, physical examination, and laboratory data that, by appropriate coding and programming, a given patient's record will be immediately and permanently recorded at a central point. Obviously such an input with a great storage and retrieval on call would have a tremendous potential for the growth of medical knowledge. Record linkage has already been applied over a limited area in Great Britain (Acheson).

While the promise of this prospect is quite overwhelming, we must anticipate the legal hurdle of privileged information that would have to be reconciled with such a coverage. More important from the standpoint of the possible impact of such an approach on the traditional patient-physician relationship is the threat of impersonality. Ogilvie spoke of "the worship of the expert" in terms of technolatry. Since automation is here to stay, eventually the computer will have a place in the actual diagnosis and treatment of disease. Under these circumstances two points must be borne in mind clearly. The machine is no more accurate than its master. Such retrieval as is available in the output will depend on the accuracy of the input. Under Dr. Edward N. Brandt we have made a sound beginning in this most important field in Oklahoma. Our staff has made conspicuous contributions to this significant area and we must protect our advantage. Futhermore the most important ingredient in the patient-physician relationship is an understanding heart. In this period of transition, your generation must maintain a delicate balance to capitalize on the technical advances as you maintain a compassionate attitude toward your sick and disabled human charges.

Osler sounded this admonition: "Medicine is an art, not a trade; a calling, not a business; a calling in which the heart will be exercised equally with the head." May God speed you.

MEDICINE BEFORE AUTOMATION

Recently *The Lancet* contained "A Dialogue of Tomorrow" by a Peripatetic Correspondent:

Sir, can you tell me the meaning of an obsolete word? I know medical history is a hobby of yours.

I'll try. What word?

Auscultation.

It meant listening.

Listening to what, Sir?

Sounds made by the human body . . . I thought you'd be puzzled. Doctors used to listen to their patients' bodies, and palpate them directly, too.

Directly? You mean they used some simpler kind of palpating machine than ours?

No, really directly . . . I see I'll have to demonstrate. Come here. Put your hand on my wrist—right on it, skin to skin.

May I really, Sir?

Yes, yes: no-one's looking. Now in the old days, if you were the doctor and I the patient, that would have been the usual thing. Television wasn't used in medicine at all; you wouldn't have been lying in your helicopter; you'd have been sitting close by your patient, probably in his home.

Sitting? Home?

Let's leave those words for another time and return to auscultation. Doctors used to listen to the air going in and out of their patients' lungs, and the heart valves opening and closing.

How could they *hear* such things?

The world was virtually silent. Ancient literature is full of references

Address to University of Pennsylvania Graduate School of Medicine, Certificate Ceremony, Philadelphia, May 19, 1961. Reprinted from *Archives of Internal Medicine* 109 (March 1962): 251–55.

to people's hearing the songs of birds and the cries of infants, and most authorities believe that such sounds literally were heard. The loudspeakers used to be turned off at night. Much of the Earth's surface was not even wired for sound. Probably everyone spoke much more quietly, and the way we are talking now would have been called shouting.

Shouting?

Speaking more loudly than is necessary.

But it is always necessary—

—To speak as loudly as possible. Yes, but it used not to be. What is more, in order to hear the lung sounds and heart sounds better, doctors used something called a stethoscope.

What was that like?

Nobody knows.

Is it true, Sir, that in those days patients used to do much better?

Do much better?

I mean, for example, was the recovery-rate from acute infections and trauma much higher? Did far fewer patients die in hospitals?

It is quite true, and the reason is simple. Microorganisms were much less virulent then.

And what about trauma?

It used to be much less violent. No other explanation is possible.

How do you know all this, Sir?

Between ourselves, I've learnt to read. I know it's frowned on as taking up time which ought to be spent on listening and learning, and certainly you young fellows have enough to listen to; but you'd be surprised what interesting things have never been electronically recorded.

Can you write, too, Sir?

Aha, my boy, now you're pulling my leg.[1]

Amusing as this light satire may be, from the standpoint of its basic significance it is later than we think. The growing interest in automatic data processing has led to many articles in the current medical literature. While most of these are premature and extravagant in their conclusions, there is a solid core of substantial evidence that computers and other forms of automation will find an increasing place in future research and the practice of medicine. From the example of scientists in other fields not only will computers fill an increasing role in resolving mathematical problems, but theoretical models may be developed to simulate biologic processes and systems with a design to resolve profound questions of physiology and pathology. The clinical application of such mechanical devices to the biologic subject, represented in the sick or disabled human being, is fraught with certain inherent difficulties. Obviously, much of the clinical data must necessarily be soft. Perforce the resolution of a symptom such as pain into appropriate

1. *The Lancet*, 1:1022 (May 7) 1960.

form for programming for the computer input will prove most difficult. Dependent upon their objectivity, physical findings may prove either hard or soft. For example, the routine temperature determinations fall well within scientific limits of error and will constitute hard data; whereas, the number and the character of the respirations might well be considered soft. In the main, laboratory data will be classified as hard. In all instances, the elicitation, interpretation, and programming of clinical and laboratory data for computer input will depend upon the accuracy and intelligence of the recorder. By the same token, the storage and retrieval as output will, in turn, find its validty in the same source.

The tremendous strides of electronic instrumentation and mechanization in medicine are discernible at a glance. The monitoring by electronic means is still largely confined to the operating rooms of certain university hospitals and advanced clinics. Telemetry has been employed in determining temperature, pulse, blood pressure, electrocardiography, and electroencephalography in certain areas; but these methods do not yet have widespread utilization. One of the most interesting of these developments is a mobile cart in which a three-purpose drift-free electronic meter is utilized to read the CO_2 and O_2 tensions directly in millimeters of mercury and the pH in units (John Severinghaus). The cardiologist is no longer satisfied to depend upon the stethoscope for the determination of heart sounds but resorts to the phonocardiogram. The string galvanometer of the electrocardiogram has been replaced by electronic devices. The most sophisticated recent development in this area has been the direct recording of electrocardiographic signals in analog form on magnetic tape at the Mt. Alto Veterans Administration Hospital, Washington, D.C. (Pipberger and Freis). These cardiac signals are then converted into digital form for automatic analysis through the use of a general purpose electronic computer. From this storage point retrieval is possible on call. The output record shows an accuracy in excess of 94 percent. The electroencephalographic apparatus is also electronically activated. Telemetry has been brought into unusual application through the use of a pressor transensor to measure the intraluminal pressure of the gastrointestinal tract at all levels (Farrar). The cathode ray oscilloscope has been transplanted from the physiologic laboratory to the clinic in widespread applications.

Singular refinement has occurred in clinical roentgenology by the use of electronic optical devices in an image intensifier. The brightness of the screen image has been increased a thousand times or more. Through this expedient fluoroscopy can now be performed under normal or subdued lighting with little or no dark adaptation. Cineradiography in the use of the television camera has taken the place of rapid change films in angiography, angiocardiography, and in certain gastrointestinal studies. As a outgrowth of the use of the cardiac monitor, electronic pacemakers have been applied in the treatment of cardiac arrhythmias attended by asystole and Adams-Stokes syndrome. Through transistor-activated electrodes, appropriately timed electrical stimulation of the myocardium insures rhythmic cardiac contraction at a rate adequate to meet the functional requirement of the patient. By this device the clinical manifestations of heart block may be controlled.

In no field of medicine has scientific advance made itself felt more fully than in the clinical laboratory. Mathematics, biophysics, biochemistry, enzyme chemistry, immunochemistry, physical chemistry, cytogenetics, and electronics are continuously reflected in clinical practice. In many instances, electronic methods are invoked in the development of the techniques and apparatus. The spectrophotometer and flame photometer are universally in demand to afford laboratory support in the resolution of clinical problems. Chromatography has found general acceptance. One of the most interesting developments in this field is the utilization of the analytrol to transfer color densities to a graphic form through electronic intermediation. A most useful recent development in the clinical laboratory is the autoanalyzer, which is gaining steadily in popularity. The Coulter counter bids fair to replace the hemocytometer in blood counting and may have a further application in screening body secretions for neoplastic cells. Electron microscopy is opening new and inviting vists in pathologic histology. Obviously the degree of magnification, thousands by this method as compared with hundreds of times by light microscopy, accounts for the great promise of its future contribution. Certainly improved measures of precision have already greatly advanced our ability to recognize earlier pathologic changes in many diseases.

With the overwhelming weight of scientific growth, aided and abetted by mechanization beyond the wildest dreams of a generation removed, comes the serious danger of an impersonalization of medical practice. Ogilvie referred to technolatry as "the worship of the expert." In an earlier day, Mitchell had decried the dementalization of physicians by gadgets. Certainly, there is an imminent danger of an inordinate dependence upon the laboratory at the sacrifice of traditional clinical methods. Jackson wrote: "Science of course is necessary; it has its justified place and each year it becomes more important to the proper practice of medicine. But neither tests nor science can fully replace the art of medicine and that is fast disappearing, though occasionally one sees shy, frightened bits peering cautiously out at a man who is ill through the maze of millimoles and hydrogen ions and tests for histoplasmosis, which mean precisely nothing."[2] A generation removed, Osler said: "Give him good methods and a proper point of view, and all other things will be added as his experience grows." We should, therefore, pause for a moment and review the established clinical methods of the recent past. The carefully elicited history frequently affords the clearest picture of the evolution of the underlying disorder. The symptoms divulged in such an exercise represent the patient's interpretation of disturbed function. Only by such a device may the physician obtain a lucid account of the natural history of disease. The physical examination, meticulously pursued with the God-given senses alert to deviations from the normal, in effect discloses the pathologic anatomy of disease. At an earlier period the laboratory was consulted largely in support of the inferred conclusions of the history and physical examination. Routine urinalyses, hemograms, bacteriologic studies, and serologic explorations were employed. Blood chemical studies did not emerge in clinical practice until the second decade of this century, and basal metabolic determinations were not a routine until the 1920s. Roentgenologic explorations were limited. Quite vividly there is recalled an interchange between Dr. Henry Pancoast, the first Professor of Radiology in the United States of America at the University of Pennsylvania and Dr. John H. Musser, Sr., Professor of Clinical Medicine (1910). At some length, Dr. Musser had presented the differential diagnosis of a superior mediastinal mass. In retrospect it was a scholarly effort. Dr. Pancoast then very quietly and simply resolved the intricate question by demonstrating the pulsation of an aortic aneurysm. Whereupon, Dr. Musser exclaimed: "There goes all of the romance of the examination of mediastinal pathology!" and stalked from the room.

The diagnostic acumen of the trained clinician of the last generation has been the subject of much deliberation and discussion. My father in medicine, Doctor David Riesman, when called to see a patient with suspected typhoid fever on the Neurologic Ward of the Philadelphia General Hospital, turned to me at the entrance of the ward and asked, "Middleton, is this the patient?" When I answered in the affirmative, he said, "He does not have typhoid fever." Thereupon, he pointed out the presence of herpes labialis which, in his experience, was negatively pathognomonic of typhoid fever. Upon examination the patient proved to have lobar pneumonia.

On another occasion, when Doctor Riesman entered the medical

2. H. Jackson, Jr. 1956, "Sermons in Stones," *N. Engl. J. Med.*, 254:910.

ward, he scanned a chart at the foot of the bed and asked, "Middleton, when did this patient develop pericarditis?" Knowing Doctor Riesman's insistence upon meticulous attention to the state of the patients on his wards, I had examined this particular patient with rheumatic fever most carefully only a few hours before. Therefore, I said quite assuredly, "Doctor Riesman, he does not have pericarditis." My chagrin was complete when examination revealed a to and fro pericardial friction rub; but Doctor Riesman, in his kindly manner, indicated to me that there were two signs upon which he laid great stress in establishing the existence of pericarditis in the patient with rheumatic fever, namely delirium and tachypnea. Long experience had taught him that tachypnea may actually precede tachycardia and elevation of the temperature in rheumatic subjects with this complication.

In Kansas City, Dr. Ralph Major stopped at the door of a patient's room and remarked, "I see you have a patient with lead poisoning." At the hands of a master clinician, the explanation was simple. He had been told that the patient suffered from severe abdominal pain; yet, as he observed the junior examiner, deep abdominal pressure elicited no expression of tenderness or pain from the patient. Furthermore, the patient's hands were deeply stained or grimy. To complete the story, physical examination revealed the lead line on the gums, and laboratory examinations disclosed the presence of many stippled red blood cells in the smears of the peripheral blood and lead in the urine and feces. The patient had been exposed to lead intoxication in breaking up electric batteries.

Conan Doyle took his professor, Dr. Joseph Bell, as the prototype for the immortal Sherlock Holmes. Deductive and inductive processes are regularly used by the physician in deriving a diagnosis from the evidence of all available sources. In obscure problems resolution by exclusion may be the essential method of approach. Diagnosis by intuition is a faculty attributed to many able clinicians, who may be hard put to explain how a brilliant conclusion is derived. Actually, in a vast majority of instances, such apparently inexplicable achievements depend upon the memories, conscious and subconscious, of an extended experience. Translated into modern language, such individuals have an unusual retrieval potential from the storage of a biologic computer, which is the human mind.

In the first half of the last century, Paris was the scene of a tremendous resurgence in clinical interest. To the French school came many foreigners to sit at the feet of such masters as Louis, Laennec, Chomel, and Andral. In 1832, the American students in Paris established the Société Médicale d'Observation. In order to maintain balance in the appropriate utilization of scientific advances in the practice of clinical medicine, the revival of such an expedient might well be employed at the present time. Better still would be the resolution of every clinician to utilize the time-honored methods of clinical practice fully and faithfully. Certainly, stabilization will be required if medicine is to escape submergence in automation. However, the two subjects of the title are not antithetic but complementary. Automation will eventually become naturally merged in medicine in the interest of the better service to mankind through improved methods of diagnosis and treatment. In our zeal to elevate the practice of medicine to its highest possible level, let us not overlook its most important ingredient, compassion. Without human sympathy and understanding medicine as a profession will perish from the face of the earth and in its stead a new breed of coldly impersonal, accurate technicians will take its place in the sun.

THE INTELLIGENT USE
OF LABORATORIES

A long experience in clinical medicine and a careful review of the developments in the laboratory support of its modern practice have emphasized certain present-day trends. I take this opportunity to share certain observations with you in the conviction that we can utilize the essential support of the clinical, roentgenologic, and radio-isotope laboratories to greater advantage.

The use of laboratories in good medical practice has greatly increased in recent years. More involved and more complicated methods have invited wider clinical utilization in the interest of more accurate diagnosis and more adequate treatment. In these objectives, every thoughtful physician would concur. We may anticipate increasing requirements with the expansion of knowledge in the basic sciences as applied to clinical medicine. With this fundamental philosophy supporting the curious-minded, highly motivated clinician in his responsibility for human life and welfare, there can be no reasonable disagreement. On the other hand, the lack of definition of an objective in enlisting laboratory support may weaken rather than strengthen the clinical attack upon a given problem. Random probing rarely attains the desired objective and it may befog the issue at hand.

Laboratory examinations may be classified as essential, desirable, and excessive to our clinical requirements. Unfortunately, trained professional and technical personnel have not multiplied in proportion to the demand imposed by newer methods and techniques. Hence, the

Reprinted from the *University of Michigan Medical Bulletin* 25 (June 1959): 190.

thoughtful clinician must perforce use ever greater discrimination in his requisitions for laboratory examinations. Every request should be carefully evaluated to avoid excessive demands and needless repetition on overworked staffs.

The interdependence of laboratory and clinical medicine bespeaks the observance of common amenities. The pathologist, roentgenologist, bacteriologist, physicist, and other associated scientists in our laboratories are essential members of the modern medical team. In their several capacities, they serve as our consultants and should be so considered. Questions that arise relative to laboratory returns are better resolved by personal conference, in the interest of professional relations and human dignity. Mere multiplication of requisitions on these laboratories may compound rather than correct real or fancied errors—to the ultimate detriment of the care of the patient.

Careful attention to the thoughtful utilization of laboratories is earnestly recommended.

THE ROLE OF
THE MEDICAL CONSULTANT

Historically the medical consultation is one of the oldest and most respected of medical traditions. On appropriate occasion it will afford the best assurance of adequate and competent care to the sick and afflicted. Admittedly as "two heads are better than one," the doubtful medical situation involving the diagnosis and the treatment of a patient may frequently be better resolved upon a conference with another physician. Under such circumstances this ethical interchange usually lends reassuring support to the patient and the family on one hand and to the attending physician on the other. Yet from time to time through misunderstanding this time-honored practice has been suspect of ineffectiveness and ulterior design. Matthew Arnold has thus voiced the attitude of some skeptics toward consultants:

> Nor bring to see me cease to live
> Some doctor, full of phrase and fame,
> To shake his sapient head and give
> The ill he cannot cure, a name.

Even the dignified Thomas Jefferson once said that "whenever he saw three physicians together, he looked up to discover whether there was not a turkey buzzard in the neighborhood." The time for a studied effort to enlighten the laity and indeed the medical and health professions on the role of the medical consultation is most opportune, if not overdue.

Appropriately the first formal consideration of medieval protocol is

Reprinted from *The Pharos of Alpha Omega Alpha* 24 (July 1961): 145–52.

ascribed to Thomas Percival (1794). To the cynical layman medical etiquette has been thus characterized: "Since it is a kind of sacred writing to him, the young doctor doesn't appreciate the humor in terming a code of ethics that little guide to propriety issued by The American Medical Association filled with trade-union rules designed to promote dignity and prosperity in the profession" (East). In a thoughtful, scholarly reprinting of Percival's *Medical Ethics*, Chauncey D. Leake (1927) performed an added service by incorporating the several modifications of the "Code of Ethics of The American Medical Association." Initially formulated by The American Medical Association in May 1847, two revisions were adopted under the title, "Principles of Medical Ethics of The American Medical Association," May 7, 1903, and June 4, 1912, respectively. The third and latest "Principles" appeared in a Special Edition of the *Journal of The American Medical Association*, June 7, 1958.

As Leake has indicated: "Medical etiquette is concerned with the conduct of physicians toward each other, and embodies the tenets of professional courtesy. Medical ethics should be concerned with the ultimate consequences of the conduct of physicians toward their individual patients and toward society as a whole, and it should include a consideration of the will and motive behind this conduct." Essentially etiquette is hedonistically oriented toward individual dignity and advancement, whereas ethics is idealistically directed toward the welfare of society.

In none of the professional relationships of the physician are the standards of personal conduct more rigidly prescribed than in his consultative capacity. The Joint Commission on Accreditation of Hospitals' "Standards on Consultation" (revised January 1955) defined the status simply as follows: "A consultant is a second physician called by the attending physician to examine and discuss his patient." Yet a century and a half before (1794) Percival had given a strict protocol of professional etiquette to guide the second physician in this situation. Except under unusual circumstances the consultant should see the patient only in the presence of the attending physician. "On such occasions no rivalry or jealousy should be indulged. Candour, probity and all due respect should be exercised towards the physician or surgeon first engaged." The same basic principles are carried into the later codes of professional conduct. As stated in the 1847 "Code," "Consultations should be promoted in difficult or protracted cases, as they give rise to confidence, energy and more enlarged views in practice." Extending this detail the 1903 "Principles" declared: "A physician who is called in consultation should observe the most honorable and scrupulous regard for the character and standing of the attending physician, whose conduct of the case should be justified, as far as can be, consistently with a conscientious regard for truth, and no hint or insinuation should be thown out which would impair the confidence reposed in the attending physician."

In general the gravity and obscurity of a clinical situation will be determining factors accepted as indicating the consultation. Certain situations, as the first Caesarian section and curettage or other pelvic procedures in known or suspected pregnant subjects, will especially require consultation for the protection of the patient and the physician. Like precautions are advisable in patients adjudged to be serious surgical risks. As stated, the physician is well advised to seek medical counsel early, where the diagnosis is uncertain or the prognosis grave. An open-minded attitude on his part will engender confidence, whereas hesitation or reluctance in seeking professional support may be interpreted as unwarranted obstinacy or pique without due consideration for the patient's welfare. It is always well for the attending physician to take the initiative under such conditions, particularly since the selection of the consultant is then usually in his hands. This decision is a responsibility second only to the choice of the attending physician. Should the request for consultation come from the patient or his family, prompt acquiescence is advisable in all except rare circumstances. If the initiative has passed out of the physician's hands, he may be placed in the embarrassing position of rejecting the suggested consultant. Wherever possible he should thereupon name two or more outstanding associates, whose training, experience and ability would add to the sum total of information in the patient affected. Only with confidence in the competency of a recommended consultant can the desired advantage to the patient and the attending physician accrue to such an interchange. Furthermore, the laity can scarcely be expected to exercise expert judgment in this area. Indeed much of the disquieting confusion of modern practice in the United States stems from the indiscriminate choice of specialists by an undiscerning public. Certain basic factors regarding the proper practice of medicine in this respect should be more widely understood by people in general. At the same time the utmost tact and discretion must be exercised to assure sound counsel.

The Golden Rule applies with singular force in this situation where a fresh viewpoint is sought. A reputation for forthright honesty and fair dealing, coupled with high professional ability and standards, is a priceless ingredient for a medical consultant. In general two types of medical consultation are recognized, i.e., formal and informal. In the formal type, the consultant is called and a definite appointment is made by the attending physician; whereupon he relates the complete record and findings, along with the conclusions, to the consultant. The therapy with its effects is outlined. After this preliminary account, the attending and the consulting physician proceed to the sick room or the examining room. Always the attending physician precedes the consultant. After appropriate introductions all are dismissed except the nurse or a responsible member of the family, if the patient be a woman. Thereupon the consultant will begin his examination by extending the questions of historical importance in indicated directions. The physical examination will be complete, with added reference to all orifices. It is unfortunately not an unusual circumstance to find such details overlooked, although I resent the definition of a consultant as one who makes a rectal examination! Let us say, the examination will be exhaustive but not exhausting.

Upon the completion of the examination the consultant excuses himself with the statement that he will return after conferring with the attending physician. Always he should leave the room before the attending physician. The conference between these two physicians must be entirely private and should candidly resolve all details disclosed at the examination. The laboratory findings, including x-rays, electrocardiograms, and other objective data, will be reviewed. Points of agreement should be observed and those of disagreement reconciled if possible. The consultant should then dictate or write and sign a complete account of his findings, conclusions, and recommendations.

Up to this point the informal consultation varies primarily in its setting and origin. Usually it is encountered in group or hospital practice. Gone are all the details of dignified protocol. A physician meets an associate in the lounge or corridor and asks him to call on a certain patient and give him his opinion and advice. Or more regularly a consultation request is submitted through channels. In either instance the same ground rules of meticulous care in the examination are evoked, usually without the presence of the attending physician. The signed report becomes a part of the permanent record. The widespread practice of assigning this function to residents and junior staff members in the hospitals cannot be condoned. Chiefs or senior members of the concerned staff should answer such calls in person as a proper courtesy to their associates seeking counsel.

Upon the conclusion of the formal conference the consultant returns to the sick room with the attending physician and imparts in general terms the conclusions derived from his study. In recent years there has been a resurgence of the belief that the patient should know the entire truth. In spite of a most thoughtful consideration of this matter, while candor usually prevails, personally I have not found this stark approach sound or helpful in many instances. Regardless of their bravado, few men or women can accept a death sentence with equanimity. Nor should the physician consider himself the arbiter of life and death. In his Valedictory Address (Harvard 1858) Oliver Wendell Holmes offered this sound advice: "Truth is the breath of life to human society. It is the food of the immortal spirit. Yet a single word of it may kill a man as suddenly as a drop of prussic acid." Or, "I think the physician may, in extreme cases, deal with truth as he does with food, for the sake of his patient's welfare or existence. He may partly, or wholly withhold it, or, under certain circumstances, medicate it with the deadly poison of honest fraud. He must often look the cheerfulness he cannot feel, and encourage the hope he cannot confidently share. He must sometimes conceal and sometimes disguise a truth which it would be perilous or fatal to speak out." In an extremely forceful passage Holmes admonished: "Plain speaking, with plenty of discreet silence"; and citing examples of the same he concluded that caution be observed "before you proclaim that homicide is always better than vericide."

In reconstructing the clinical picture the consultant will utilize every available bit of evidence. When the canvas is completed, he will turn it tinted in its brightest hues to the patient who has waited the verdict with alert anticipation. This step in communication may be singularly difficult. A famous British cardiologist saw a brilliant contemporary statesman in consultation. To me the physician expressed unusual satisfaction in the results of his study. The private physician of the statesman gave a somewhat different version. He said after the consultation his patient had exploded. "All that examination and not a blasted word from him!" Silence may be even more distressing than words. Holmes again had a watchword for the physician: *"Breviter, sauviter, caute.* Say not too much, speak it gently, and guard it cautiously." Milton wrote:

> Gently hast thou told thy message,
> Which might else in telling wound.

Notwithstanding a distinct reservation regarding the wisdom of unmitigated candor in dealing with the patient whose will to get well must be reinforced, the attitude toward the family must perforce be forthright. The entire family should be brought together in a single group with the attending physician. There is a distinct loss of effective emphasis if the same report is repeated two or more times to straggling members. The consultant will do well to outline the natural history of the disease in question. In terms that can be clearly understood the evolution of the process should be delineated. If the diagnosis has been confirmed or derived by agreement between the consulting and the attending physicians, its significance should be carefully explained to the family or its responsible representatives. Where added laboratory examinations are required to bring the picture into sharper relief, their purpose should be explained. To the family the prognosis is perforce the most important element of the report at this juncture. Hippocrates wrote: "And he will manage the cure best who has foreseen what is to happen from the present state of matters." Extended clinical experience with careful weighing of all evidence accumulated in the study of the patient against the natural history of the disease will afford the best basis for the judgment of the outcome. Remember always that a guardedly unfavorable prognosis that is succeeded by recovery is inevitably better received by the family than a favorable outlook that terminates fatally. Wherever possible, the hand of the attending physician will be strengthened. Wherever applicable, a common approach has been: "Had I been in attendance from the outset of this illness, there is not one detail of management I would have changed." When an altered treatment is recommended, it is important to explain that the earlier medication was indicated at the time of its prescription, but that another mode of action is now desired. If a sharp difference of professional opinion has developed between the consulting and the attending physicians and no reconciliation is possible, the consulting physician will withdraw with the advice that a third physician be called. Under no circumstances should the consulting physician assume the care of this patient, unless the attending physician with the consent of the family so requests. As Holmes said, "Thou shalt not covet thy neighbor's patients." Particular observance of this admonition applies in the instance of referral when the temptation may be overemphasized by the expressed desire of the patient for a change of medical attendants. Under such compromising circumstances the consultant should protect the prerogatives of the referring physician by declining to accept the patient.

The referred patient, seen under any circumstance, is basically a subject for consultation and should be so considered. As stated, the sanctity of the referring physician's rights will always be honored. Not only does this provision apply to the return of the patient, but the concurrence of the attending physician should always be obtained before an added consultant is called. Where such additional counsel is deemed necessary, his preference should prevail. The courtesy of this approach will strengthen the professional bonds regardless of the ultimate selection of the second consultant. A common basis for criticism of the consulting physician is his tardiness in the transmission of his report of and recommendations for the referred patient. If the condition of the patient be emergent or if an unavoidable delay in reporting be foreseen, a preliminary report by telephone will spare much anxiety to the patient and his family and great discomfiture to the referring physician. Neglect of this amenity may alienate the family counsellor, whereas its simple observance in prompt and cogent advice will assure continued professional rapport. The final report should be comprehensive and directional without recourse to inconsequential minutiae that befog the issue. Bear in mind the referring physician is a busy man looking for assistance in a perplexing clinical situation. Do not hesitate to admit the limitations of your information. In so doing you will grow in professional stature and respect.

Personal experiences in consultation crowd from memory's spring. My first consultation came as an undergraduate at the University of Pennsylvania. Our practical training in obstetrics was obtained at the Southeastern Dispensary in the slums of Philadelphia. A classmate, considerably my senior in years, had left on an earlier call for a home delivery. Several hours later he called in great perturbation and asked me to come to his assistance. The baby had been delivered and what he suspected to be a ruptured cord of a twin presented at the vulva. To my relief it proved to be merely a rolled strip of retained amniotic membrane. Reassured on this point the fond parents were most relieved and, I am certain, accepted me as the father of three children upstate, as my classmate had introduced me!

As his house officer in Blockley (Philadelphia General Hospital) my father in medicine, Doctor David Riesman, undoubtedly exercised the greatest influence on my subsequent career in medicine. Many of my later clinical practices stemmed from that formative period, when I was clay in the hands of a master. No problem was trivial; no patient, a case. His sedulous attention to details was to be a lasting lesson. The consultation was in response to a personal appeal for advice from a medical peer. Each day was a revelation; each examination, a lesson in observation. In his quaint humor he would say: "Middleton, store that in your memory pigeonhole. It will come in handy some day." And so they have a thousand times; but over and above those isolated facts has come recurrently the vision of the erudite, thoughtful, meticulous clinician, whose every examination was a model of perfection.

The Wisconsin scene lent itself to a steady clinical growth in a salubrious academic atmosphere. An interest in pneumonoconiosis led to frequent consultations. Industrial medicine was in its infancy; but since the Wisconsin Industrial Commission was one of the first to make silicosis a compensable disease, I was called in consultation in such situations in increasing frequency. By choice the status of a friend of court was elected; but this was not always possible. Moreover, it became increasingly apparent that a witness who was on the Medical Faculty of the University of Wisconsin, created an obvious bias. Eventually the staff of the University of Wisconsin Medical School, on the advice of the Regents, took action that practically eliminated them from such controversial cases, unless they were in actual attendance upon the involved person as a patient at the Wisconsin General Hospital.

In the medical community of Madison a very reserved Norwegian-trained physician practiced a high grade of medicine. A fellow-countryman, a prominent figure in Chicago medicine, had told me something of his stature in Norway. I was flattered when he asked me to see a patient in consultation with him at her home. He had diagnosed pleurisy with effusion (left). Upon examination I confirmed his diagnosis. When he requested that I perform the thoracentesis, I proceeded by the conventional eighth interspace posterior approach. After withdrawing 500 cc. of clear, straw-colored fluid, I was taken aback to feel the cardiac systole through the needle. Listening anteriorly a to and fro friction rub synchronous with the heart beat had appeared and convinced me that I had unwittingly done my first pericardial paracentesis!

Shortly before leaving Madison I was called to see the father of a former student in consultation at Beaver Dam. The patient had had a cerebral vascular accident. After the completion of the examination I suggested that a lumbar puncture should be done. The son said: "I knew you would want a spinal puncture and I have the tray ready for you." Although I had not done a lumbar puncture for almost twenty years, my mind raced back to my initial lessons at Norristown State Hospital (1909–10) and I was confident that the simple technique would not elude me. The first thrust was successful; but it left me wondering how many equally simple procedures can be lost through disuse.

Perhaps my most unusual experience in consultation came during World War II. As a member of General Hawley's staff at the Headquarters of the Zone of Communications, European Theater of Operations, I received a call from the American Embassy. "Would you be available to see a French civilian in consultation with a French physician?" With General Hawley's approval I agreed to make myself available. The embassy then said: "We will let you know as soon as we clear with the State Department in Washington." All of these details arranged, I was taken to the apartment of Dr. Alexis Carrel. It will be recalled that by reason of his reception of certain Germans during the occupation of Paris he had been accused of collaboration. I had known him only casually in the United States. When he saw me, he was quite overwhelmed. "Ah! America remembers. My friends are there. I should never have left New York!" My examination confirmed all details of the diagnosis and prognosis. Dr. Carrel suffered from cardiac decompensation on the basis of hypertensive cardiovascular disease and his days were numbered. When I asked whether there were anything I could get for him, he said, "Oranges." I made a careful search of our hospitals in the Paris area but could find none. I did take him four quarts of orange juice and he was most grateful.

Not all of my experiences in consultation have been as fraught with human tragedy. During the closing days of preparation for Overlord I was called to see a Lieutenant General entrusted with a most responsible role in the invasion. A sufferer from chronic duodenal ulcer, he had had a severe gastrointestinal hemorrhage. Having completed my study, I said: "General, my reputation is not so good that I can assume the care of an ulcer patient who chain-smokes cigarettes. Either you give them up or you find another doctor." When I saw him the following day, he said: "I awakened at four this morning and lit a cigarette and then I said, 'Am I a man or a mouse? And who in the hell is this man Middleton anyway?' And I put out my cigarette."

Granting the acknowledged place of the traditional consultation in the practice of medicine, its present form presents certain apparent defects. These weaknesses may be viewed from three aspects, the patient, the party of the first part, and at least two physicians, the parties of the second part. In a more complete analysis still a third element, the family and friends of the patient must be considered. The latter group, naturally concerned for their loved one and in wider contact with solicitous enquirers, will frequently be the first to express fears for the sick. By direction or indirection their doubts are transmitted to the attending physician, in whom the patient has still the greatest confidence. Rarely in the face of discouraging progress or obvious loss of ground the patient may initiate the suggestion of a consultation. The subjective and emotional aspects of the situation outweigh the practical factors in many instances. Too frequently the request for a consultation is an agonal gesture, "doing everything possible" for the dying friend or kinsman. The attending physician may be entrapped in his own defensive meshwork of protection for the sick one and the family. His sympathetic viewpoint may have spared the family at the expense of their confidence in his capabilities. The unresolved diagnostic problem should rarely pose any doubt in his mind as to the wisdom of the prompt counsel of a trusted consultant. The guarded prognosis may more easily mislead.

In approaching the clinical problem presented by his confrere the consultant must consciously attempt to exchange places with him. Without obsequiousness he must first view the clinical situation from the attending physician's point of reference. Realizing the advantage of a fresh look at a more fully developed period of the disease, he will attempt to trace the stages by which the present condition has been derived. With due humility he will evolve his independent opinion with deference to the judgment of the attending physician in some unimportant details but with firm adherence to his own convictions in serious issues involving the health and the life of the patient. Mutual back-scratching creates an atmosphere of insincerity that robs the consultation of its true proportions and dignity.

In many instances the professional fee for consultation is established by the local custom or agreement among physicians. Again the distance and time involved will be determining factors; but, as in any other schedules, extenuating circumstances may modify the fee in any direction. Personally, when I was actively engaged in consultation practice, I encountered several specific problems. In the first place, I found great difficulty in reconciling myself to a sliding scale of fees based on the financial status of the patient, graphically described as the Robin Hood approach. The conventional custom of charging exorbitant fees to the rich to compensate for the charity extended the poor was distasteful to me. To meet my personal problem my fees for consultation were set, after conferring with the attending physician, at a level that would not embarrass the family with modest means; but I refrained from imposing a disproportional level for the wealthy. My experience over the years justified this position with one possible exception, which should receive especial attention. As a member of the medical faculty my status was "geographic full time." By the terms of such an appointment, consultation and referred practice was limited by time, academic duties, and a fixed level of income from this source. Although this widespread practice among medical schools has distinct advantages in rendering the services of skilled staff members available to the public at large and the medical profession in particular and in keeping the clinicians of the medical faculty in intimate contact with the problems of practice, the point of potential friction is the financial question involved. Without entering into this matter, which is handled in different fashions by the several schools, the involved clinician of the medical faculty must conduct himself with discretion in the exercise of his privilege. On one hand, he must not exploit his position; but by the same token he should not disrupt the prevailing fee schedule of the community by too sharp limitation of his charge for professional services.

Recapitulating, the consultation should be one of the strongest links in the modern practice of medicine. To this end the medical profession must be carefully indoctrinated in its utilization to the mutual advantage of the patient and themselves. Very importantly the laity should be assiduously instructed in the role, significance and value of the consultation. With the advances in medical science and practice in recent years the giants of old who stood out conspicuously above their fellows are singularly missing. Since a higher plateau of practice has developed, there are fewer peaks and fewer valleys. The development of a caste of consulting physicians is as undesirable as it is unnecessary. Certainly the conventional group practice or so-called clinic does not answer the specific question. Yet in every medical community there will arise certain physicians, who by reason of their professional stature and personal integrity, engender confidence and invite counsel. In the finest tradition of medicine these chosen few will always be called in consultation by their colleagues. In their ultimate refinement they will even be known as physicians' doctors!

"LET'S GIVE THE HOSPITAL BACK TO THE PATIENTS!"

Historically derived, the hospital originally served as a refuge for weary and disabled travelers. Later, its functions in the care of the ill and handicapped received their greatest impetus in the Christian era, but even the most visionary of earlier generations could not have pictured the hospital of the twentieth century as we know it. Almost inevitably, in the mechanization and sophistication of this complex organization that we term the modern hospital there has risen a certain impersonality that threatens its greatest service to humanity. Hence, when one of my associates, Dr. J. Herbert Smith, recently gave vent to his feelings with the expression, "Let's give the hospital back to the patients!", I realized that he spoke from the heart. Upon reflection, many circumstances serve to reemphasize the growing concern of many friends of medicine in this significant matter.

With illness, not infrequently one encounters a new or a renewed sense of dependence upon the part of the patient. Pain is a great leveler. Varying degrees of stoicism may modify the given individual's reaction to this most common complaint. The appearance of symptoms foreign to the common experience creates a sense of doubt and insecurity in the mind of the patient, which finds augmentation when the patient is left to his own devices to resolve the intangible manifestations of disease. At night the shadows magnify the psychologic hurdles and these questions are multiplied. Singularly, illness enhances both

Reprinted from the *Medical Annals of the District of Columbia* 31 (February 1962): 103–5.

the strengths and weaknesses of a given patient. In general, however, dependence upon the physician or the medical attendant is accentuated, and to this end the dislocation from normal daily activity and human interchange lends added weight.

Transported to the modern hospital for stay and care, the patient meets with the receptionist and members of the staff. Undoubtedly, the most important link in this transition is the first one who greets the patient upon entrance to the hospital. The reaction at this critical moment may determine a ready acceptance or a resistance amounting to actual hostility to his surroundings. Hence, it is extremely important that easy rapport be established at this point. The heart of the hospital will be adjudged both by the patient and the family from the human warmth of the admitting office and the sick room (or ward). No pains should be spared in the selection and indoctrination of staff members who will meet these simple but vital functions. In this strange atmosphere, the patient will be prepared for bed, and all personal belongings will be checked for safekeeping. From the austerity of the common hospital room, some coldness has been removed by warmer, less conventional furniture, and softer colored draperies, and pastel-tinted paints.

Regardless of these minor concessions in the interest of the patient's comfort, hospital routines have fallen into certain scheduled hours that are entirely foreign to the habits of the patient. For example, the waking at five to six o'clock in the morning for the routine taking of the temperature, pulse, and respiration, washing of the hands and face, brushing of the teeth and combing of the hair, presumably sets the schedule for the seven o'clock breakfast. Thereupon, after appropriate baths and bed-making, the floor is in order for the visits of the attending physicians. The luncheon and dinner hours are again set according to a formula that does not consider the patient's accustomed manner of life. In general, the nutriments and drinks that are served with and between meals are designed to meet the dietetic requirements of the given patient; but little advance has been made in affording attractive meals and appropriate portions to the taste of the individual. From personal observation over many years, the acceptance of hospital diets is largely overlooked, if one may judge from the rejections. This circumstance should be a responsibility not only of the dietitian but of the physician and nursing attendants.

To add to the indignities of the patient, the use of the unnatural bedpan and urinal is imposed. The latter may prove a convenience; but little advantage has ever been ascribed to the teetering bedpan, the control of which presupposes certain acrobatic abilities in the user. Indeed, recent studies have established the greatly increased physical effort that is employed in its use as compared with the bedside commode. Notoriously, physicians have paid scant heed to the wastage of time and patience in the waiting rooms of their offices; but it is almost inconceivable that such inefficiency should be tolerated in the x-ray and other special laboratories of a modern hospital. To compound this patent fault, the entire institution and its maximal operation are geared to the forty-hour week with the occasional concession of an added half-day on Saturday. Illness and disability know no moratorium in time. Patients are ill twenty-four hours a day, seven days a week, 365 days a year. Of course, emergencies over the weekend are regularly met by cadres of key personnel in all well-run hospitals, but the curves of occupancy, admissions, and discharges in the vast majority of the hospitals tell an eloquent tale of ineffectiveness and wastage that is receiving renewed attention in certain quarters.

In a hypercritical vein, Robert Ruark wrote: "You will see signs all over the hospital which read, 'Quiet.' The patients are quiet. But the staff is about as quiet as New Orleans during Mardi Gras. The nurses are all rude, orderlies scream and yell, the swill is better than the food, and the service pure Mills Hotel." Granting the excesses of reportorial license, certain of these points are valid and by the same token ready of correction. The quiet and peace of the sick room should permeate the corridor, nurses' stations, and service areas. The several mobile carts and chairs require periodic greasing to minimize irritating squeaks. In many hospitals, plastic or rubber mountings have silenced the clatter of waste baskets and cans; but too frequently anxious patients await the din of garbage collection in hospital courtyards at the break of each day.

As these circumstances are reviewed and our reciprocal responsibilities are brought into focus, it becomes increasingly apparent that many of the details of the hospital care are determined in the primary interest of the staff without due consideration for the comfort and convenience of the parties of the first part, the patients. Obviously, each and every one of these details should be subjected to careful study and evaluation. Where the staff is primarily involved and the patient inconvenienced, they should be modified or corrected. Furthermore, such practices as would lead to the added comfort of patients without serious dislocation of their own care and of the staff activities should be initiated in the interest of the former.

With few notable exceptions, hospitals of whatever order—sectarian, private, or governmental—are constructed in the interest of the health of the community from private or tax funds. While members of the medical profession pay their share in these respective sources, there is no justification for the position that the ultimate buildings that constitute the hospital should be our vested interest. By reason of the technical order of our profession and its co-professional supporting staffs, physicians must play a major role in the operation of hospitals; but we should bear in mind that the health of the people and its projection are not an exclusive prerogative of medicine. In the interest of balance and sustaining support, far-sighted physicians have generally encouraged the active participation of public-minded citizens on hospital boards of directors. And this is the natural state of mutual respect that should exist in a democracy.

Resolved to least common denominators, "Medicine exists for the benefit of the afflicted and not the afflicted for the benefit of medicine." With the astounding growth of the modern hospital, new problems and perplexities have arisen. Not the least among these has been an oversight of our primary responsibility to the patient. Quantitatively and qualitatively, this movement has been relative but appreciable. The time is ripe for a careful review of every procedure involving patient care by every member of the hospital staffs throughout the length and breadth of the land. The leading question should be: "How does this procedure or arrangement affect the patient?" Where his human dignity and his physical or psychologic comfort have been sacrificed in the interest of some inconsequential or unproved advantage to the staff, it should be amended without delay. Then and then only will the medical profession and its co-professional supporting cast take their proper positions as servants, not masters, of their patients.

"Let's give the hospital back to the patients!"

RANDOM REFLECTIONS

FOREWORD TO DOCTOR
DAVID RIESMAN'S ESSAYS

"Happy is the man that findeth wisdom, and the man that getteth understanding."

PROVERBS 3:13

Ten thousand people had gathered in the Field House of the University of Wisconsin, June 21, 1937, to attend the Commencement exercises which reached their fitting climax in the granting of the honorary degrees. In response to the summons a slight but arresting figure in turn occupied the center of the stage. For the faculty Professor Weaver declaimed the following citation: "Upon the recommendation of the faculty and by vote of the Regents, I present to you for the honorary degree of Doctor of Laws, David Riesman, Professor of Clinical Medicine in the University of Pennsylvania. Profound scholar; active member of many learned societies; skillful physician; master clinician; inspiring teacher; humanist of wide influence outside and within his own profession."

In a felicitous vein President Dykstra concluded: "David Riesman, statesman in the field of medicine, whose lectures and clinics have been the source of deep and abiding values to multitudes of students, among them members of our own medical staff, by virtue of the authority vested in me by the Regents, I admit you to the degree of Doctor of Laws, honoris causa."

At that moment came the poignant realization that Doctor David Riesman must live for posterity through his spoken and written words as disseminated by his devoted students, house officers, and associates. To future generations will be lost the engaging personality, the charm-

Reprinted from *High Blood Pressure and Longevity and Other Essays Selected from the Published Writings of David Riesman* (Philadelphia: The John C. Winston Co., 1937; repr. 1938).

ing intimacy, and the sustaining force of his friendship that no painter nor biographer may hope to capture for the canvas or the printed page. Gone, too, will be the quiet assurance of the ideal clinician, the unobtrusive dignity of his every word and act, and the calm voice of authority that is never raised in fruitless argument. Missing also the deeply sympathetic understanding and the intuitive human touch that characterize his every contact with the sick and the afflicted, putting to shame a counterfeit bedside manner. Further will his saving grace of humor, droll rather than robust, escape them. Withal the encompassing kindliness and devotion to his students and friends will probably be the most elusive of his personal attributes.

The breadth of his activities and the catholicity of his interests amaze even his most intimate friends. Abreast of every advance in medical science he nevertheless finds relaxation in astronomy and atomic physics. Medical history, particularly relating to the medieval period and the Dublin School, has received his close attention. He is a student of Shakespeare and yet finds time to delve into papal history and the Italian renaissance. Even admitting Doctor Riesman's superior intellect one must look to other sources to explain such an unusual measure of cultivation. To those fortunate enough to enjoy the hospitality of the Riesman home a partial explanation is immediately forthcoming, for the dinner table always carries the stimulating mental pabulum of enlightened conversation as well as the accustomed articles of calorific value. To his brilliant and engaging wife then Doctor Riesman owes much of his mental breadth. Into his advice that a young physician "should choose an understanding wife, for no man needs one more," may be read his personal experience. With characteristic insight he wondered "why any woman would want to marry a doctor."

Fortunately Doctor Riesman will live through his teachings. Indeed, it would be impossible to draw a picture of the man without this relationship. No man of our period has more adequately fulfilled the Hippocratic pledge, "By precept, lecture, and every other mode of instruction, I will impart a knowledge of my art to my own sons; and those of my teachers, and to disciples bound by a stipulation and oath according to the law of medicine, but to none others."

Doctor Riesman's qualities as a teacher (and teacher he will be to the end) combine many fundamental attributes that may with profit be analyzed. Disdaining all tricks of pedagogics he relies almost exclusively upon a fine mastery of his subject. Yet there is not the slightest semblance of pedantry in his clinics or lectures. Students of every station, undergradaute or graduate, are held attentively by a master in organization. Citations from his vast clinical experience enrich every presentation and their effectiveness is greatly enhanced by the natural-ness of their introduction. Here many are for the first time introduced to the fine heritage of medicine. Insidiously the fascinating story of our medical past is woven into the clinical presentation and almost imper-ceptibly the student is induced to extend his vista into the cultural aspect of medicine. Encyclopedic though his general and medical infor-mation upon a given subject may be, Doctor Riesman holds his teaching responsibilities too seriously to attempt the spectacular extemporaneous approach. Never would his native caution and keen sense of propriety stoop to the fickle appeal of such demonstrations; hence the telephone call of the evening prior to each clinic to arrange all details. Nor is this practice a mark of clinical ineptitude or lack of assurance, for his bed-side opinion based upon a logical and analytical approach is respected through the length and breadth of the land.

Deeply grounded in pathology, Doctor Riesman has not allowed this advantage to warp his clinical approach. As a part of his singular mental endowment a curiosity as to the newer developments in medical science has made each new method a part of his own diagnostic and therapeutic armamentarium. It follows that his presentations lack the dogmatism of the pragmatic instructor but the thinking listener soon senses a sounder philosophy in the contemplative teacher who has more than one string to his bow. Gifted with a faculty of apt expression, his bedside discus-sions have a lasting quality. As the years pass one is struck by the fre-quence with which lessons learned by strikingly clear demonstrations at Doctor Riesman's hands have become an integral part of one's practice. The bruit over the eye balls in Graves' disease, the soft eye ball of diabetic ketosis, the tachypnoea and delirium in rheumatic pericarditis, the preicteric pruritus of the eyelids, and the absence of herpes in typhoid fever are among the gems that are quickly "recalled from the mental pigeonhole" where he placed them years before. As a mark of his influence almost forgotten drugs, such as apocynum and aspido-spermin, are still rescued by his former students to bridge therapeutic gaps. His instruction is at one time both practical and profound. More-over its provocative quality excites a desire for a greater familiarity with the subject under discussion and recourse to the literature is inevitable. This end is facilitated by his kindly interest in all men.

Unstintingly Doctor Riesman has given of his time and energy to several institutions in Philadelphia, but a lion's share of his interest has always been diverted to the Philadelphia General Hospital. "Every great institution is the lengthened shadow of a single man." It would be hyperbolic to attribute such a relation for Doctor Riesman to so ancient an institution as Blockley; but the fact remains that much of the soundness of its present medical service may be clearly traced to his devotion to its welfare. When his vision of semi-private pavilions for the sick of moderate means is here consummated through public or private support, they should in propriety bear his name.

At the complimentary dinner to Doctor Riesman on the occasion of his seventieth birthday he remarked in explanation of his sustained mental vigor: "I have maintained contact with 'young men' of all ages." There flashed to mind an episode of some years past. A senior medical student at Pennsylvania had written to Doctor Riesman suggesting a deviation of the arterial blood from the diseased kidney through the inferior suprarenal branches of the renal arteries to the adrenal bodies in explanation of the hypertension of nephritis. The reply (May 19, 1911) is so typical of the inherent thoughtfulness and kindliness of the man that it is reproduced to essential detail:

> Your theory is very ingenious. I am sorry that you did not advance it during one of my ward classes or public clinics, as I should have been much interested to have had it discussed by the other students. (Then follow several pertinent quotations from the literature.)
>
> It would be interesting to follow the question up experimentally and at the autopsy table. I do not know whether anyone besides yourself has fully appreciated the significance of the vascular relation between the kidney and the suprarenal gland. Come and see me some morning, and let us talk the matter over.

The idea itself proved fruitless; but another medical student came under Doctor Riesman's spell. The favored group that has felt the stimulus of his friendship and the warmth of his guiding hand is relatively large. Students, interns, and associates swell the number. Then, too, Doctor Riesman has been one of the most effective speakers in medical gatherings throughout the country, but unfortunately these contacts lack the intimacy that fully measures the man. In widely scattered journals and textbooks some 200 articles on a host of medical topics have been published by Doctor Riesman. All of them bear the mark of clinical insight and some are medical classics of lasting merit. A representative group of these publications is herein assembled to preserve them for posterity.

To you, our beloved Chief, this volume is dedicated by your "professional children" in the hope that it may carry some measure of your beneficent influence to a wider circle of medical men of the present and the future.

SPEAKING FOR POSTERITY

As I listened to certain of our speakers, Mark Twain was reenacting the scene of the returning bedraggled young pirates. Tom Sawyer, Joe Harper, and Huck Finn were enjoying their own obsequies in the church. However, I do not hear "Old Hundred" and this is a thoroughly joyous occasion. After the afternoon's experience, I would add that I have some reservations regarding the Regents' relaxation of the ban on the designation of University buildings for living individuals!

However, with the psalmist, I can humbly say, "My cup runneth over."

As I contemplate this magnificent edifice and quietly wander through its inviting spacious quarters, my thoughts race across the tedious years of our travail. There pass in review a host of men and women of Wisconsin, who have given most generously of their time, thought, and substance to its consummation. In the preliminary stages of planning, that sage senior statesman, Regent Frank J. Sensenbrenner, lent his moral and material support to the project. At that time an estimate of $350,000 was set for the incorporation of the proposed Medical Library into the Service Memorial Institutes. When the proposal took renewed life and form under Mischa Lustok and his able conspirators, a goal of $1,000,000 was fixed as the objective of the Wisconsin Medical Alumni; whereupon I recommended a lumbar puncture for Mischa! Certainly Hammerstein must have had this group in mind when he wrote: "Climb ev'ry mountain, ford ev'ry stream, follow ev'ry rainbow till you find

Text of the response made at the dedication of the William S. Middleton Medical Library, University of Wisconsin—Madison. Reprinted from *Wisconsin Medical Alumni Quarterly* 7 (Summer 1967): 26–27.

your dream." I salute you, sons and daughters of Wisconsin, for the vision and pertinacity that won *your* dream.

No perceptive individual would question the vital position of the library in education. On the official acceptance of the Widener Library, Professor George L. Kittredge said if every building in Harvard Yard were to be destroyed by fire and the library spared, there would still be a University. Its importance is, if possible, even greater in medical education. "Books are the lifestream of the Medical School and the Library is its heart" (Middleton). During the years of our passage through the Slough of Despond, the hope of brighter days ahead lightened the burden. Yet, Miss Helen Crawford, her staff and their predecessors labored under unspeakably inadequate conditions. Only their unconquerable souls maintained the high esprit de corps and standards of service that have earned the admiration and gratitude of the students, medical faculty and University. And from here —

MacLeish wrote: "The American journey is not ended. America is never accomplished. America is still to build; for men, as long as they are truly men, will dream of man's fulfillment. So, changes in many fields are in progress and prospect. Yet change is ever viewed with reservation and suspicion by many people. Now automation, as a new way of life, is upon us. Indeed, an upheaval that will dwarf the Industrial Revolution of the last century is brewing. Singularly there persists a lag in the sociological adjustment to scientific advance. Society is earth-bound, while science soars in the stratosphere. Hence, with the application of electronic and computer techniques to librarianship, certain dislocations may be anticipated.

Obvious advantages of some newer methods obtrude themselves. Photography and duplication by Xerox and other means have greatly expedited the dissemination of information. By the same token these measures have eliminated the burden and hazard of the shipment of the original sources. Much of the purely mechanical functions of cataloging, indexing, distribution, recording, budgeting, and movement of personnel lends itself to more rapid and more accurate data processing. MEDLARS is the harbinger of greater things to come, for the constructive evolution of which we may trust Dr. Martin M. Cummings and the staff in the National Library of Medicine. Miniaturization will vastly increase the interlibrary movement of books. The conservation of precious space in the stacks will also be served by this device. Already regional depositories for the less-used volumes have been activated; but they must not be deemed tombs for tomes.

Inevitable though these radical departures may prove to be, conventional librarianship naturally views newer developments with some misgivings. In effect, engineering and mechanical science are threatening its cultural foundations. Certainly the prospect of a bottle of Coke, an IBM 1040 and a printout by an electric typewriter is less alluring and romantic than:

> A Book of Verses underneath the Bough,
> A Jug of Wine, a Loaf of Bread and Thou
> Beside me singing in the Wilderness —
> Oh, Wilderness were Paradise enow.

The captious philosophy of "creative Federalism" has a potentially ominous overtone. Should the fountains of intellectual productivity in the peripheral libraries be thereby dried, we will have admitted a Trojan horse to our camp in the guise of central control. Yet so great is the reservoir of scientific and medical literature that the federal government alone can and must afford direction and support in its dissemination. Such central leadership will insure an equitable flow of information through regional and local libraries. Accepting these material partners of the new order as fellow servants in a common cause, medical librarianship will experience a new lease on life in even greater contributions to scholarly advance.

Our Medical Library is the living symbol of the faith of the alumni and friends of the University of Wisconsin Medical School. Its brick and mortar are the physical evidence of your loyalty. Over and above this external demonstration, the surpassing spirit that moved you to undertake this major enterprise and to carry it to a successful conclusion, will be a shining example to Wisconsin men and women for generations to come. Never let it wither or fade.

From the bottom of my heart, I thank you.

THE DESTINY
OF THE AMERICAN COLLEGE
OF PHYSICIANS

"Your young men shall dream dreams; your old men shall see visions."
JOEL 2:28

By Roman law the collegium was a corporation established for the control and administration of medicine. In the Middle Ages the College of Physicians of Rome, composed of highly representative physicians, assumed complete supervision of all practitioners of the healing arts and allied activities in that city. Florence was the scene of a college's most effective operation in Italy. From this city the movement infiltrated the rest of Europe and Great Britain with certain deviations in form and function determined by local or national circumstances. In Central Europe the guilds prevailed and the professional college never won sustained support. The French colleges were multiplied; but the dominance of the Faculté de Médecine effectively prevented the continued growth of a college of physicians in Paris.

As our lineal prototype, the College of Physicians of London naturally arrests the attention. Never was it more truly said, "Every great institution is the lengthened shadow of a single man." Thomas Linacre (1460–1524) attended the cathedral school of Canterbury under William Celling, who later (1472) became the prior of Canterbury. When Henry VIII named Celling his envoy to the papal court, the latter in turn invited Linacre to accompany him to Italy. Linacre left Oxford

Presidential Address, Thirty-Second Annual Session, American College of Physicians, St. Louis, Missouri, April 9, 1951. Reprinted from *Annals of Internal Medicine* 35 (July 1951): 1–7.

and went with his old master as far as Bologna. He later moved to Florence to improve his educational opportunities. His medical degree was taken with honors at Padua. Returning to Oxford he surrounded himself with a coterie of learned and scholarly associates, illuminated by the brilliant light of the Italian Renaissance. Linacre found favor in the royal household and was called to court to tutor Prince Arthur. Upon the accession of Henry VIII to the throne (April 22, 1509) he was made king's physician. His private practice was likewise highly successful. Yet his vision was undimmed. He retained a clear picture of the fine contribution of the Florentine College to the standards of medical practice, and aspired to emulate this worthy example in London. Through his unselfish influence, Henry VIII granted the charter of the College of Physicians of London in 1518. Nor was Linacre satified with this regal formality. He gave the College its first meeting place, served as its first president, and established its library through the gift of his books. The debt of medicine to this scholarly physician, humanist, and devout churchman can never be discharged.

Traditionally the College of Physicians of London ("Royal" designation added later) incorporated three functions; namely, academic, administrative, and medico-political. In the absence of well-organized departments of medicine in the universities, the College encountered no early opposition to its academic programs of teaching, examining, and awarding diplomas and degrees. However, the preemption of the authority to contest the adequacy of training in the universities eventually led to sharp conflict and acrimonious civil suits between the College and the medical faculties. From the administrative angle, the College was admittedly in a strategic position to regulate the practice of medicine and medical ethics. Through the years this function has brought great credit to the corporation. The medico-political activities have fluctuated widely from time to time. In the main they have been confined to advice to the government on matters pertaining to health, but on occasions the College has embarked upon discussions of more involved policy.

The chronicle of the Royal College of Physicians of London is literally a record of the ideals, ambitions, and achievements of Anglo-Saxon medicine. Its traditions afford a worthy charter for similarly motivated bodies the world over. Yet at one period, its provincialism, which excluded all save residents within seven miles of the center of London and graduates of medical schools other than Cambridge and Oxford, almost sealed the doom of the College. Indeed, Lord Justice Mansfield saw fit from the bench to caution against so restricted a policy, "which might exclude even a Boerhaave." Reason prevailed.

The universities took their proper place in medical education. With certain liberalization, the qualifications were broadened and the standards of Fellowship in the College maintained. Artificial strictures were removed to admit physicians of superior attainments and responsibilities from all parts of Great Britain and the British Empire.

A proper chronological account of the Royal College of Physicians of London, fascinating though it is, falls beyond the present purview. However, certain details of organization and operation may to advantage be noted. The president is elected annually, but he may stand for reelection without limitation. Sir Henry Halford, Bart., presided for twenty-four years (1820–1844). Two presidents (John Caius and Sir George Baker, Bart.) were each reelected twice at intervals after their first presidency. The College accepts its civic responsibility by naming its Fellows to membership on many public committees and councils. The Royal College of Physicians of London is thereby a vital element in the body politic as well as the body medical of Great Britain. Nor will such a venerable institution escape the marks of its years in fixed customs and traditions. Among the most cherished of its possessions is the Gold-Headed Cane. The Trusts of the College constitute a fine legacy from the past and offer security for the future. William Harvey (June 26, 1656) gave his patrimonial estate in Kent to the College to afford the Censors a monthly collation and the Fellows an annual feast. The sums involved reflect better times. The Hamey Trust dates from Dr. Baldwin Hamey's munificence in saving the College building in Amen Corner from confiscation (1651). He made other provisions in the interest of the College; but characteristic of this institution is the preservation of the Spanish oak wainscoting of the previous building, supplied by him, to line the Censor's Room of the present home (Pall Mall East). The Sadleir Trust has an interesting history. Dr. William Croone, F.R.C.P., provided for two lectureships in his will (1684), one of which was to be delivered annually before the College. Dr. Croone afforded no support in endowment; but his widow, who later married Sir Edwin Sadleir, Bart., fulfilled her husband's design by demising the King's Head Tavern in Lambeth Hill (September 21, 1706) to her second husband for life, and, upon his death, four-fifths interest to the College of Physicians. Apparently the legacy was a profitable one, since the Sadleir Trust not only supports the Croonian Lectures, but several other less favored trusts as well. The Tavern was sold to the corporation of the City of London (1915). A study of these ancient and more recent trusts is most illuminating. The encouragement and support of research are increasingly evident in later grants and bequests. More infrequently the Royal College of Physicians is cooperative with other agencies in wide areas of human and scientific endeavor. Even the Almanac and Calendar of the College carry the reader back through its history; viz., "5 September, College House, Amen Corner, burnt down in the Great Fire, 1666," or "30 September, Harvey present for the last time, 1656." Neither devastating fire, death, nor enemy bombing has submerged this proud institution.

Fate made Dr. Heinrich Stern its instrument during a visit to London in 1913. His attendance upon a meeting of the Royal College of Physicians stirred him deeply and he resolved to initiate a similar organization in America. Returning to his foster home in New York, he found little encouragement for the project. Persisting, he finally enlisted sufficient support to obtain the legal incorporation of the American College of Physicians, May 11, 1915. The first constitution defined the purposes of the American College of Physicians in these words: "To promote the advancement of the science and practice of medicine, to further the study of biological medicine among its members, to elevate the standard of preliminary education of physicians and a standard of medical education, and secure the enactment of just medical laws by the state and federal government, and of a federal law providing for a national medical license, to attain the establishment of a national board of health, to promote friendly intercourse among physicians, to enlighten and direct public opinion in regard to great problems of health and medicine, and to afford recognition to distinguished achievement in medicine." These objectives followed in different accents the Royal College of Physicians of London's academic, administrative, and medico-political prerogatives.

The American College of Physicians committed the first error of provincialism that had so seriously threatened the Royal College. The early Fellowship was geographically restricted to the environs of New York City. Internecine strife scarcely waited for the death of the founding spirit, Dr. Stern (May 23, 1918). The long tenure of office, which might operate advantageously or disadvantageously to the College, led to serious disaffection and was abolished (1920). With the foundation of the American College of Physicians, there was developed an associated American Congress of Internal Medicine. This organization was responsible for the conduct of the annual scientific sessions and clinics. From its rather nebulous ranks, candidates were nominated to Fellowship in the College. The Congress was administered by its own president and vice-president, but it was under the administrative control of the Council of the College. This anomalous situation was terminated by a merger of the two bodies under a revised Constitution and Bylaws in 1926.

The present Constitution of the American College of Physicians outlines its objectives as follows:

> The object of the American College of Physicians shall be to establish an organization composed of qualified internists of high standing who shall meet from time to time for the purpose of considering and discussing medical and scientific topics, and who through their organization shall attempt to accomplish the further purposes of:
> (a) Maintaining and advancing the highest possible standards in medical education, medical practice and clinical research; (b) perpetuating the history and best tradition of medicine and medical ethics, and (c) maintaining both the dignity and efficiency of Internal Medicine in its relationship to public welfare.

The academic functions of the Royal College have by time and changing circumstances been largely delegated to the medical schools of Great Britain. So well entrenched was undergraduate medical education in the United States and Canada upon the establishment of the American College of Physicians, that the conflicts with faculties of medicine, such as had marred the relationships on the Continent, and to a lesser degree in Great Britain, never arose. Yet the American College has carved for itself an important and growing responsibility for postgraduate medical education. Utilizing the facilities of the medical centers, the College has acted as a catalyst in bringing the recipient into contact with adult education. This function promises to grow steadily in effectiveness through careful planning.

The Annual Sessions of the American College of Physicians have grown in importance and significance. Not only the quality of these programs, but the continued study to improve their scope and usefulness characterizes the effort. The most recent exploration in this direction has been the introduction of television to extend the effective range of clinics and demonstrations in removed hospitals and laboratories. Perhaps most distinctive among the educational devices of the College is the Regional Meeting. From humble beginnings, these sessions have grown remarkably in strength and effectiveness. The programs, arranged by the several Governors, afford an intimate insight into the practice of a given community. No two programs are alike, but there is a studied effort to encourage the participation of the younger Associates, or prospective Associates in these communions of the spirit.

The *Annals of Internal Medicine,* as the official organ of the College, vastly extends its educational horizon. Its growth is a brief for the demand and the reception by the medical profession. Its standards have well earned its present enviable leadership among journals of like objectives. By the same token the prestige accruing to the College through its sponsorship of the *Annals* is an imponderable asset.

Viewed in the light of the long-term investment, perhaps the most important of the College activities is its program of Research Fellowships (April 15, 1934). Many young men sustained by this support have fulfilled the promise of their earlier period, and have risen to positions of responsibility and eminence in medicine. More recent has been the embarkation of the College on the Latin American Fellowships (March 1949). Collaborating under a subsidy from the W. K. Kellogg Foundation, the American College of Physicians takes the responsibility for placing outstanding young teachers of Latin American countries in appropriate clinics and medical centers in the United States. The reciprocal advantage of such interchanges cannot be overestimated. In a materialistic period of human history, even a small contribution on the scales of international amenity may well swing the balance in favor of mutual understanding and peace among nations.

Traditions are not firmly fixed in thirty-six years. The Royal College of Physicians of London, with its wealth of stimulating and colorful tradition, was almost 400 years old when the American College of Physicians was born. Yet, there are certain straws in the wind of ultimate development in this College. To be sure, the lectureships are few, and the Trust Funds limited in number, but they are significant in their memorial origin and effective utilization. It is a healthful sign that the American College should use a considerable portion of the income of its Endowment Fund for the advancement of research. A further good prognostic index is the munificent contribution of one of its living Fellows to a Traveling Scholarship (A. B. Brower). This donation has been matched by the College for the same worthy purpose.

The founding fathers of the American College of Physicians anticipated some measure of administrative responsibility, if we may judge from the original constitution. However, the organization of American medicine in undergraduate training and licensure made such a provision presumptuous, and the later revisions of the Constitution contain no reference to such control of medical practice. However, the College has a vested interest in graduate and postgraduate medical training and continues its moral responsibility for the ethical practice of its members.

The Royal College of Physicians of London has maintained its medico-political activities at varying levels through the centuries of its existence. Its representation in important government bodies for advice and direction is an hereditary prerogative. In matters of public health, there has rarely been a dissident vote as to the propriety of its participation. Where political policy is involved, the support of the Fellowship of the Royal College has been divided. The first Constitution of the American College of Physicians clearly envisioned a parallel position of medico-political influence to that of the mother College. With the evolution of our College, this position was modified but not abrogated. The "further purpose" (of) "maintaining both the dignity and the efficiency of Internal Medicine in its relationship to public welfare" is a constitutional mandate for the participation of the College in any good work in the public weal. Traditionally, the College has remained aloof from entanglements in controversial administrative and medico-political issues. Yet, when upon due deliberation the die has been cast, the College has lent its complete support to the accepted decision. One notable example presents itself. The participation of the College in the examination of candidates for certification in internal medicine was strongly resisted as an administrative function until a careful study established its soundness and inevitability. Then the College gave not only its moral, but also its material weight to the movement, and its Fellows have contributed and will continue to contribute to the sustained growth of the American Board of Internal Medicine.

In our complex civilization new and divergent demands will perforce be made upon the American College of Physicians. The material advancement of the College has been astounding. Measured in terms of numerical strength in Fellowship, assured position in internal medicine, and comparative contributions to its growth, the American College of Physicians is one of the most powerful medical organizations in the world. Nor may the College abrogate its hard-won leadership. With this position come increasing responsibilities for medical guidance in national affairs. Without a sacrifice of dignity, official representation of the College on governmental committees and councils is as desirable as it is inevitable in the fulfillment of our mission.

By careful planning for the future, we must consolidate our position. The support of research and of exchange fellowships is a most commendable project, which should be steadily expanded. The growth of the *Annals of Internal Medicine* augurs well for the future. The Annual Sessions and the Regional Meetings are splendid efforts, but they are not enough. Mere material advantage does not suffice; the American College of Physicians of tomorrow must be a spiritual force that permeates every city, town and hamlet on this continent. In Gloucestershire late in the eighteenth century, five physicians banded themselves together for social and professional interchange. Their gatherings at Fleece Inn (Rodborough) and Ship Inn (Alveston) were convivial occasions; yet from these meetings of kindred spirits came the first ac-

count of the vaccination against smallpox (Jenner), and an early association of angina pectoris with coronary atherosclerosis (Jenner; Parry).
Their example is a challenge to every one of us. With the blessing of
the American College of Physicians, and without stultifying protocol,
small informal groups under the guidance of inspired Fellows and
Associates may well bring a resurgence of clinical medicine and human service in our day.

"Make no small plans; they have no magic to stir men's souls."

DEANS AND DIENERS

An American young woman was enjoying her holiday in North Wales when another group of fellow countrywomen joined company. Upon remarking the coat of arms of the Prince of Wales, one of them exclaimed: "I do so want to learn as many Welsh expressions as I can, while I am over here. What does, 'Ich dien', mean?" The tour conductor said: "Sorry, madam, I can't say." When the inquisitive one had left, he remarked: "Little I could have told her about Welsh; I am English myself."

The subject, "Deans and Dieners," admits of a logical approach and a ready resolution. By derivation the term 'dean' implies the chiefship over the men. Dignified usage finds the perpetuation of such a connotation in the clergy and in the diplomatic service. In Cambridge and Oxford the dean supervises the junior students in their preparation for graduation. In this country his function range from registry and college representation at the university level to complete administrative responsibility. In certain academic circles the last named status affords virtual autonomy.

When I assumed the administrative direction of the Medical School, President Glenn Frank permitted no exalted illusions as to my altered status. He asked, "Bill, do you know what is a dean?" I answered, "No, I have been attempting to answer *that* question for the three days since you offered me the position." President Frank said, "A dean is a fellow who is too dumb to teach and too bright to be president." In the

Remarks made on Student Field Day, University of Wisconsin—Madison, May 10, 1948. Reprinted from the *Wisconsin Medical Alumni Bulletin* 4 (Summer 1964): 17–19.

thirteen years of my tenure as dean of the Medical School I have modified this point of view appreciably. I am convinced that a dean is the
whipping boy for the faculty and the administration and the wailing
wall for prospective and ill-starred medical students. And at Wisconsin
—WE CAN TAKE IT!

The University of Wisconsin has known but three deans of the Medical School. The first of these recalls an almost forgotten part of University history. When Governor Nelson Dewey signed the act incorporating the University of Wisconsin (July 26, 1848), medicine was specifically named as one of four basic departments. Dr. Alfred E. Castleman
of Delafield was the leader in the effort to implement this provision.
Eventually eight men were named to the faculty that never functioned.
As dean of this paper faculty, after many frustrating experiences,
Castleman gave up the fight and recommended its abandonment—
ostensibly because of housing shortage!

Dr. Charles R. Bardeen came to Wisconsin in 1904. By reason of the
alphabetical listing he was the first graduate of the Johns Hopkins
Medical School. In his lighter moments he maintained that his degree
was granted on the condition that he would never practice medicine.

He brought to Wisconsin the rich tradition of the graduate teaching
of anatomy learned at the hands of Professor Mall. Already he had introduced the method of tissue study by frozen section. As professor of
anatomy his inquisitive mind took him into the intimate study of myology, bodily stature, heart size, and other fields. As dean his academic
lot was not an easy one. For a number of years the two-year status of
the Medical School found many of its students under the ultimate control of the College of Letters and Science in the granting of the bacca-
laureate degree. The vision of Dean Bardeen in selecting the first medical faculty continues to bear fruit in productive scholarship and research.

My first introduction to Dean Bardeen was unfortunate in a minor
particular. On my arrival to join the medical faculty in the Department
of Student Health (1912) I was invited to dine with the Van Valzahs.
After dinner Van walked back with me to the Cornelius house (next to
the Business Office of the University), which then served as the Student Health Clinic. On State Street we met Dean Bardeen, as he was
leaving the University Club. When Van introduced us, after the Pennsylvania custom I tipped my hat. Chuck's obvious amusement taught
me a lesson. I never again took my hat off to a Midwestern campus administrator.

Upon Dean Bardeen's death (1935) the present incumbent was

named to this high office. The less said of his efforts the better. Apparently he still thinks that *the primary mission of the School is to teach medicine, and its major product, physicians.*

I understand that he continues to practice medicine, a heinous offense. He is said to hold classes, which is unforgivable, particularly if he teaches anything. Aside from the observance of certain military punctilio, correcting grammar and spelling, picking cigarette butts and paper from the floor, his major activities consist in handball, tennis, and the protection of the morals of callow youth. At least he has no delusions of grandeur.

An assistant dean has been described as a mouse that aspires to be a rat. Dr. Meek has none of the characteristics of either rodent. A splendid teamworker, he finds time for basic research and proves himself a master teacher and counsellor to a host of students.

Turning to a more profitable subject, by definition a diener is a male servant or attendant. The German verb, *dienen,* affords a fine dignity in the translation—to serve, to be of service to, to do service, to be good for, useful to. The recent death of Clarence Rowley brought vividly to mind the stalwart company of dieners and orderlies with whom it has been my privilege to work at Wisconsin. A bronze plaque in Science Hall commemorates the services of George Willet in the Anatomy Laboratory. His dedication and high sense of moral values left their imprint on generations of Wisconsin medical students and staff members. William Young was a self-taught chemist whose meticulous attention to supplies and apparatus made him the trusted associate of Dr. Loevenhart, Dr. Tatum, and all of their associates and graduate students.

EVERYTHING BUT THE SQUEAL

On one occasion I incurred his displeasure by holding a special thermometer, by which I was checking thermocouple readings of alterations in the esophageal temperature, longer than he had anticipated. In Dr. Bunting's laboratory Arthur Otis ruled supreme. Certainly he was another of our most worthy collaborators. How he could sharpen a knife. His warm and cheery morning greeting is missed in our midst. On one occasion in mild protest against my acknowledged proclivities in affording pathological materials for section, he said, "Doc, this time you brought back everything but the squeal!" John Mullen is his worthy successor and he plays a good game of handball!

Clarence Rowley operated effectively for forty years in the Department of Physiology, trusted and respected by his fellow workers and legions of medical students. In his unobtrusive fashion he would speed laggard staff members as well as students when the clock crowded five o'clock.

In many ways James Hipple tops this outstanding group. A mechanical genius, he has the most capable hands I know. Possessed of one of the most clearly analytic minds I have ever encountered, he intuitively goes to the basic principles of every problem. He never fails to improve upon the original design of a staff member. Mechanical ingenuity of a remarkable order is his forte. On one occasion he constructed an Edelman electrocardiographic apparatus with the original as his sole guide. His grasp of all technical devices continues to amaze his associates of the faculty.

The establishment of our hospitals, Bradley Memorial Hospital, Student Infirmary, and State of Wisconsin General Hospital, introduced a new and vital member to our team, namely, the hospital orderly. Many of our clinical staff had their hospital training in large hospital centers of the East and elsewhere. With my derivation from the Philadelphia General Hospital (Blockley), with them I was prepared to greet the proverbial hospital tramp. Irresponsible and undependable, he was driven from one hospital to another over the land by addiction to the bottle or needle. You may imagine my surprise and gratification when men of sound mind and sterling character filled these important positions in the University. It has been a privilege, to which I would publicly testify, to work with Bill Lazear, Gene Gerfen, Nick Pfeiffer, Carl Skrenes, and a host of other splendid orderlies in the past twenty-eight years. I hold them in high esteem as teammates.

In a special category I place Wilhelm Kaplan, for he not only serves as orderly (or general factotum) in surgery; but he has charge of the Laboratory of Animal Surgery. Dr. Erwin Schmidt rendered a signal service to the Medical School when he brought Wilhelm to us. Each morning I am greeted by a familiar, "How are you, Doctor Middleton?" "Fine—and you, Wilhelm?" "Parfait, Doctor Middleton, parfait." I salute them all.

These men have been and are an integral part of the University of Wisconsin Medical School and its tradition. The University of Wisconsin with its Hospital is richer for their presence and their service. In this sick world, we, as medical men and women, can take a significant lesson from their example and face the daily task and the challenge of practice with the watchword, "Ich dien."

FORWARD!

Four and a half years have passed since that shocking, fateful Sunday at Pearl Harbor. Stunned by the patent unpreparedness of our defenses at a most vulnerable point in our perimeter, the fall of Corregidor completed our humiliation six months later, four years ago. Grimly the American people set itself to the task at hand. "Blood and sweat and tears"—prophetic words. Tense effort, wanton expenditure of life and treasure, the anguish of mind and body are vivid memories of the world-wide travail. Just a short year removed, the vaunted Nazi war machine disintegrated in unconditional surrender in the European Theater of Operations. The momentary exultation of victory was pardonable in the release of V-E day, but sober reflection soon took its place.

In this hour of remembrance we are met to pay humble but proud tribute to the sons and daughters of Wisconsin who "gave the last full measure of devotion." Of 12,500 students and graduates of the University who answered the call, 485 succumbed. May our lives be enriched by their sacrifice.

War has ever been a grisly, brutal business. Yet man from the earliest historical era has attempted to perpetuate the illusion of chivalry in arms. If ever it existed, the intrusion of invention and science into the conduct of war has long since effaced every semblance of decency and regard for humanity. Only in the individual devotion to duty, self-sacrifice, and mercy may we have an amelioration of the common psychological decline. The very thesis of war is unholy. Only self-preservation condones it.

Delivered at University of Wisconsin—Madison Convocation, May 8, 1946.

274

Retaining all of its ancient horrors, modern warfare has multiplied its capacity for destruction and devastation. Jungle warfare saw deception and savagery at a premium. On the other hand aerial movements and motor transportation vastly speeded the tempo of military operations. In this area the psychology of the combat soldier changed perceptibly. Mechanization largely impersonalized warfare. With amazing inconsistency the hideous flamethrower was retained in World War II, while the lethal gas was eschewed. With diabolical thoroughness the rocket and mass bombing grew in effectiveness against combatants. *Total* warfare became a horrible reality in robot, jet-propelled, and atomic bombs. To complete the ring of terror there was lacking only jet propulsion of atomic destruction through the stratosphere from a remote continent, an arresting thought for warmongers.

To meet this challenge our Wisconsin recruit went to war. In a democratic manner he volunteered or answered the call of Selective Service. With obvious abstraction he packed his prized possessions, closed his desk, and bade his reluctant farewells. With commendable application he adapted himself to the routine and rigors of military life. His physical fiber tightened, his reaction time speeded, teamwork and high degrees of technical skill became his part in the evolution of a modern machine of war, indeed the greatest machine of war in history. Then as his assurance grew, mere training began to irk him. Finally his impatience was answered; he was alerted for overseas duty. After months of preparation he was to have the test of fire in one of the many elements of the Army, Navy, or the Marines, in far-flung foreign theaters of operations.

Following him from the classroom, office, farm, and shop we found him fundamentally unchanged. He worked hard, played hard, fought hard. Physically he was fit; he was keen; his eyes were clear. He was perhaps a bit subdued and suddenly mature. He was singularly thoughtful. For the first time international affairs arrested his attention. He spoke gravely of the folly of isolationism and pondered over the loss of the peace after World War I. He was profoundly interested in America's place in the post-war period. He had no illusions. His victory might also be lost as was his father's in World War I. Almost overnight he became a seasoned veteran. A score of murderous beaches, rigors of combat, treachery of the jungle where every shadow might hide a lethal danger, the cross fire of the hedges, mountain passes, deadly landing operations, suicidal naval assaults, and, to cite a single example, high-level daylight bombing such as was carried out in the European Theater of Operations, made of him an effective fighter. On the land, in the air, on and under the sea, he met a desperate, resolute foe and beat him at his own game. He encountered strange diseases in strange lands. He was in constant combat with the elements. Campaigns were carried out under unbelievable physical and geographic handicaps. The heat of the tropics contrasted with the cold of the Arctic and the Ardennes Bulge. He endured the march from Bataan and the Golgotha of Buchenwald. Such fortitude gave complete denial to the charge of soft living. Whatever the hardship, whatever the hazards of his mission, always an abiding faith in home and in you, his people, sustained him. Then the rendezvous—and yet by the strange alchemy of death he is forever young!

To us his torch is passed. To him we owe devotion to the cause of freedom for all peoples throughout the world. And yet a year spent and no peace. Domestic strife and misunderstanding shake the very pillars of the temple. Shallow demagogues prate of the American standards and way of life. Idle words, and they would trade our spiritual heritage for material advantage. Confusion, doubt, yes, open suspicion tincture our international relations. These thunderheads must not be permitted to precipitate disruption. Candor will resolve most of the current differences among nations. We must not risk the peace for which he paid so dearly. Nor is it too late to regain the lost ground; with vision we may reach the plateau of mutual confidence and permanent security among the peoples of the world.

Then and then only may we close ranks with our Wisconsin sacrifice, and eyes front, chins up, march proudly into eternity.

MILITARY MEDICINE: ITS ROLE IN WORLD HEALTH

Through the ages, vague suggestions of wonders to come have been vouchsafed by all manners of men. The power of prophecy is reserved for a limited few. Justly famous for his painting and sculpture, the incomparable Leonardo da Vinci (1452–1519) was one of these rare spirits. An engineer-architect, mechanician, and natural philosopher, his design of a flying machine comes as no surprise, when one finds his brilliant intellect anticipating Bacon's explorations into experimental science. Failing in his aeronautic machine, da Vinci said: "There shall be wings. If the accomplishment be not for me, it is for some other. It shall be done." In the realm of fancy, Jules Verne (1825–90) took his avid youthful readers *"Vingt mille lienes sous les mers"* years before submarine navigation became a commonplace mode of transportation. In a letter to Joseph Priestley, Benjamin Franklin (1706–90) prophetically wrote, "The rapid progress that true science now makes, occasions my regretting sometimes that I was born too soon. It is impossible to imagine the height to which may be carried, in a thousand years, the power of man over matter. We may perhaps learn to deprive large masses of their gravity, and to give them absolute levity for the sake of easy transport. Agriculture may diminish its labours and double its produce; all diseases may be by sure means prevented or cured and our lives lengthened to pleasure even beyond the antediluvian standards."

While Franklin's predictions for aeronautics and agriculture have

Keynote address of the 74th Meeting of the Association of Military Surgeons, Washington, D.C., November 20, 1967. Reprinted from *Military Medicine* 133 (April 1968): 257–64.

been exceeded through the acceleration of research and development in these fields, his optimistic prospect for the control of diseases bids fair to fall short of his timetable. Yet health is the birthright of every human being and medicine is dedicated to its attainment. At first glance, war is scarcely a climate in which the advancement of the health of its participants might be considered a primary objective. Of its baser elements, Erasmus (1466–1536) wrote:

> One war springeth of another. . . . There is agreement among poisonous serpents. But unto man, there is no wild or cruel beast more hurtful than man. . . . Moreover, when the brute beasts fight, war is one for one, yea and that very short. . . . When was it ever heard that an hundred thousand brute beasts were slain at one time fighting and tearing one another? . . . Now if man will weigh, as if it were in a pair of balances, the commodities of war on one side and the incommodities on the other, he will find that an unjust peace is far better than a righteous war.

From a different approach, the issues raised may thus be analyzed: "As we view the ledger dispassionately, measuring the anguish of mind and body and the material cost of war against certain apparent gains, one circumstance emerges vividly. The major advances have represented an acceleration of normal growth, in which the pooling of experience and the teaming of experts have been the determining factors. War is a catalyst, and the trickle of essential knowledge which distills from this horrible cauldron, adds little to the vast flood of science" (Middleton).

Nevertheless the health of combatants and the supporting civilian population may swing the tide of battle. History is replete with examples of the decisive effect of disease and epidemics in conflicts of the past. Moreover, the contributions of military medicine, past and sustained, afford a brilliant chapter in medical history. Regardless of their immediate impact on military personnel, this circumstance is especially evident in areas removed from the trauma of battle and related to the welfare of mankind in general. A conspicuous example is the fundamental study of the physiology of digestion by William Beaumont, an Army surgeon (1785–1853). The product of the prevailing preceptor-house pupil system, he never attended a medical school. Yet, when the thoraco-abdominal gunshot wound of Alexis St. Martin fortuitously resulted in a gastric fistula, Beaumont seized the opportunity for his remarkably objective studies. With meager facilities, this research was pursued in frontier army posts from 1825 to 1833. His *Experiments and Observations on the Gastric Juice and the Physiology of Digestion* (1833) brought prestige to American medicine and undying fame to its author. A measure of Beaumont's philosophy may be gathered from this passage. "But we ought not to allow ourselves to be seduced by the ingenuity of argument or the blandishment of style. Truth, like beauty, when 'unadorned is adorned the most'; in pursuing these experiments and inquiries, I believe I have been guided by its light. Facts are more persuasive than arguments, however ingeniously made, and by their eloquence, I hope to be able to plead for the support and maintenance of these doctrines."

Bacteriology was in swaddling clothes when George M. Sternberg (1838–1915) isolated the pneumococcus (1880). He had distinguished company, for Pasteur reported his discovery of this organism in the same year. Sternberg's publications, including the first American textbook on bacteriology, enjoyed a wide circulation. Sternberg's professional status was recognized by his appointment as Surgeon General of the Army (1893). Enteric infections have been the bane of military medicine from the beginning of recorded history. In fact, military operations in the field have repeatedly been impaired or immobilized by diarrheal and dysenteric epidemics. Lacking knowledge of their etiology and epidemiology, sanitary provisions for the protection of military personnel were by modern standards quite lax. Although Eberth isolated the typhoid bacillus in 1880, the incidence of typhoid fever in our army in the Spanish American War (1898) was appalling. Certain French and German workers had contributed materially, but Almoth Edward Wright (1861–1947) was the real father of typhoid vaccination (1896). As professor of pathology in the Army Medical School, Netley, England, he directed the vaccination of all British troops in South Africa and India. His further studies on opsonins and other immunological phenomena marked him as a leader in the field. Frederick F. Russell of the United States Army initiated the typhoid vaccination program of our troops in 1909. This experience was consolidated by its application to 20,000 soldiers on the Mexican border (1912). Thus, military medicine led the successful attack against typhoid fever in Great Britain and the United States. The lessons of sanitation to combat enteric infections in the field have been more difficult of achievement.

An interesting linkage brought Walter Reed (1851–1902) into a key position for the study of yellow fever in Cuba that was to write a dramatic page in military medicine and human progress. Major Reed had done commendable work on typhoid fever in the laboratory of Professor William H. Welch at the Johns Hopkins Medical School. When the Army Commission for the investigation of yellow fever was established (1900), he was named its chairman. His associates were Aristide

Agramonte, James Carroll, and Jesse W. Lazear. Several detached observations directed their immediate attention to the probable vector, *Aëdes (Stegomyia) aegypti* (Finlay, 1881, among others). Carroll survived an experimentally induced attack of yellow fever, whereas Lazear succumbed to an accidental infection. By convincing evidence, the cause of the disease was proved to be a filterable agent transmitted by the mosquito. Thus the Army Commission laid the foundation for the eradication of yellow fever and, in turn, for the exploitation of tropical resources hitherto denied by its ravages.

From the public health standpoint, the immediate dividends from these surpassing discoveries were realized in the control of epidemics of yellow fever in New Orleans, Rio de Janiero, and Mexico. The most telling conquest was in Cuba, the scene of the Army Commission's basic observations. Assigned as chief sanitary officer to Havana, Major William C. Gorgas (1854–1920) initiated a plan for the protective screening of the yellow fever patients and for the eradication of mosquitoes. Speaking of the remarkable success of the program, Gorgas wrote, "The results were better than we dared to hope. . . . Yellow fever rapidly decreased, and on September 28, 1901, the last case of yellow fever occurred in Havana, and since that time—now more than two years—not a single new case has developed in the city. I think it is evident that the disappearance of yellow fever from Havana was due solely to this mosquito work. Remember that it was an every-day disease in Habana, and had been so for more than a hundred years." The arrival of patients with suspected or proved yellow fever constituted no unusual problem. In their transportation from the city wharf to the yellow fever hospital, Gorgas said: "The only precaution taken is to see that Habana mosquitos do not get an opportunity to bite him."

The scene changes. Disregarding the international events that made the construction of the Panama Canal an essential undertaking for this country, the tremendous health hazards of the zone rendered the odds for its successful completion almost prohibitive. Already the French, with the able de Lesseps as leader, had forsaken the task under the unceasing onslaughts of malaria and yellow fever (1880–89). The morbidity and mortality from these diseases fully earned the designation "White Man's Grave" for the area of operations. To Gorgas was given the stupendous task of making life and working conditions in this pestridden area livable and sufficiently healthy to get on with the job. Encountering obstinate resistance from his superior officers of the line, he was fortunate to have the influence in high places to prevail in the execution of the essential measures of preventive medicine. Great then as was the engineering feat of constructing the Canal (1914), even greater credit must be accorded the preventive measures and the indomitable will of William C. Gorgas, who made them stick. His subsequent career as Surgeon General of the Army (1914) and in the worldwide prevention of disease cast added luster on military medicine.

Clearly malaria was more devastating than yellow fever in Panama. Its clinical description antedates Hippocrates (460–370 B.C.) who gave a clear account of its manifestations. To this day, it remains the leading creditor against health and life over a wide sector of the globe. While drainage, cultivation, and the eradication of mosquitoes have limited its zone of endemicity, still to military operations and civilian life in such areas it poses problems of grave significance and great magnitude. While serving as a surgeon in the French Army in Algeria, Alphonse Charles-Louis Laveran (1845–1922) discovered the plasmodium of malaria (1880). For his contributions in tropical medicine, Laveran was awarded the Nobel Prize in 1907. Under the stimulating guidance of Sir Patrick Manson, Ronald Ross (1859–1932), while in the Indian Medical Service, recognized the anopheline mosquito as the vector for malaria. With remarkable brilliance he traced the sexual and the asexual cycles of these parasites in the vector and in the human host. His fundamental research and his practical plans to destroy the mosquito won the Nobel Prize (1902).

Still, malaria constitutes a major medical problem to the present day. Prematurely, as events were to prove, quinine was relegated to a subsidiary role in the control of malaria in World War II. Atabrine, chloroquine, primoquine, and other agents proved to have certain advantages in the prophylaxis and treatment of malaria. Indeed, so great was the confidence in the new drugs that the huge stockpile of quinine from World War II was deemed surplus to the foreseeable military requirements and considerable quantities were sold. History has repeated itself in Vietnam. Infestation with *Plasmodium falciparum* is common. Among these malarial patients resistance to certain of the newer agents has developed quite regularly. Quinine has regained a measure of dependability. The several Medical Services of the Armed Forces are exerting every effort to close the gap. Independently and with the cooperation of medical schools and private foundations, some 65,000 drugs have been screened and over 2,000 synthesized. Diaminodiphenylsulfone (DDS) has proved a promising suppressive agent. Quinine with other drugs, as pyrimethamine, apparently prolongs the usefulness of each component and reduces the incidence of relapses. The establishment of the susceptability of certain primates to human strains of *Plasmodium falciparum* offers an experimental model of great potential value for the trial of test drugs. From this approach, much time and human exposure may be spared.

So the stream of military medicine that will naturally flow into civilian practice, steadily grows. Unusual interest stems from the remarkable progress in studies of the blood and blood processing for transfusion in the Armed Forces. Basic studies (Army) have been directed to the genetics of the erythrocytes and iron metabolism. The life span of the platelets has been fixed at 2.2 days. Under Army contract, workers at Michael Reese Hospital (Chicago) have conducted an experiment of unusual promise. The removal of the stroma of the erythrocytes abolishes their antigenic properties. As a hemoglobin concentrate, such a preparation affords a ready transport and exchange for oxygen without disturbance of the oncotic pressure of the plasma. Fort Knox studies have established a prolongation of the erythrocyte survival period from twenty-one to forty-two days upon the addition of adenine. The Naval Blood Research Laboratory, Chelsea, has continued its program of frozen blood. In Vietnam, a wounded Marine, who received ninety-three units of blood, forty-one of them frozen, survived without adverse reactions. The frozen blood is still held as a reserve for the normal supply of acid citrate dextrose blood. One of the most impressive medical lessons of the current hostilities is the advantage of the prompt delivery of skilled attention to the wounded combatants. Early evacuation by helicopter facilitates the prompt correction of shock. The Military Blood Program Agency (July 1962) coordinates the plans, policies and procedures of this effort in the Army, Navy, and Air Force under the Surgeon General of the Army. In a national emergency, this Agency would assume immediate responsibility for the procurement, processing, and distribution of blood for civilian as well as military requirements. Another healthy sign of the times is the close coordination of far-flung laboratories over the world with the parent laboratories in the United States. For example, the interchange between a field laboratory at Da Nang, Vietnam, and the key laboratories at Bethesda and Chelsea is paying large dividends. Schooled in the shock units of World War I, the sophistication of the present-day treatment of traumatic shock in forward areas, with continuous or repetitive checks on many physiological parameters, is a miracle of modern medicine.

Nor are the impacts of military medicine necessarily removed from the civilian population. The Clinical Investigation Program of the Air Force covers a broad spectrum of subjects. A careful analysis assigns a general applicability of sixty-four of seventy-eight projects to civilian as well as military medicine. Naval Medical Research Units have answered the call for medical support for such emergencies as poliomyelitis in Kwajalein, Marshall Islands (1963), famine in Southern Iranian ports (1963), cholera in Iran and Afghanistan (1965), meningitis in Morocco (1966), and malaria, filariasis, and yellow fever in Ethiopia. A singular example is encountered in the *Journal of the American Medical Association*, October 2, 1967. The leading article, "Congenital Abnormalities Following Gestational Rubella in Chinese," gave J. F. Grayton of the United States Naval Research Unit, Taipei, Taiwan, as the first of the several authors. His part was a major contribution to international amity. Throughout the world, representatives of the several Medical Services are earnestly engaged in independent or cooperative efforts with native agencies to meet health problems. For example, small research laboratories are maintained by the Army at Kuala Lampur, Malaysia, and Saigon, Vietnam. In cooperation with Thailand, the Army supplies certain key personnel in the SEATO laboratory in Bangkok. The Naval Research Units in Cairo, Egypt, and Taipei, Taiwan, have had distinguished records. The Dental and the Veterinary Services have been especially diligent and effective in their international exchanges.

One of the most rewarding programs is the Preventive Medical Technician Course given to foreign students at the Naval Hospital, Oakland. Through 1965, this twenty-two-week program had been given to 1,000 young representatives from the Republic of China, Republic of Korea, Pakistan, Republic of Vietnam, and Latin American countries. On the recommendation of the Latin American Surgeons Conference, March 1963, another prototype educational program was initiated at the United States Air Force School for Latin America (now the Inter-American Air Force Academy), Albrook Air Force Base, Canal Zone. This project was funded by the Military Coexistence Program and certain operational sums. From the on-job training of personnel from Latin American Air Forces in the medical facilities of the United States Air Force, there evolved the program of training five-man teams from Latin America in medical service, laboratory, aeromedicine, and public health. Upon completion of these courses, such teams return to their native countries as assistants to physicians. In this role, they bring medical and sanitary support to backward areas. A total of 170 students from fourteen countries (Central and Latin America and the Dominican Republic) have taken this six-month course. Expanding this philosophy to the field, Mobile Training Teams (six United States Air Force and two representatives from the host country) have visited remote areas upon invitation. Apart from the professional services and guidance given by these intimate exchanges, there is an opportunity to evaluate at first hand the fruits of the training program. The acceptance and response of the recipients is whole-hearted. Sanitation and water supplies have been greatly improved. Certainly the official evaluation should be a matter of public record. "The Preventive Medicine Civic Action Program greatly contributes to hemispheric solidarity and assists the U. S. Air Force missions and the host Air Forces in achieving many of their medical, counter-in-sur-gency, and nation-building objectives" (McConnell).

Were a precedent sought, the letter of General George Washington to General Smallwood, captor of the "Symmetry," should serve the purpose. Particularly does the issue stand in sharp relief when we realize that the Commander in Chief was writing from the encamp-ment at Valley Forge in the Winter of Despair, 1777–78. Furthermore, he was interceding for the enemy:

> A few days ago I received a letter from Doctor Bayes, Surgeon of the 15th British Regt. requesting me to return some valuable manuscripts taken in the Brig Symmetry. He says they are packed in neat kind of portable library and consist of: Dr. Cullen's lectures on the practice of medicine, 39 or 40 vols., Cullen's lectures on the Institutes of Med. 18 vols.; Anatomical lectures, 8 vols., and Dr. Black on Chemistry, 9 vols.; the whole in octavo. If they can be found, I beg that they be sent up to me, that I may return them to the Doctor. I have no other view in doing this, than in showing our enemies that we do not war against Sciences.

Military medicine has perforce always been interested in nutrition. James Lind (1716–94) has been termed the father of nautical medi-cine. A surgeon in the Royal Navy, he wrote a classical thesis on scurvy (1754), in which he established the protective virtue of lemon juice. Although the Royal Navy was very tardy in its adoption of Lind's sug-gestion, his further contributions to naval and prison hygiene mark him as an original thinker. Certainly, all men who "go down to the sea in ships" owe Lind a debt of gratitude for his clinical acumen in the protection of naval personnel against vitamin C deficiency.

The experience in Korea and Formosa (1952–54) emphasized the importance of nutrition among the allied native forces. Regardless of motivation, we would obviously profit immeasurably by the improved stamina and performance of such men when brought to good physical standards. An externally altruistic motive might thus prove ulterior in practice. Some idea of the magnitude of the problem may be deduced from the fact that of three billion people in the world today, one and one-half billion are malnourished. Of this number, one-half billion are always hungry. Twenty-five million die each year from malnutrition (Kern). The fragmentary approach was eventually resolved by the organization of the Interdepartmental Committee on Nutrition for National Defense (1955). The composition of this Committee (Frank B. Berry, Defense; W. H. Sebrell and Harold R. Sandstead, Public Health Service; Howard T. Karsner, Navy; and Stanhope Bayne-Jones, Army) assured high standards of planning and achievement. The Departments of Defense, State, Agriculture and Health, Education and Welfare, and later the Atomic Energy Commission had representation on this Committee, to which were called specialists in nutrition, biochemistry, food technology, agriculture, and medicine as consultants. As a basic policy, the Committee conducted its surveys only upon the request of a sovereign nation. Early, such approaches were made by Iran, Pakistan, and Turkey. The supporting funds were supplied by the United States Mutual Defense Assistance Program. Each survey was designed to cover a large group of subjects in the significant elements of nutrition and a statistically adequate, but smaller, number in depth. Although these studies involved only the military personnel of the host nation, with such a broad sampling of the adult population natural inferences could be drawn for the entire people of the country. Significantly, native counterparts in survey personnel matched the team from the United States and the logistical and laboratory support came from the host country. These arrangements assured a continuity of interest and constructive action on the recommendations of the teams that called heavily upon the federal and academic ranks of experts for the execution of this important task. The average duration of a survey was seventy to eighty days and the cost of each study to this country was $53,000. Since its organization, the International Committee on Nutrition for National Defense (now the Nutrition Section, Office of International Research, National Institutes of Health) has conducted surveys of nutrition in twenty-eight developing countries, as well as in Alaska and in the Blackfeet and the Fort Belknap Reservations in Montana. In all, the nutritional status of over a quarter million people has been studied. In the last analysis, the most tangible measure of the success of this carefully planned and implemented movement is the sustained effort of the host countries to surmount their formidable problems of malnutrition. In each of these host nations there has been established either a high level Interdepartmental Committee on Nutrition or a national Institute for Nutrition. "Food becomes the so-called first line of defense" (Berry and Schaefer). This has been a truly magnificent achievement.

Two of our most illustrious generals appreciated the importance of military medicine in civilian health. In Cuba, General Leonard Wood demonstrated his medical background and his perspicacity in naming William C. Gorgas the chief sanitary officer of Havana. His judgment bore fruits in the astounding restoration of healthful living to this notorious pest spot of the Western Hemisphere. General of the Army Douglas MacArthur showed similar wisdom in his medical organization of Japan after the surrender of August 14, 1945. Under the immediate supervision of Brig. General Crawford F. Sams of the Army Medical Service, programs for the control of smallpox, tuberculosis, cholera, typhoid fever, and typhus fever were initiated and effectively pursued. With the complete cooperation of the Japanese, patterns of preventive medicine and hygiene were extended on such a comprehensive scale as to constitute a major medical-political weapon (Friedman). In both instances, the action of the commanding general in advancing the welfare of a foreign people redounded to the credit of our nation and to the stabilization of the occupied country. Even if ulterior motives were assigned to this activity, careful attention to the health of the affected alien population afforded commensurate protection to our own forces.

World War II saw several detached operations in the interest of civilian health through the assignment of medical personnel and materiel from the Armed Forces. With closer international relationship came new real or implied obligations. Opportunities for medical assistance saw the assignments of personnel to control rabies in Korea and Thailand. Tuberculosis testing of cattle in Ireland and the Republic of the Philippines was undertaken. Foot and mouth disease was studied by the veterinarians of the Air Force in Argentina and Brazil. However, a change in the official attitude has become evident in recent years. Instead of indiscriminate grants to emerging countries for reckless expenditures without let or hindrance, the outlined medical plan is designed to help the less fortunate to help themselves.

Confronted with the overwhelming requirements for medical assistance to the military and civilian populations of Vietnam, certain decisive factors presented themselves. The language barrier was apparent. The historical, religious and ethical backgrounds of her people differed from American patterns. Values of our civilization were divergent in many details. The national political situation was unclear. The central government of South Vietnam was insecure. Several other Free World nations were supporting medical units in the country. Unrelated civilian agencies in the United States were actively affording medical relief missions in the land. Emotionalism outweighed reason. But health conditions in South Vietnam were appalling. Certain figures are convincing: 800,000 children with hookworm infestation;

100,000 lepers; certain epidemics of smallpox with 92 percent mortality, at birth a life expectancy of thirty-five years. Dengue, malaria, rickettsial diseases, leptospirosis, melioidosis, cholera, plague, Group B arthropod-borne encephalitis, hepatitis, and tropical sprue are rampant in Vietnam (Gilbert and Greenberg).

The situation called for a close coordination of medical support. Medical Civic Action took official form through a memorandum of the Deputy Secretary of Defense, May 14, 1965. This communication directed the Assistant Secretary of Defense (Manpower) and the Assistant Secretary of Defense (Health and Medical) to develop the policy and to coordinate the activities of six mobile medical teams (three Army, two Air Force, one Navy). Their operations at the Vietnam level were through the Military Assistance Command, Vietnam, with appropriate liaison between the Embassy of the United States and the Ministry of Health of the Republic of Vietnam. The approaches have taken several forms. Under MEDCAP I (Medical Civic Action Program) after basic indoctrination, eight teams of medical personnel of the United States Army Forces assisted, trained, and advised their opposites of the Republic of Vietnam in the care and treatment of civilians. MEDCAP II has broader terms of reference. For example, each Air Force Base participated under a full-time Civic Action Officer. In turn, this officer maintained contact with the District Chief, MACV adviser, Army, Navy, and the Free World Military Assistance Forces counterparts, base commander, and local civilian officals. Through the District Chief, appropriate proposals are identified and programmed under the Revolutionary Development Project. If one is accepted, it is assigned to a given Service. Thereupon, all details are evolved by the Medical Coordinator and the Civic Action Officer of the designated unit. On the scene, the hamlet chief selects the site of meeting; but the foregathering of the prospective patients grows from curiosity to actual suffering. MEDCAP II is designed to bring medical care to native Vietnamese; but its continuity and sustained force must derive from the people. The unit distributions of military personnel to this project are eight Army, seven Air Force, and six Marine Corps. The participants from the United States Armed Forces have found the assignment most rewarding. The most recent form of participation of the Medical Services in Civic Action in Vietnam is MILPHAP (Military Provincial Hospital Augmentation Program). After a three weeks' indocrination in the political, military, sociological, and life elements of Vietnam, the team of four officers and twelve enlisted men (skilled technicians in the main) is assigned to a provincial hospital. They furnish all hospital equipment and are functionally supplemental to the existing establishment. They are, however, immediately responsible to the provincial chief and the senior provincial medical officer. Certain tactical and official obstacles have been encountered. If these hindrances to the delivery of superior medical care are overcome, MILPHAP may measure up to its promise. Following the best traditions of medicine, medical officers in Vietnam have privately and unofficially rendered attendance on orphanages and homes. This unsung charity keeps the medical officers in the stream of life and strengthens the ties with the common people. "Medical aid to the underprivileged has become more than a humanitarian movement, it is a potent instrument in the struggle for the minds and loyalty of men" (Ellingson).

Military medicine has kept the faith. Its tradition of service to mankind has bridged the years and the changing tides of history. Its contributions to the advancement of medical science and practice constitute a proud hallmark of the Medical Services of the Armed Forces. In the current crisis, its force for the improvement of mankind has been conspicuously effective. To paraphrase the Holy Writ, by their works our medical confreres in Vietnam are worthily fulfilling its charge— "that they might have [health] and that they might have it more abundantly" (John 10:10).

FOREWORD,
MEDICAL SCHOOLING IN SOUTH CAROLINA

Pride in achievement and the design to preserve historical continuity usually determine the chronicling of events and circumstances that attend human affairs. With Shakespeare, we would agree:

All the world's a stage,
And all the men and women merely players.

While the validity of this observation is obvious in general history, it is eminently applicable to medical education, where personalities obtrude at every pass. Too frequently their piquancy is lost in the detachment of years and distance. In effect, one hopefully exchanges the intimacy of personal interplay for the perspective of time and judgment. Nor can this hiatus be entirely filled by the common recourse to contemporary media that too frequently convey the animus of the moment. Hence, the recorder must depend upon every scrap of available information, weigh its significance to related individuals and situations and weave the data into a fabric that we term history. Always, whether in the glare of the footlights or in the background, the leading actors and their supporting cast will afford the drama of human endeavor. Rare fortune finds the ultimate leader the historian in this instance.

To paraphrase President Harnwell, "[The Medical College of South

Foreword to Dr. Kenneth M. Lynch, *Medical Schooling in South Carolina* (Columbia, S. Car.: R. L. Bryan Co., 1970).

Carolina] is both a captive and a product of its history and reflects it in its organizational development." A medical school in South Carolina was first proposed by President Thomas Cooper of South Carolina College to the Medical Licensing Board and the Medical Society of South Carolina (1821–22). His suggestion apparently stirred the medical profession to action. The Medical College of South Carolina was chartered in 1823 by the Legislature and its first session began November 8, 1824. Its problems were manifold from the outset and the chronicler has done them full justice. Perhaps most significant, if the harassing question of its location be reserved for the text, was its proprietary control by the private practitioners of Charleston. Not until February 19, 1913, after the survival of many crises, did it pass to the ownership of the State. Private and detached medical schools had been established in a number of other centers and Charleston, with its commercial and cultural advantages of the period, promised a successful prospect for the Medical College of South Carolina. The author affords a faithful account of the vicissitudes that attended its course.

Significant was the fact that all of the original faculty of the Medical College of South Carolina, except for Stephen Elliott, LL.D., professor of natural history and botany, were graduates of the University of Pennsylvania. In his famous "A Discourse upon the Institution of Medical Schools in America," John Morgan (1765) said:

> Perhaps this Medical Institution, the first of its kind in America, though small in its beginning, may receive a constant increase of strength and annually exert new vigor. It may collect a number of young men of more than ordinary abilities, and so improve their knowledge as to spread its reputation to distant parts. By sending these abroad duly qualified, or by exerting an emulation amongst men of parts and literature, it may give birth to other useful institutions of a similar nature, or occasional rise, by its example, to numerous societies of different kinds calculated to spread the light of knowledge through the whole American continent wherever inhabited.

So Samuel Henry Dickson, James Ramsay, Henry Rutledge Frost, Thomas Grimball Prioleau, John Edwards Holbrook, and Edmund Ravenel, graduates of Pennsylvania, fulfilled Morgan's prophecy in sowing the seed of medical education in South Carolina.

Conspicuously missing from the original faculty of the Medical College of South Carolina was James Moultrie, Jr., one of the foremost medical statesmen of his day. However, he became professor of physiology on the reconciliation of certain differences with the second medical school in Charleston (1832). His "Memorial on the State of Medical Education in South Carolina," delivered before the South Carolina

Society for the Advancement of Learning (1835), is a masterly analysis of the situation that merits a place with Morgan's "Discourse" among the classical essays on medical education in this country. With calm objectivity, he outlined the weaknesses and deficiencies of the existing program. Anticipating by twenty-four years the institution of a sequential approach to medical education, he said: "Let the period of learning be extended to six or eight months and let each student be compelled to attend three or four courses." Not only did Moultrie urge more searching examinations for graduating students, but he invoked the same principle in recommending that "each applicant for a professorship shall give a *practical* or *demonstrative* proof of his abilities and competence to fill the situation."

Moultrie also indicated the paucity of clinical facilities that was to haunt the Medical College of South Carolina. The author of this history stresses the tenuous relationship with local hospitals through the years. Indeed, the Medical College continued to function on a precarious scale through the latter half of the nineteenth century in no small measure by reason of the lamentable state of medical education in the country at large. The stage was set for the Flexner Report (1910) that shook American medicine to its roots.

Obviously, there are few instances in history of the emergence of a single individual as the determinant in human events. Certainly the author would be the last one to accept the thesis that "Every great institution is the lengthened shadow of a single man"; but Kenneth Merrill Lynch appeared on the Charleston scene at a critical period in the existence of the Medical College (1913). Except for a short period of detachment in private practice (1921–26), his entire professional career has been in this academic community.

My qualification to assess "Dale" Lynch as a physician, teacher, administrator, and man may be laid primarily to a friendship that has stood the test of time since 1911. As fellow housemen in Blockley (Philadelphia General Hospital), our associations were intimate; but there was a further common bond in the shared guidance of Professor Allen J. Smith, Chairman of the Department of Pathology in the University of Pennsylvania School of Medicine. Dale's ties with Professor Smith were close, since he worked in his department. A former Dean of the University of Texas Medical School, Professor Smith was a lodestone for interns and residents from that state. By tacit understanding, anyone whom he befriended was an Allen J's man. Dale and I were so favored.

Naturally, Dale's research at Blockley interested me greatly. He had undertaken the difficult task of studying the transmission of leprosy.

You can imagine my amazement when I found fastidious Dale Lynch collecting bedbugs (*Cimex*) from the cots in the attic at Blockley! My curiosity carried me further. Since there had been a report of leprous lesions induced by the injections of suspensions of histologically established leprous tissues into cold-blooded animals, Dale set up an ingenious model to circumvent the bedbug's aversion to cold-blooded animals. Shaving a rabbit, he removed thin sections of its skin. He applied these segments of rabbit skin to the frog. The bedbug, which had been exposed to leprous tissue, bit through the rabbit skin; but no characteristic lesions developed in the frog. Any man who would go to such extremities to fool a bedbug was a marked individual in my book!

This foreword is not a biographic sketch of Dale Lynch, whose attainments in pathology and parasitology have given him an international stature, but his place is preeminent in the historical evolution of the Medical College of South Carolina. After eight years as Vice Dean with Dean Robert Wilson, a cultured gentleman of the old school, Dale succeeded to the Deanship in 1943. The master plan of the Health and Medical Educational, Service and Research Center was evolved with advice from many quarters (1943). Federal funds (Hill-Burton) with legislative support expedited its construction. The steps in the evolution of this modern complex of buildings, with each acquisition of land and the transformation of a marsh into a beautful and useful campus dedicated to human service, may be traced in the stirring account of the trials and tribulations that have eventually been crowned with success. Significant was the dedication of Medical College Hospital (May 10, 1955), since for the first time in its history the Medical College of South Carolina had complete control of adequate hospital facilities. The later construction of the Veterans Administration Hospital in an adjacent site assured adequate expansion for clinical instruction. So this magnificent Center emerges through the pages of this chronicle as a tribute to its master architect, Kenneth Merrill Lynch, who is eminently qualified to record each step of this glorious achievement, and to the everlasting credit of all of his supporters and collaborators.

> Last scene of all,
> That ends this strange eventful history.

UNACCUSTOMED AS I AM

The ancient cliché, "unaccustomed as I am to public speaking," is rarely heard nowadays. Indeed, the very expression is a breach of a basic principle of public address: never introduce a speech with an apology. The spoken word is the common possession of normal human beings and language is the recognized medium of communication. The interchange between peoples of the same language anticipated the written word. While codes were introduced for telegraphic and early radio messages, the telephone, radio, and television now transmit the spoken voice to the listener without essential distortion. The more sophisticated methods of communication have vastly extended the range of the spoken voice. Instead of reducing the demands for public speakers, these media have greatly increased the same.

The physician has a singular responsibility in this area. The opportunity to inform the lay public and to educate the profession is boundless. As physicians, we must meet the varied invitations to address lay and professional groups with intelligent perspective. It would appear most presumptuous of any individual without training in public speaking to advise his fellows in this important matter. Yet, from necessity, certain lessons may be learned by personal experience. Close attention to the playing back of a recorded paper or speech will disclose personal faulty accent, emphasis, and timing. In my hands this expedient in self-criticism has been invaluable. Realizing early the exactions of an academic position in this direction, I have made a close, sustained study of public speakers. In time one may draw relatively accurate estimates

Reprinted from *The Journal of the American Medical Association* 178 (October 21, 1961): 308–311.

of a given speaker's depth, substance, soundness, and effectiveness. Weaknesses are especially patent. Sources of strength fix themselves upon the attentive, analytic listener with experience. Only from such a background would one have the temerity to express his thoughts in so involved a subject. In this instance, praying your indulgence, may I ask that you do as I say, not as I speak.

PREPARATION OF THE SPEECH

Regardless of the occasion, every speech deserves careful preparation. In most instances this phase represents the actual writing of a paper. In others, the notes that have been accumulated need only be arranged by headings. In either event, an outline of the subject matter will bring order out of a mass of diversified materials. Carefully, then, the relevant data are drawn under the several headings. When this stage is reached, order and organization by topics will follow naturally. In the implementation of this end reading and rereading of reference cards or notes, to which letters or numerals are affixed for guidance, will insure their inclusion under the appropriate headings of the outline. Before the final stage of the incorporation of the data, careful study to define sequence, direction, and conclusion should precede the actual first draft of a paper. In general, this element will be written in longhand unless the author is perchance adept in typing. In simpler papers the first draft may be read to a dictating machine for transcription. From experience, a rough, double-spaced typed copy will afford the best working base upon which corrections may be made. The editing of this copy should be most careful. Corrections, deletions, and insertions should follow a recognized pattern to facilitate secretarial collaboration.

The preparation of a given paper affords the author an unexcelled opportunity to gain a commanding grasp of the subject. Its orderly evolution has become a part of his conscious thinking for days and weeks. In his leisure moments he will have arranged and rearranged its substance to gain greater effectiveness. The time and the occasion will naturally modify the plans for presentation. Walshe wrote: "A good speech is a work of dramatic art, carefully prepared and appropriate in form and substance to its end. The speech that wasn't worth preparing can scarcely be worth listening to. . . . Our audiences don't expect much, and our speakers have a mysterious confidence in their ability to be coherent and amusing without topic or preparation."

Regardless of the method of presentation the speaker must avoid talking down to his audience. Simple rather than involved sentences will hold the attention and permit closer adherence to the order of the presentation. Ponderous phrases and overweighed figures of speech are relics of a departed day; but even then Wolcot wrote:

> I own I like not Johnson's turgid style
> That gives an inch th' importance of a mile;
> Casts of manure a waggon-load around
> To raise a single daisy from the ground.

PRESENTATION

Three manners of presentation are offered to the speaker. He may read his paper, he may use notes, or he may speak without reference either to his paper or to notes. Each method has its advantages and its followers. If the paper is read, the speaker must never lose sight of the fact that the assembly and not the paper on the lectern is his audience. He must have as much familiarity with its contents as though he were to present it without reference to the text. Singularly, there are comparatively few good public readers. Apparently, in many instances, from the standpoint of the audience, punctuation is ether lacking or ignored. Perhaps the most disconcerting custom is the reading of figures or statistics without the support of a visual aid. Some of the best public speakers are cultivated readers. With heads up and voices well controlled they have so trained themselves that even with careful observation it is difficult to discern that they are actually reading. A widely accepted compromise with reading the complete paper are notes. With a carefully evolved list of headings the speaker can give his undivided attention to the audience, the real target of his presentation, without perceptible reference to notes. His train of thought, as directed by his notes, will permit an orderly evolution of his subject to its logical conclusion.

Keith said: "I preferred listening to the imperfect word coming spontaneously to the lips of the speaker rather than to the most finished of read phrases." From the standpoint of the listeners, undoubtedly the free-wheeling" of speakers is preferred to reading. Its exercise is the most exacting form of presentation. It requires complete command of the subject without recall or redress. By the same token, it is the most subtle flattery of an audience, in that the speaker must perforce prepare himself to the fullest degree to deliver his message. A carefully organized text is resolved to a broad outline with appropriate capitals for emphasis. Three or four major headings will usually suffice to bring the subject to a clear conclusion. These headings will be memorized and collateral reading will be appropriately adapted without conscious commitment. Avoid too involved and laborious quotations. Spontaneity and warmth of expression are invaluable adjuncts. When one has mastered the method, deep personal gratification will be earned in this form of delivery.

The place on a stated program will have a definite influence on the reception of a given paper. The opening position in the morning program usually finds the confusion of a gathering audience. The first place in the afternoon is commonly greeted by a somnolent group with obvious splanchnic rather than cerebral plethora. The introduction by the chairman is too commonly an ordeal both to the speaker and the audience. It may range from a perfunctory announcement of the title of the paper and the name of the speaker, to a fulsome, lengthy account of his curriculum vitae and qualifications. In the latter instance, a favorite story is occasionally recounted. Reluctantly, the famous actor, Wilton Lackaye, had accepted the invitation of an amateur dramatic society to address their meeting on the condition that its entire proceedings would last not longer than thirty minutes. Overwhelmed by the stature and the luster of the distinguished guest, the chairman embellished his introductory remarks in flights of flowery laudation. After an interminable exhibition of gaucherie he turned to Lackaye and said, "The guest of honor will now give his address." With studied deliberation, the guest rose and said, "My address is the Lambs Club," and took his departure.

Certain physicians are splendid raconteurs. To these chosen few should be reserved the privilege of story-telling in medical meetings. The set stories, particularly if off-color, lend nothing to the dignity of our sessions. In many instances, they detract immeasurably from the effectiveness of a scientific paper. A professional audience, although superficially amused by such diversions, would elect other performers and platforms of entertainment other than their scientific sessions.

The manner of presenting the paper will have an important bearing upon its success. The studied attitudes of professional actors and public speakers have little place for the physician. Yet one of the best contemporary medical speakers was an actor in an amateur theatrical troupe of an eastern university in his undergraduate days. Another excellent physician-lecturer was a concert baritone. Regardless of the individual experience each public appearance is a period of stress. As a matter of principle, do not bet on a placid horse. The best speaker, like the spirited horse, will show a certain tautness before his introduction. Like football player's, this tension passes with the kickoff. Otis Skinner recounted a trying experience of "going stale" in Pittsburgh. After a long run and many single night showings on the road his mind suddenly went blank on familiar lines in his part. This threat is accentuated by a complacent frame of mind. The extreme tenseness of certain individuals may manifest itself in marked tremors. Easy deep respirations may control these disconcerting movements. Many years ago a singing teacher in a small town in eastern Pennsylvania recommended rising on the balls of the feet with the hands loosely clasped behind the back to ease the tension of singing and speaking. This inconspicuous maneuver is very effective in controlling tremors. The dangling hands may prove most troublesome. Instead of placing them in the pockets, rest them singly or together on the lectern or, as stated, clasp them behind the back.

The speaker is naturally the cynosure of his audience. The clothes should be inconspicuous. The well-modulated voice with particular emphasis on clear enunciation will hold the undivided attention of the listeners if the message is noteworthy. From time to time speakers in medical meetings have demonstrated misguided instruction in public speaking by affectations of the voice and by extravagant movements of the arms and body. A prominent eastern surgeon shocked his hearers at a midwestern medical school by a speech reminiscent of religious exhortation. By contrast, years ago the famous John B. Murphy came to Philadelphia as the chief speaker at the annual meeting of the Undergraduate Medical Association of the University of Pennsylvania School of Medicine. Of commanding presence, his voice was by contrast high pitched and squeaky. Yet a critical audience was held spellbound by the brilliance of his message. Perhaps the most effective medical lecturer of my acquaintance was Dr. George A. Piersol, Professor of Anatomy at the University of Pennsylvania School of Medicine. Although his subject was far from exciting, he held the close attention of his classes by the clarity of his diction, the simplicity of his rhetoric, and his remarkable command of the English language. An ease of manner on the part of the speaker by the same token puts the audience at rest. The speaker can establish better rapport by fixing an individual or a segment of the assemblage in his gaze. Smooth movements of the hands and arms may be used for emphasis; but jerky, irregular motions may be very disconcerting to the audience. Personal mannerisms are always diverting and should be eliminated at any cost.

VISUAL AIDS

The meeting room should always be studied by the speaker before his scheduled appearance. Particularly will he be interested in the seating arrangement and acoustics. Long, narrow halls present immediate handicaps. It is unusual to gain audience response in the rear of such rooms. The public address system should be inspected and tested personally before the meeting. If this is impossible, the speaker will be well-advised to observe the efforts of his predecessors on the program in its use.

Visuo-auditory aids are increasingly used to supplement or illustrate scientific and quasi-scientific talks. The augmentation of the auditory impressions by visual means has long been recognized as an effective expedient by teachers at every level of education. The slate and blackboard of our childhood school days bore early witness to this basic principle. All visual aids require unusual care in their preparation. The conventional lantern slide, while the most useful of demonstration adjuncts, is still the most abused medium of illustration. While standards are widely publicized, their observance is the exception rather than the rule. Overcrowding, illegibility, and impropriety of subject matter are some of the common faults in the preparation of slides. A standing order of no slides rather than inadequate ones, should prevail. Indeed, in fairness to the audience, one of the ground rules of a medical meeting should permit the chairman to disqualify a speaker whose slides are nonacceptable. The same precautions apply to color slides and to motion pictures with and without sound tracks. The speaker must remember that his side or back is turned to the audience when he demonstrates at the blackboard or screen. The use of a pointer or electric light beam will serve to keep the audience abreast of the demonstration. At all times he must assure himself of the adequacy of the public address communication. The reading of the legends and the substance of materials on the projected slides by the speaker is a bête noirê to many listeners. As advantageous and helpful as these visual aids are, the essayist must avoid such dependence as to render himself helpless if they are misplaced. Again, speakers using projectors of any type should assure themselves of their performance before the scheduled meeting. At an international medical meeting in the East several years ago, the presentation of a foreign guest was completely ruined by the inability to project his slides. His chagrin after the transatlantic voyage may well be surmised.

Certain amenities are due the scheduled discussers of papers, if they are opened for such comment. Usually a copy of the prospective paper is afforded these individuals; but this courtesy is not universal. In general the British are more direct in their criticism than the Americans. William Harvey referred to the "candor of cultivated minds." Trotter commented: "At no time has the astringent tonic of critical writing been more necessary for the health of medicine." Professor Anton J.

Carlson once pungently commented on a paper before the American Physiological Society: "What we need is more dogs, less words." Walshe struck a similar note when he wrote: "Indeed there is a striking contrast between the strong and priceless tradition of literary criticism and the poverty of criticism in medicine and the medical sciences. Yet, surely science must benefit by the strong fresh wind of criticisms blowing through laboratories, clinics, and studies and keeping the atmosphere therein free from the mildew of mythology and orthodoxy that so easily infect and stunt our thinking." The same strictures should apply to the spoken as to the written word. Intellectual honesty and candor would dispel the clouds of patent insincerity that too frequently befog the discussion of medical papers. In keeping with local custom, at times abstracts of papers are requested for press releases. This expedient undoubtedly has a salubrious effect in solidifying public relations. Where closely monitored it will unquestionably assure a minimum of distortion of the inadequately understood medical information. From whatever cause, the press accounts of medical affairs have been vastly improved in recent years—a healthy sign of the times.

AUDIENCE-SPEAKER RELATIONSHIP

Finally we turn to the audience-speaker relationship. Up to this point the attention has been strictly directed to the speaker's responsibility to his audience. By the same token the assemblage may be expected to observe certain amenities. Many of the present-day medical meetings have concurrent programs of great interest. The inability to synchronize or to dovetail these sessions to meet the diversified requirements of many physicians in attendance has led to an increasing movement on the floor. At a panel discussion in a recent national meeting the constant ebb and flow of seething humanity was evident from my vantage point. To a few speakers of the group, this inattention was manifestly repugnant and only with effort could they maintain their own train of thought. There can never be recourse to barred doors; but two expedients for remedying this situation are available to all. In the first place the interims are regularly spaced in most meetings. Then, too, the darkening of the room for the projection of slides affords a natural occasion for movement. In justice to the speaker and the remaining audience this consideration should be accorded. Public speaking is a two-way street. Every experienced public speaker feels the response of his audience. Restlessness, unnecessary movement, and ill-concealed conversation reflect inattention and may adversely influence the delivery of the speaker. Conversely, he may rise to his full stature and effectiveness when close rapport is indicated by quiet attention and the lightening of the faces of his listeners as his points go home. The applause that conventionally follows his paper is small reward for its preparation and delivery; but every tried speaker will know whether he has gotten his message across from his own personal reaction. Public address is here to stay. This medium affords the medical profession a widely acceptable channel of communication. It, follows, therefore, that the individual physician must studiously develop his full potential in this important direction.

DESIGNED

BY SYLVIA SOLOCHEK WALTERS

COMPOSED, PRINTED, AND BOUND

BY IMPRESSIONS, INC., MADISON, WISCONSIN

TEXT LINES ARE SET IN CALEDONIA, DISPLAY LINES IN OPTIMA

Library of Congress Cataloging in Publication Data
Middleton, William S/Values in Modern Medicine
Includes bibliographic references
1. Medicine—Addresses, essays, lectures
I. Wisconsin Medical Alumni Association. II. Title
[DNLM: 1. History of medicine, Modern
2. Physicians. WZ 59 M629v 1972]
R114.M5/610′.8/72–1379
ISBN 0–299–06220–1